D0846269

ATLAS OF
ECHOCARDIOGRAPHY

SECOND EDITION

ERNESTO SALCEDO, M.D.

Head, Cardiac Function Laboratory
Department of Cardiology,
Cleveland Clinic Foundation, Cleveland, Ohio

W. B. SAUNDERS COMPANY

*Philadelphia / London / Toronto / Mexico City /
Rio de Janeiro / Sydney / Tokyo*

W. B. SAUNDERS COMPANY
Harcourt Brace Jovanovich, Inc.

The Curtis Center
Independence Square West
Philadelphia, PA 19106

Library of Congress Cataloging in Publication Data

Salcedo, Ernesto E.
    Atlas of echocardiography.

Includes bibliographical references and index.
1. Ultrasonic cardiography—Atlases.   I. Title.
    [DNLM: 1. Echocardiography—atlases. WG 17 S162a]

RC683.5.U5S24   1985   616.61′207543   84–10544

ISBN 0–7216–7899–8

Atlas of Echocardiography   ISBN   0–7216–7899–8

Last digit is the print number: 9   8   7   6   5

TO MY WIFE, SYLVIA

PREFACE

In response to the vast advances that have occurred in echocardiography in the past few years this edition has been completely revised and expanded. As in the first edition of the *Atlas of Echocardiography,* the information is presented in a pictorial and simple format. M-Mode and two-dimensional echocardiography represent different modes of the same tool and should be considered as complementing one another. Descriptions of both techniques are given to highlight their interdependent roles.

A clear understanding of cardiac anatomy is required for adequate echocardiographic study and interpretation. Numerous illustrations of the cardiovascular system in the chest and tomographic sections of the heart are included in the introductory chapter. The echocardiographic examination technique is presented through numerous photographs and illustrations.

Each of the sections describing the echocardiographic abnormalities is organized in a similar and systemic way. Extensive use of titles and subtitles should facilitate identification of the most important facts as well as the localization of information. References cited within the text are listed at the end of the book according to chapter and section to aid the reader in locating an article referring to any specific topic. A general introduction is presented at the beginning of most chapters. This serves to emphasize the clinicopathologic findings of the topic under consideration. This general introduction is followed by a detailed discussion of the different echocardiographic abnormalities. A review of the differential diagnosis and pitfalls completes the text of most chapters.

Representative echocardiograms and illustrations accompany the text. Particular care was taken to select illustrative cases of good diagnostic quality. The M-mode and two-dimensional echocardiograms are presented independently to bring out their special qualities or together to expose their similarities. All of the echocardiograms are labeled to facilitate recognition of the different structures under study. A side-by-side presentation is used when further clarification is needed. Each illustration is accompanied by a legend that includes a title, a summary of the clinical data relative to the patient's problem, and a detailed description of the echocardiogram.

All of the echocardiograms were obtained in the cardiac function laboratory of the Cleveland Clinic Foundation, Cleveland, Ohio. As in the first edition, the presentation of the experience of one institution should provide cohesion and make the analysis of the material simpler and easier to follow.

Echocardiography is a prime example of the mixture of art and science in medicine. An echocardiogram of good technical quality has a definitive aesthetically pleasing effect in addition to its diagnostic value. It is hoped that this Atlas will be of value on these two levels, scientific and aesthetic, to all who are interested in echocardiography.

Ernesto E. Salcedo, M.D.

ACKNOWLEDGMENTS

Writing this second edition of the "Atlas of Echocardiography" required considerable time and effort. It also was very enjoyable, particularly because of the outstanding support I had from many people who assisted me in bringing this work to light.

This work would not have been possible without the support and encouragement from my colleagues in the Department of Cardiology at the Cleveland Clinic Foundation. A special note of thanks goes to all of them. Our cardiology fellows provided the academic atmosphere for the development of this Atlas. They served as collaborators and constant sources of stimulation.

Many technicians worked diligently in our Cardiac Function Laboratory, where all the echocardiograms in this book were obtained, but I must give special recognition to our Senior Technicians: Terri Castle, Rona Baker, and Helga Lombardo.

I am also indebted to Ms. Kathleen Jung, who created all the art work and to Ms. Ann Paladino from our Photography Department, who supervised the reproduction of all the echocardiograms.

My personal thanks to Ms. Jo Ralph, who typed, collated, and edited this Atlas. Her patience and skill and the long hours she spent in this work, are gratefully acknowledged. I wish also to address an individual note of thanks to Ms. Mary Jo Cranley. Her cheerful and expert assistance in organizing all the references and the bibliography, as well as doing the proofreading of the text, is warmly appreciated.

Additional and valuable secretarial assistance was provided by Ms. Kyra Weber and Ms. Joan Becker. Their assistance is sincerely acknowledged.

It is a pleasure to recognize the editorial assistance from Ms. Suzanne Boyd and Ms. Lorraine Kilmer of the W. B. Saunders Company. Their support and guidance is deeply appreciated.

Finally, I want to express my gratitude to my most important collaborators, my wife Sylvia and my children Ernesto, Sylvia, and Marco. Their love, patience, and confidence in the outcome of my efforts was the strongest inspiration I had in completing this work.

ERNESTO E. SALCEDO, M.D.

CONTENTS

1 ECHOCARDIOGRAPHIC ANATOMY 1

The Heart in the Chest 1
Echocardiographic Windows 1
Cardiac Valves 1
Tomographic Anatomy of the Heart 1
    Long-Axis Sections 2
    Short-Axis Sections................................ 2
    Four-Chamber Sections 2

2 ECHOCARDIOGRAPHIC EXAMINATION AND MEASUREMENTS... 9

Two-Dimensional Echocardiography 9
    Left Parasternal Transducer Position 9
    Apical Transducer Position......................... 10
    Subcostal Transducer Position 11
    Suprasternal Transducer Position.................. 11
Combined M-Mode and Two-Dimensional Echocardiography 12
M-Mode Echocardiographic Measurements.......................... 13
    Mitral Valve....................................... 13
    Aorta and Aortic Valve 13
    Left Atrium.. 14
    Left Ventricle..................................... 14
    Pulmonic Valve 14
    Right Ventricle 14
Two-Dimensional Echocardiographic Measurements 15
    Parasternal Long-Axis Views 15
    Parasternal Short-Axis Views....................... 15
    Apical Four-Chamber View.......................... 15

3 ECHOPHONOCARDIOGRAPHY AND ECHOCARDIOGRAPHIC FINDINGS WITH ALTERED ELECTRICAL ACTIVATION 51

Echophonocardiography 51
    First Heart Sound.................................. 51
    Second Heart Sound................................ 52
    Third Heart Sound 52
    Fourth Heart Sound 52
Systolic Time Intervals................................... 52
Altered Electrical Activation 52

4 MITRAL VALVE DISEASE 63

Mitral Stenosis.. 63
    Echocardiographic Findings........................ 63
    Severity of Mitral Stenosis........................ 64
    Surgical Considerations 65

Differential Diagnosis 65
Echophonocardiography 66
Mitral Insufficiency... 66
Secondary Echocardiographic Abnormalities.................... 66
Rhematic Mitral Insufficiency 67
Mitral Valve Prolapse 67
Echocardiographic Abnormalities............................... 67
Maneuvers to Enhance Diagnostic Accuracy 67
Conditions Obscuring Diagnosis 68
Secondary Mitral Valve Prolapse 68
Ruptured Chordae Tendineae 68
Echocardiographic Abnormalities............................... 68
Echophonocardiography 69
Papillary Muscle Dysfunction 69
Mitral Annulus Calcification 69

5   AORTIC VALVE DISEASE 105
Valvular Aortic Stenosis 105
Echocardiographic Findings in Calcific Aortic Stenosis........ 105
Severity of Aortic Stenosis 106
Conditions Complicating the Diagnosis 106
Echophonocardiography 107
Aortic Insufficiency... 107
Echocardiographic Diagnosis 107
Severity of Aortic Insufficiency 108
Conditions Complicating the Diagnosis 109

6   THE AORTA AND DISEASES OF THE AORTA 127
Anatomic Considerations 127
Echocardiographic Examination of the Aorta...................... 127
Aneurysms of the Aorta... 128
Arteriosclerotic Aortic Aneurysms................................. 128
Syphilitic Aortic Aneurysms 128
Aortic Dissection 128
Aneurysm of the Sinus of Valsalva 129
Marfan's Syndrome... 129
Cardiovascular Abnormalities................................. 129
Echocardiographic Findings.................................... 130
Ankylosing Spondylitis 130

7   TRICUSPID VALVE DISEASE 143
Tricuspid Stenosis.. 143
Tricuspid Insufficiency 143
Tricuspid Valve Prolapse 144

8   PULMONIC VALVE AND PULMONARY ARTERY................. 151
Pulmonary Hypertension 151
Primary Pulmonary Hypertension 152
Pulmonic Stenosis.. 152
Pulmonic Insufficiency.. 152
Pulmonary Artery Dilatation 152

9   INFECTIVE ENDOCARDITIS 161
General Considerations 161
Echocardiographic Findings... 161
Mitral Valve Vegetations.. 162
Aortic Valve Vegetations.. 162

Tricuspid Valve Vegetations...163
Pulmonic Valve Vegetations...163
Nonvalvular Endocarditis..163
Valve Ring Abscess...163

10 PROSTHETIC VALVES 175

Classification 175
General Echocardiographic Findings 175
Caged-Ball Valves...176
Caged-Disc Valves 177
Tilting-Disc Valves 177
Björk-Shiley 177
Lillehei-Kaster 177
Bileaflet Valves..177
St. Jude Medical 177
Homografts (Allografts) 178
Heterografts..178
Porcine Valves 178
Bovine Valves 178
Autograft Valves 178
Prosthetic Valve Endocarditis 179
Conduits 179
Carpentier Ring 179

11 THE LEFT VENTRICLE 197

Left Ventricular Size and Function 197
Ventricular Dimensions...198
Derived Left Ventricular Volumes 198
Left Ventricular Mass 199
Ejection Phase Indices 200
Ventricular Pressures...200
Analysis of Segmental Wall Motion 201
Left Ventricular Hypertrophy...202
Left Ventricular Size and Function in Systemic Hypertension 203
Left Ventricular Size and Function in Athletes 203
Cardiomyopathies 203
Congestive Cardiomyopathy 203
Differential Diagnosis 204
Hypertrophic Cardiomyopathy 204
Differential Diagnosis 206
Echophonocardiography 206
Restrictive Cardiomyopathy 206
Cardiac Involvement in Systemic Diseases 207
Neurologic and Neuromuscular Diseases 207
Collagen Diseases...207
Physical and Toxic Causes 208
Left Ventricular Masses 208

12 CORONARY ARTERY DISEASE...................................249

Coronary Artery Visualization...249
Left Ventricular Function in Coronary Artery Disease..............250
Acute Myocardial Infarction...251
Myocardial Scar...251
Left Ventricular Aneurysm 251
Left Ventricular Pseudoaneurysm....................................252
Ventricular Septal Rupture 252
Papillary Muscle Dysfunction 252

Mural Thrombus... 252
Right Ventricular Infarction 253

13 THE LEFT ATRIUM.. 263

Left Atrial Enlargement 263
Left Atrial Myxoma... 263
    Conditions Complicating the Diagnosis 264
    Echophonocardiography 264
Left Atrial Thrombus.. 264
Coronary Sinus.. 264
Congenital Aneurysm of the Left Atrium 265

14 THE RIGHT ATRIUM AND THE RIGHT VENTRICLE.............. 281

Right Atrial Enlargement... 281
Right Atrial Masses... 281
Venous Catheters 281
The Eustachian Valve and the Chiari Network 281
Right Ventricular Volume Overload 282
Increased Right Ventricular End-Diastolic Pressure................ 282
Right Ventricular Hypertrophy....................................... 282
Right Ventricular Tumors... 283
Right Ventricular Thrombus.. 283

15 DISEASES OF THE PERICARDIUM................................. 293

Pericardial Effusion.. 293
    Echocardiographic Differentiation of Pleural from
      Pericardial Effusion 294
Cardiac Tamponade 294
Constrictive Pericarditis.. 295
Pericardial Metastases.. 295

16 CONGENITAL HEART DISEASE 307

Deductive Echocardiography 307
    Atria.. 307
    Atrioventricular Valves 307
    Ventricles.. 307
    Great Vessels 308
    Semilunar Valves 308
Cardiac Malpositions.. 308
Abnormalities of the Interatrial Septum............................ 308
    Atrial Septal Defect... 308
    Common Atrium 309
    Patent Foramen Ovale.. 309
    Atrial Septal Aneurysm 310
Abnormalities of the Interventricular Septum 310
    Ventricular Septal Defects 310
    Ventricular Septal Aneurysms 311
Endocardial Cushion Defects.. 311
Straddling Atrioventricular Valves 312
Anomalous Pulmonary Venous Return.............................. 313
    Classification 313
    Echocardiographic Abnormalities.............................. 313
Patent Ductus Arteriosus.. 313
    Echocardiographic Findings.................................... 313
Left Ventricular Inflow Obstruction 314
Congenital Aortic Stenosis... 314
    Congenital Valvular Aortic Stenosis........................... 314

Biscuspid Aortic Valve.. 315

Subvalvular Aortic Stenosis 315

Supravalvular Aortic Stenosis.................................. 316

Coarctation of the Aorta... 316

Pulmonic Stenosis.. 317

Ebstein's Anomaly.. 317

Tricuspid Atresia 318

Conotruncal Abnormalities 318

Fallot's Tetralogy 318

Pulmonary Atresia with Ventricular Septal Defect.................. 319

Persistent Truncus Arteriosus.. 319

Transposition of the Great Arteries 319

Double Outlet Right Ventricle....................................... 320

Single Ventricle... 320

REFERENCES.. 355

INDEX.. 375

1 ECHOCARDIOGRAPHIC ANATOMY

1.1 THE HEART IN THE CHEST

The heart lies within the pericardium, in the mediastinum, behind the sternum and ribs, between the lungs, and in front of the spine. It is suspended at its base by the great vessels and inferiorly is supported by the diaphragm. It occupies an asymmetrical position with its apex directed primarily to the left anteriorly, and slightly inferiorly. The base of the heart is directed toward the cardiac apex perpendicular to the long axis of the heart. The left cardiac border is formed by the left ventricle, and the right border is formed by the right atrium. The left atrium is positioned directly posteriorly in front of the spine and esophagus. The right ventricle is the most anterior chamber, lying directly behind the sternum (Figs. 1–1, 1–2).[1]

1.2 ECHOCARDIOGRAPHIC WINDOWS

Much of the heart is covered by bony structures or lung, which make it inaccessible to ultrasound. The echocardiographic windows (Fig. 1–3) are areas in which the heart lies underneath the chest surface without such interference. These areas are:

1. Left parasternal area
2. Apical area
3. Subcostal area
4. Suprasternal area
5. Supraclavicular area

1.3 CARDIAC VALVES

The cardiac valves can serve as landmarks to the echocardiographer, so their identification is very helpful not only to detect valvular abnormalities but to orient the echocardiographic examination (Fig. 1–4). The pulmonic valve is the most superior valve, lying behind the junction of the third costal cartilage and the sternum. The aortic valve is situated inferiorly, anteriorly, and to the right in relation to the pulmonic valve. The mitral valve is positioned immediately posteriorly, inferiorly, and to the left in relation to the aortic valve. The tricuspid valve is situated the most inferiorly and the farthest to the right.

1.4 TOMOGRAPHIC ANATOMY OF THE HEART

The three-dimensional structure of the heart can be understood best and related to echocardiography by study of and familiar-

1

ity with the tomographic anatomy of the heart.[2-5] Instead of using the classic dissection of the heart, in which the heart is opened according to the direction of blood flow, the tomographic approach uses a bisection method whereby the heart is divided into two pieces by one plane of section. Sections in three orthogonal planes can be made (Fig. 1–5).

Long-Axis Sections

Anteroposterior sections of the heart in a plane parallel to its long axis provide anatomic information regarding the inflow and outflow tracts of the left ventricle, as well as the septum, posterior wall, and apex (Fig. 1–6). The relationship between septum and aorta is clearly seen in this section. Parts of the right ventricular outflow tract appear directly in front of the left ventricle. The left atrium is also included in this cut and appears behind the aorta.

Short-Axis Sections

Anteroposterior sections of the heart in a plane perpendicular to its long axis provide cross-sectional anatomic views of the heart that can extend from its apex to the great vessels (Figs. 1–7 to 1–12). With this type of cut the circular shape of the left ventricle can be observed in cross section. The right ventricle is situated anteriorly and to the right; the more basal the cut the more anterior the position of the right ventricle becomes.

A similar relationship between the centrally located aorta and the pulmonary artery that surrounds it can be observed at the level of the great vessels.

Four-Chamber Sections

This method involves sectioning the heart from apex to base, along the acute margin of the right ventricle and the obtuse margin of the left ventricle, including the atria (Fig. 1–13). In this cut, the heart is seen divided in four by the interatrial and interventricular septa in the mid longitudinal plane and by the mitral and tricuspid valves in the mid transverse plane.

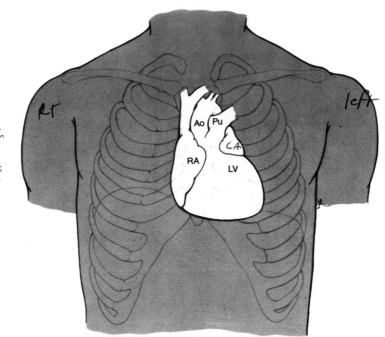

FIGURE 1–1
THE HEART IN THE CHEST
Anterior view. LV = left ventricle; RA = right atrium; Ao = aorta; Pu = pulmonary artery.

left cardiac border

right border

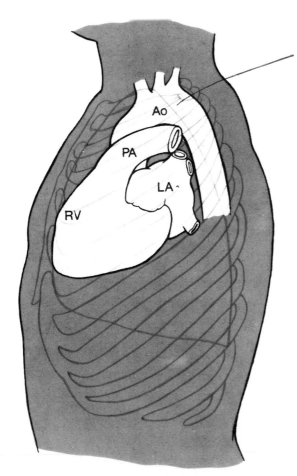

PSLAX view   AORTA — The heart lies w/F pericardium, in the mediastinum, behind the sternum and ribs, between the lungs, in front of spine. It is suspended at its base by great vessels and inferiorly supported by diaphragm

FIGURE 1–2
THE HEART IN THE CHEST
Lateral view. RV = right ventricle; PA = pulmonary artery; Ao = aorta; LA = left atrium.

most anterior chambers lying directly behind the sternum.

positioned directly posteriorly in front of spine & esophagus

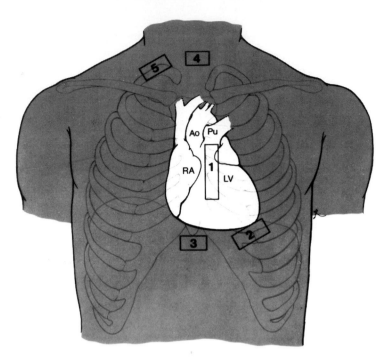

FIGURE 1–3
ECHOCARDIOGRAPHIC WINDOWS
(1) Left parasternal; (2) apical; (3) subcostal; (4) suprasternal; (5) supraclavicular. For definitions of abbreviations see legend for Figure 1–1.

FIGURE 1–4

CARDIAC VALVES, ANTERIOR VIEW
The pulmonic valve (PV) is the most superior and farthest left in position. The aortic valve (AoV) is immediately inferior and to the right. The mitral valve (MV) is inferior to and sightly to the left of the aortic valve. The tricuspid valve (TV) is the most inferior and farthest right of the cardiac valves. SVC = superior vena cava; RA = right atrium; RV = right ventricle; LV = left ventricle.

CARDIAC VALVES, LATERAL VIEW
This diagram highlights the anterior and superior position of the pulmonic valve (PV), the medial position of the aortic valve (AoV), the posterior position of the mitral valve (MV), and the inferoanterior position of the tricuspid valve (TV).

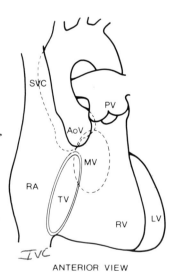

ANTERIOR VIEW

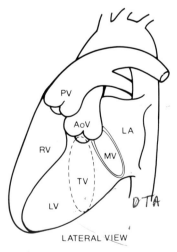

LATERAL VIEW

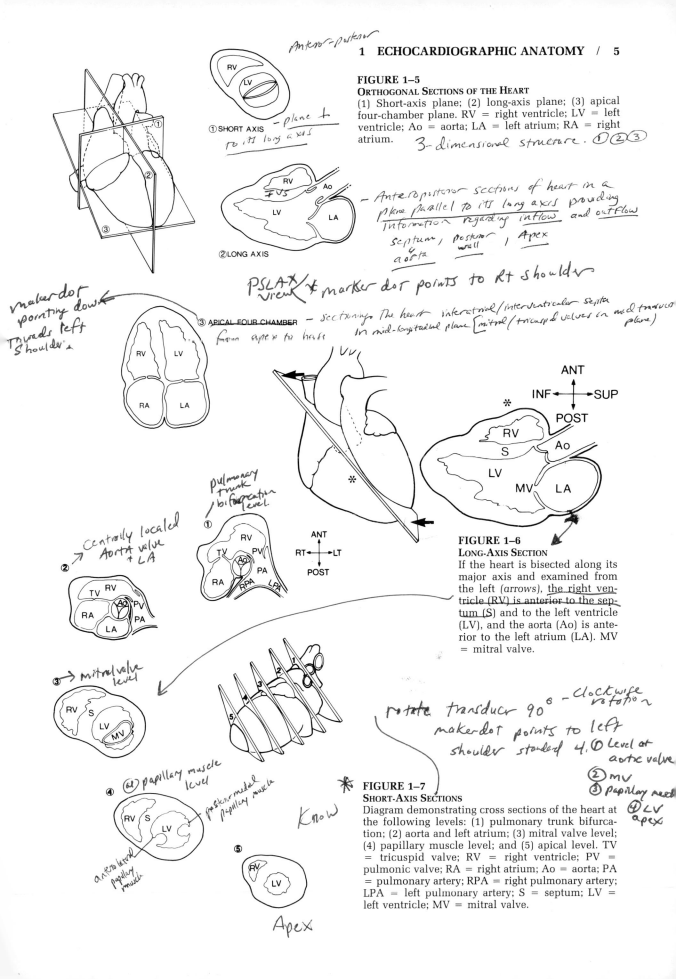

Antero-posterior

① SHORT AXIS *- plane ⊥ to its long axis*

② LONG AXIS

③ APICAL FOUR CHAMBER

FIGURE 1–5
ORTHOGONAL SECTIONS OF THE HEART
(1) Short-axis plane; (2) long-axis plane; (3) apical four-chamber plane. RV = right ventricle; LV = left ventricle; Ao = aorta; LA = left atrium; RA = right atrium. *3-dimensional structure. ①②③*

- Anteroposterior sections of heart in a plane parallel to its long axis providing Information regarding inflow and outflow septum, posterior wall, Apex & aorta

PSLAX view ✳ marker dot points to Rt shoulder

- sectioning the heart interatrial/interventricular septa in mid-longitudinal plane [mitral/tricuspid valves in med transducer plane]

from apex to base

marker dot pointing down towards left shoulder

Centrally located Aorta valve + LA

mitral valve level

pulmonary trunk bifurcation level

ANT
INF ↔ SUP
POST

ANT
RT ↔ LT
POST

FIGURE 1–6
LONG-AXIS SECTION
If the heart is bisected along its major axis and examined from the left (arrows), the right ventricle (RV) is anterior to the septum (S) and to the left ventricle (LV), and the aorta (Ao) is anterior to the left atrium (LA). MV = mitral valve.

rotate transducer 90° - Clockwise rotation makerdot points to left shoulder started 4. ① Level at aortic valve ② MV ③ papillary muscle ④ LV apex

④ (a) papillary muscle level

posteromedial papillary muscle

anterolateral papillary muscle

Know

FIGURE 1–7
SHORT-AXIS SECTIONS
Diagram demonstrating cross sections of the heart at the following levels: (1) pulmonary trunk bifurcation; (2) aorta and left atrium; (3) mitral valve level; (4) papillary muscle level; and (5) apical level. TV = tricuspid valve; RV = right ventricle; PV = pulmonic valve; RA = right atrium; Ao = aorta; PA = pulmonary artery; RPA = right pulmonary artery; LPA = left pulmonary artery; S = septum; LV = left ventricle; MV = mitral valve.

Apex

RPA lies behind the aorta.

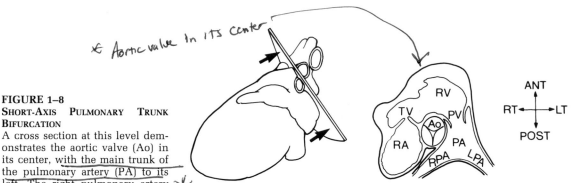

Aortic valve In ITs center

FIGURE 1–8
SHORT-AXIS PULMONARY TRUNK BIFURCATION
A cross section at this level demonstrates the aortic valve (Ao) in its center, with the main trunk of the pulmonary artery (PA) to its left. The right pulmonary artery (RPA) lies behind the aorta. The left pulmonary artery (LPA) is to the left. Note that at this level the left atrium is not visualized. RV = right ventricle; RA = right atrium; TV = tricuspid valve; PV = pulmonary valve.

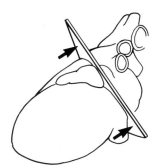

FIGURE 1–9
SHORT AXIS, AORTA, LEFT ATRIUM
At this level the aorta (Ao) is in the middle of the sector scan. The left atrium (LA) is immediately behind, and the main pulmonary artery (PA) is to the left. RV = right ventricle; TV = tricuspid valve; RA = right atrium; PV = pulmonic valve.

FIGURE 1–10
SHORT AXIS, MITRAL VALVE
The right ventricle (RV) is anterior to and to the right of the septum (S) and the left ventricle (LV). The anterior and posterior portions of the mitral valve (MV) are seen in cross section, with the posteromedial commissure at about 7 o'clock and the anterolateral commissure at about 3 o'clock of the left ventricular circumference.

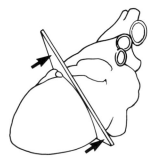

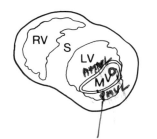

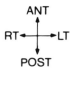

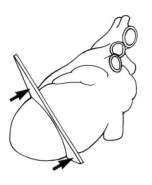

FIGURE 1–11
SHORT AXIS, PAPILLARY MUSCLES
At this level the right ventricle (RV) is more to the right than anterior to the septum (S) and the left ventricle (LV). The postero-medial papillary muscle is seen at about 7 o'clock and the anterolateral papillary muscle at about 3 o'clock of the ventricular circumference.

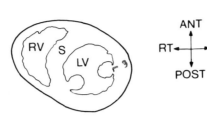

Circular shape of the left ventricle can be observed

FIGURE 1–12
SHORT AXIS, APEX
At this level little or no right ventricle (RV) is visualized. The papillary muscles can no longer be distinguished. LV = left ventricle.

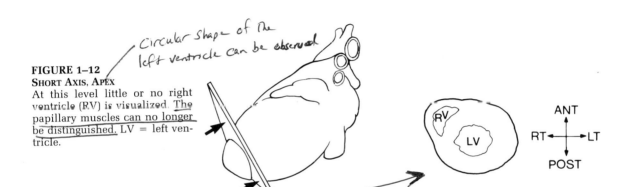

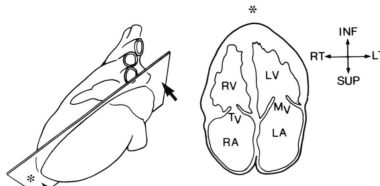

FIGURE 1–13
FOUR-CHAMBER SECTION
The heart is sectioned from apex to base along the acute margin of the right ventricle (RV) and the obtuse margin of the left ventricle (LV). The heart is divided in four by the interatrial and interventricular septa and by the mitral (MV) and tricuspid (TV) valves. RA = right atrium; LA = left atrium.

2 ECHOCARDIOGRAPHIC EXAMINATION AND MEASUREMENTS

2.1 TWO-DIMENSIONAL ECHOCARDIOGRAPHY

For the two-dimensional examination of the cardiovascular system a number of standard transducer positions and imaging planes are used, as described here.[1-3]

A. Left Parasternal Transducer Position

This is the usual starting area for the echocardiographic examination (Fig. 2–1). The patient is placed in the semilateral position with rotation of the chest at about 30 degrees and the left arm held above the head. The transducer is then placed in the third, fourth, or fifth intercostal space in the left parasternal region and perpendicular to the chest. The following imaging planes can be recorded from this area:

   1. Long-Axis Left Parasternal Views. With the transducer positioned as described, the sector plane is directed so that it transects the heart along its long axis (Fig. 2–2). There are two variants of this view.

   a. LONG AXIS OF THE LEFT VENTRICLE. In this view, the sector plane transects the left ventricle along its long axis (Fig. 2–3). The

right ventricular free wall and the right ventricular cavity are the most anterior structures. Behind these, the middle third and base of the interventricular septum can be seen. The left ventricular cavity lies behind the septum, and the posterior wall of the left ventricle, between the papillary muscles, is the most posterior structure.

The interventricular septum is seen to continue with the anterior aortic wall. The aortic root is observed in its long axis from this view. At its base the right coronary aortic cusp and the noncoronary aortic cusp are seen to open and close during the cardiac cycle. Behind the aorta the left atrium can be visualized.

The mitral valve is seen in its long axis, with the anterior leaflet originating from the posterior aortic wall and the posterior leaflet originating at the level of the posterior atrioventricular groove (Fig. 2–4). Frame-by-frame analysis of the cardiac cycle allows for detailed study of the motion of the mitral and the aortic valves, as well as measurement of chamber dimensions (Figs. 2–5, 2–6).

This view generally does not permit imaging of the true apex. The anterior and posterior walls of the left ventricle may

(see Fig. 17)

9

curve toward each other and meet in the middle of the scan, but this area may not represent the true apex of the left ventricle, only a foreshortened apex (Fig. 2–7). To record the apex of the left ventricle in the long-axis view, the transducer must be displaced to a lower intercostal space and directed more toward the left. In this position, the aorta is usually not seen.

b. LONG AXIS OF THE RIGHT VENTRICULAR INFLOW TRACT. With the transducer in the left parasternal region, aligned to the long axis of the heart, a slight angulation of the sector scan toward the right brings into the image the inflow tract of the right ventricle (Figs. 2–8 to 2–10). This view also allows visualization of the right atrium and the anterior and posterior tricuspid leaflets.

2. Short-Axis Left Parasternal Views. With the transducer in the left parasternal region, if the sector plane is rotated 90 degrees clockwise from the long-axis view, short-axis views are obtained of the left ventricle (Fig. 2–11). Five short-axis views can be recorded.

a. PULMONARY TRUNK BIFURCATION. With the transducer in the left parasternal position, the sector plane is aligned to the short axis of the heart by rotating the probe 90 degrees from the long axis. The imaging plane then is angulated superiorly until the pulmonic valve is visualized as a fine structure at about 2 o'clock of the aortic circumference. By further superior angulation, the pulmonary trunk and its bifurcation come into view (Figs. 2–12, 2–13).

The pulmonary trunk is to the left of the aorta. The right pulmonary artery is to the left and behind it. In front of the aorta is the right ventricular outflow tract, and to its right is the right atrium.

b. AORTA AND LEFT ATRIUM. By angulating the sector plane slightly inferiorly from the pulmonary bifurcation position, the left atrium can be visualized behind the aorta (Figs. 2–14, 2–15). The bifurcation of the pulmonary artery is no longer apparent. The aorta and aortic leaflets appear in the center of the picture. The right coronary cusp is the most anterior, the left coronary cusp is posterior and to the left, and the noncoronary cusp is posterior and to the right. With each systole these structures move toward the aortic walls (Fig. 2–16). The interatrial septum originates from the posterior wall of the aortic root at about 7 o'clock and runs posterior and to the right. The right atrium

is seen to the right of the aorta; its most anterior margin is formed by the tricuspid valve. The medial tricuspid valve originates at about 9 o'clock of the aortic circumference.

c. MITRAL VALVE LEVEL. Further inferior angulation of the transducer brings into the image the base of the left ventricle with the mitral valve funnel (Figs. 2–17 to 21). The left ventricle in this view has a doughnut shape. The right ventricle appears to the right and anterior to the left ventricle. The interventricular septum forms the anteromedial walls of the left ventricular circumference.

d. PAPILLARY MUSCLE LEVEL. Additional inferior angulation of the probe takes the sector image to the level of the papillary muscles (Fig. 2–22). These muscles appear as round structures within the left ventricular cavity. The posteromedial papillary muscle is situated at about 7 o'clock, and the anterolateral papillary muscle is at about 4 o'clock of the ventricular circumference. The right ventricle at this level is more to the right than in the anterior direction. The left ventricular cavity appears smaller (Figs. 2–23, 2–24).

e. APICAL LEVEL. To record the apex in the short-axis view, the transducer needs to be moved one or two intercostal spaces below the former views (Fig. 2–25). The left ventricle at the apical level appears as a small round structure with a small cavity in the center. The right ventricle, if seen at all, is to the right of the left ventricle and is no longer anterior (Fig. 2–26).

B. Apical Transducer Position

With the patient in the left lateral decubitus position, the transducer is placed directly over the apical impulse of the left ventricle and is oriented parallel to the long axis of the heart (Fig. 2–27). Four imaging planes are selected from this position.

1. Apical Four-Chamber View. With the transducer in the cardiac apex and directed superiorly and parallel to the major axis of the heart, the sector plane can be positioned so that it transects the heart at the level of its maximal side-by-side dimensions (Fig. 2–28). This plane encompasses the left ventricle and atrium, the right ventricle and atrium, the mitral and tricuspid valves, and the interatrial and interventricular septum. This view permits visualization of the long axis of the left ventricle, the interventricular septum in its entire longitude, and the free lateral wall (Fig. 2–29). The left ventricular apex is also seen.

2. *Apical Five-Chamber View.* This view is obtained with the transducer in a position similar to that used for the four-chamber apical view. The transducer is then angulated slightly anteriorly toward the anterior chest wall. This brings into the image the left ventricular outflow tract, the aortic root, and the aortic valve (Fig. 2–30). Hence, it is possible to image the four cardiac chambers plus the aortic root, which becomes the fifth chamber (Fig. 2–31).

3. *Apical Two-Chamber View.* The apical two-chamber view is obtained by rotating the transducer 90 degrees clockwise from the apical four-chamber view (Fig. 2–32). The two-chamber view records only the left ventricle and the left atrium with the interposed mitral valve. This plane is orthogonal to the four-chamber view and provides a long-axis view of the left ventricle (Fig. 2–33). The anterolateral and posteromedial left ventricular walls are visualized.

4. *Apical Long-Axis View.* The apical long-axis view is obtained by rotating the transducer 45 degrees clockwise from the apical four-chamber view (Fig. 2–34). This view is similar to the long-axis left parasternal plane except that it includes the true apex. Besides the apex, it encompasses the interventricular septum, the posterior ventricular wall, the left atrium, the aortic root, the aortic valve, and the mitral valve (Fig. 2–35). This view is equivalent to the angiographic right anterior oblique view.

C. Subcostal Transducer Position

This position was initially used in patients with chronic obstructive lung disease in whom the parasternal window was obliterated by the hyperinflated lung (Fig. 2–36). Now it is obvious that this position permits optimal visualization of a number of cardiac structures. It is the view preferred for evaluating the interatrial septum and the inferior vena cava. Many congenital abnormalities can be studied best from this region. Three important imaging planes are recorded from this area.

1. *Inferior Vena Cava and Hepatic Veins.* With the patient in the decubitus position, the transducer is placed in the subxiphoid region, and its head is tilted

inferiorly and slightly to the patient's right. The probe is rotated until the liver parenchyma, hepatic vessels, and vena cava come into the image. Both the short axis and the long axis of the inferior vena cava can be recorded by rotating the transducer 90 degrees from one position to the other (Figs. 2–37, 2–38). The hepatic veins can be seen to drain into the inferior vena cava. The drainage of the inferior vena cava into the right atrium is also apparent in this view.

2. *Subcostal Four-Chamber View.* When the transducer is positioned to image the inferior vena cava in its short axis, tilting the transducer superiorly will bring into the image the subcostal four-chamber view (Fig. 2–39). The two atria and the interatrial septum are best visualized by this view. The tricuspid and mitral valves, as well as the right and left ventricles, also can be seen. A portion of the liver is usually recorded between the transducer and the cardiac silhouette (Fig. 2–40).

3. *Subcostal Right Ventricular Outflow Tract.* From the subcostal four-chamber view the transducer can be rotated clockwise about 90 degrees and tilted slightly superiorly to obtain the plane of the right ventricular outflow tract (Fig. 2–41). In this view, the left ventricle is visualized in the short axis, and the entire right ventricular outflow tract can be observed (Fig. 2–42).

D. Suprasternal Transducer Position

With the transducer in the suprasternal notch, it is possible to image the aortic root, the aortic arch, the origin of the aortic branches, the descending aorta, the right pulmonary artery, and the left atrium (Figs. 2–43, 2–44).

The transducer is placed in the suprasternal area and is aimed inferiorly, then rotated until the aorta, which lies almost immediately beneath the transducer face, is visualized. Two views are of interest in this region.

1. *Long Axis of the Aortic Arch.* To obtain a view of the long axis of the aortic arch from the suprasternal position, the sector plane must be oriented posteriorly and to the left. The aortic arch appears in the middle of the image, with parts of the ascending aorta as well as the descending aorta in both ends of the image. The vessels going to the neck are seen to emerge from the major curvature of the aortic arch. The right pulmonary artery is seen medial to the aortic arch, and the left atrium is visualized inferiorly and somewhat anteriorly (Fig. 2–45).

2. Short Axis of the Aortic Arch. Rotating the transducer 90 degrees from the prior position brings the aortic arch into the short axis and the right pulmonary artery to its long axis. The superior vena cava also can be registered from this position. This is done by angulating the transducer anteriorly and rotating it counterclockwise (Fig. 2–46).

2.2 COMBINED M-MODE AND TWO-DIMENSIONAL ECHOCARDIOGRAPHY

A complete echocardiographic study should include both M-mode and two-dimensional techniques so that the advantages of each method can be maximized. The most desirable way of obtaining this type of study is by the simultaneous use of M-mode and two-dimensional imaging. This is best done by using a multi-element cross-sectional transducer that produces a two-dimensional picture. One element can be chosen for simultaneous recording of the M-mode echo in a selected region of the heart.

The principal advantage of two-dimensional echocardiography over the M-mode technique is the ability of the former to provide information of motion and shape in two planes rather than in only one. This allows for a better spatial definition and hence better anatomic characterization. However, because of the relatively slow sampling rate (approximately 30 frames per second) of two-dimensional echocardiography, M-mode echocardiography offers advantages with regard to axial resolution and timing of events. For every patient, the author performs a two-dimensional study, which is stored on video tape, and a two-dimensional derived M-mode echocardiogram from which routine measurements are taken. With the two-dimensional study, a complete anatomic analysis of the heart is obtained, and with the M-mode technique, a fine detailed analysis of selected areas is performed.

The M-mode recordings derived from the two-dimensional format look the same when they are obtained from either the short- or the long-axis cross sections (Fig. 2–47). At the left ventricular level, the long-axis parasternal view allows selection of the area of interest for the M-mode recording below the tip of the mitral valve and above the papil-

lary muscles. This can be particularly helpful in doing serial studies when left ventricular size is to be measured in the same area. Obtaining the M-mode tracing from the short axis of the left ventricle permits localization of the area of interest between the papillary muscles.

1. Examination of the Mitral Valve. To examine the mitral valve, the transducer is positioned perpendicular to the chest at the left parasternal border in the fourth or fifth intercostal space; the sector scan is aligned to the long axis of the left ventricle; and the M-mode beam is directed toward the mitral valve, in which it transects the anterior and posterior leaflets to exit through the posterior wall of the left ventricle (Figs. 2–48, 2–49). At end-systole, both leaflets are close together (Fig. 2–50). During early diastole, as the mitral valve opens, the anterior leaflet moves closer to the transducer and thus inscribes a superior motion in the echocardiographic recording (Fig. 2–51). As the rapid filling period of the left ventricle begins, the mitral valve moves back to a semi-closed position (Fig. 2–52), is reopened by atrial systole (Fig. 2–53), and finally closes with the beginning of ventricular systole (Fig. 2–54). The posterior leaflet moves in a similar manner but in an opposite direction and with lesser amplitude. During systole, both leaflets remain closed, inscribing a slight anterior motion related to mitral ring excursion. As mentioned before, the M-mode tracing of the mitral valve can be obtained from either long-axis (Fig. 2–55) or short-axis (Fig. 2–56) sector scans.

2. Examination of the Aorta and the Aortic Valve. With the sector scan aligned to the long axis of the left ventricle and the M-mode line directed superiorly, the echocardiographic beam transects the right ventricular outflow tract, the anterior aortic wall, the aortic valve, and the posterior aortic wall. The beam exits through the posterior wall of the left atrium after passing through the left atrial cavity (Figs. 2–57, 2–58). The motion of the aortic root is characterized by two parallel lines that move anteriorly during systole and posteriorly during diastole. Within the aortic root, the right and noncoronary cusps of the aortic valve move in opposite directions during systole—the right coronary cusp moves anteriorly and the noncoronary cusp posteriorly. They remain separated throughout systole and come together at the center of the aortic root with the beginning of diastole (Figs. 2–59, 2–60). The posterior wall of the left atrium has a slight systolic posterior motion. The M-mode tracing of the aortic valve can be obtained from the long-axis (Fig. 2–61) or short-axis (Fig. 2–62) sector scans.

3. *Examination of the Left Ventricle.* Direction of the M-mode line inferiorly from the mitral valve position brings the echocardiographic beam toward the left ventricle. At this level, the right ventricular cavity, the interventricular septum, and the posterior wall of the left ventricle are transected by the echocardiographic beam (Figs. 2–63, 2–64). During ventricular systole, the right ventricular wall and the interventricular septum move posteriorly, whereas the posterior wall of the left ventricle moves anteriorly (Fig. 2–65). Opposite motion of the ventricular walls occurs during diastole (Fig. 2–66). The M-mode tracing obtained from either the long axis (Fig. 2–67) or the short axis (Fig. 2–68) looks the same.

4. *Echocardiographic Scan.* A continuous recording made while the M-mode line is moved from the aorta and passed through the mitral valve and then into the left ventricle allows for continuous visualization of these structures in a strip chart recording (Fig. 2–69).

5. *Examination of the Tricuspid Valve.* To examine the tricuspid valve, the transducer is placed at the left sternal border in the third or fourth intercostal space and is angulated inferiorly and to the right. The sector scan plane is aligned to the inflow tract of the right ventricle. The M-mode line is directed to transect the tricuspid valve. The motion of the tricuspid valve is similar to that of the mitral valve. During diastole, the tricuspid valve moves anteriorly toward the transducer. The posterior leaflet is visualized moving in the opposite direction (Fig. 2–70).

6. *Examination of the Pulmonic Valve.* The echocardiographic examination of the pulmonic valve is done by placing the transducer at the third intercostal space and orienting the sector plane to the short axis of the aorta. The M-mode line is directed to the left, toward the pulmonary artery. Inside the pulmonary artery, one of the pulmonary valve leaflets can be seen. The diastolic motion of the valve is best observed as it moves away from the transducer, inscribing an inferior motion during early diastole. At end-

diastole a negative atrial wave is recorded that is immediately followed by the aperture of the leaflet, which remains open throughout systole (Fig. 2–71).

2.3 M-MODE ECHOCARDIOGRAPHIC MEASUREMENTS[5]

A. Mitral Valve

1. *E to F Slope.* Measured in centimeters per second, this is the slope of the anterior leaflet of the mitral valve during its partial closure in early diastole (Fig. 2–72). The normal measurement is 7 to 15 cm per second.

The slope is decreased in mitral stenosis and conditions with decreased compliance of the left ventricle.

2. *Valve Excursion.* Measured in centimeters, this is the vertical distance from point D to point E of the mitral echogram (Fig. 2–72). The normal distance is 2 to 3 cm.

Valve excursion is decreased in nonpliable mitral stenosis, in decreased cardiac output, and in conditions with decreased compliance of the left ventricle. Valve excursion is increased in mitral valve prolapse and in conditions with increased flow through the mitral valve.

3. *Septal-Mitral Valve Distance.* Measured in millimeters at the beginning of systole (point C), this is the distance from the mitral valve to the interventricular septum (Fig. 2–72). The normal measurement is 3.4 mm (2.9 to 4.1 mm range).

The distance is decreased in idiopathic hypertrophic subaortic stenosis and ostium primum atrial septal defect and increased in the presence of a dilated left ventricle.

B. Aorta and Aortic Valve

1. *Aortic Valve Leaflet Separation.* Measured in centimeters, this is the vertical distance from the right coronary to the noncoronary cusps at the beginning of systole (Fig. 2–73). The normal measurement is 1.7 to 2.5 cm.

The distance is decreased in aortic stenosis and conditions associated with decreased stroke volume and increased in aortic insufficiency.

2. *Left Ventricular Ejection Time.* Measured in milliseconds, this is the time from aortic cusp opening to closure.

3. Aortic Root Dimension. Measured in centimeters at the level of the aortic valve at end-diastole, this is the vertical distance from the outer edge of the anterior aortic wall echo to the inner edge of the posterior aortic wall echo. The normal measurement is 2.1 to 4.3 cm.

The distance is increased in aneurysm of the aorta and aortic insufficiency.

C. Left Atrium

1. Left Atrial Diameter. Measured in centimeters, this is the vertical distance from the inner edge of the posterior wall of the aorta to the posterior wall of the left atrium at end-systole (Fig. 2–74). The normal measurement is 2.3 to 4.4 cm.

2. Ratio of Left Atrium to Aortic Root Dimension. This measurement is obtained by dividing the left atrial diameter by the aortic root dimension. The normal value is 0.87 to 1.11 cm.

D. Left Ventricle

Left ventricular measurements that are routinely obtained by M-mode echocardiography are end-diastolic diameter, end-systolic diameter, fractional shortening, and end-diastolic septal and posterior wall thickness. A more detailed discussion of left ventricular size and function is presented in Chapter 11. See Figure 2–75.

1. End-Diastolic Diameter. Measured in centimeters at the peak of the ventricular complex (QRS), this is the distance from the left endocardial surface of the interventricular septum to the endocardial surface of the posterior ventricular wall. The normal measurement is 4.6 ± 0.54 cm.

2. End-Systolic Diameter. Measured in centimeters, this is the distance from the left endocardial surface of the septum to the endocardial surface of the posterior wall of the left ventricle at the time of nadir of septal motion. The normal measurement is 2.9 ± 0.5 cm.

3. Percentage of Shortening of the Internal Diameter. This value is calculated from the formula

$$\% \text{ shortening} = \frac{\text{EDD} - \text{ESD}}{\text{EDD}} \times 100$$

where EDD is end-diastolic diameter and ESD is end-systolic diameter.

4. Septal Thickness. Septal thickness is measured at end-diastole as the distance from the right to the left endocardial surfaces of the interventricular septum. The normal thickness is 0.97 ± 0.06 cm.

Septal thickness is increased in idiopathic hypertrophic subaortic stenosis and asymmetric septal hypertrophy and decreased in coronary artery disease.

5. Posterior Wall Thickness. Measured at end-diastole, this is the distance from the endocardial surface to the epicardial surface of the posterior wall of the left ventricle. The normal measurement is 0.94 ± 0.09 cm.

Posterior wall thickness is increased in left ventricular hypertrophy.

E. Pulmonic Valve

1. E to F Slope. Measured in millimeters per second, this is the slope of the diastolic motion of the pulmonic valve (Fig. 2–76). The normal measurement is 36.9 ± 25.4 mm per second.

The slope is decreased in pulmonary hypertension.

2. a Wave Amplitude. Measured in millimeters, this is the posterior displacement of the pulmonic valve observed after atrial systole. The normal value is 2.7 mm.

The a wave amplitude is decreased in pulmonary hypertension and increased in pulmonic stenosis.

3. Amplitude of Opening. Measured in millimeters per second, this is the slope of the pulmonic valve opening in early systole (BC slope). The normal value is 2.1 ± 12.7 mm per second.

The amplitude is increased in pulmonary hypertension.

F. Right Ventricle

1. End-Diastolic Diameter. Right ventricular end-diastolic diameter is measured in centimeters at the peak of the R wave of the electrocardiogram as the vertical distance from the endocardial surface of the anterior right ventricular wall to the right endocardial surface of the interventricular septum (Fig. 2–77). The normal measurement is 0.7 to 2.3 cm in the decubitus position and 0.9 to 2.6 cm in the left lateral position.

End-diastolic diameter is increased in right ventricular volume overload.

2.4 TWO-DIMENSIONAL ECHOCARDIOGRAPHIC MEASUREMENTS

A. Parasternal Long-Axis Views

1. Aorta. The aorta is measured at end-diastole at the valve plane perpendicular to the walls of the aortic root (Figs. 2–78 to 2–80). The normal measurement is 2.9 cm (2.2 to 3.6 cm range).

2. Left Atrium. The left atrium is measured at the aortic valve plane, also perpendicular to the aortic root (Figs. 2–78 to 2–80). The normal measurement is 3.6 cm (2.7 to 4.5 cm range).

3. Left Ventricular Minor Axis. This dimension is measured at the level of the chordae tendineae, perpendicular to a hypothetical major long axis of the left ventricle (Figs. 2–78 to 2–80). The normal measurements are 4.8 cm (3.5 to 6 cm range) at end-diastole and 3.1 cm (2.1 to 4 cm range) at end-systole. The percentage of fractional shortening is 36 per cent (25 to 46 per cent range).

4. Right Ventricular Minor Axis. This dimension is measured at the same level as the left ventricular minor axis dimensions parallel to this measurement (Figs. 2–78 to 2–80). The normal measurement is 2.8 cm (1.9 to 3.8 cm range).

B. Parasternal Short-Axis Views

1. Aorta and Left Atrium. The aorta and left atrium are measured at the center of the sector scan in their anteroposterior dimensions (Figs. 2–81, 2–82). The normal measurements are 3 cm (2.3 to 3.7 cm range) for the aorta and 3.6 cm (2.6 to 4.5 cm range) for the left atrium.

2. Left Ventricular Minor Axis Dimension at Chordae Level. This dimension is measured at the vertical distance from the septum to the posterior wall endocardium at the level of the chordae tendineae (Fig. 2–83). The normal values are 4.8 cm (3.5 to 6.2 cm range) for end-diastole and 3.2 cm (2.3 to 4 cm range) for end-systole. The percentage of fractional shortening is 34 per cent (27 to 42 per cent range).

3. Left Ventricular Minor Axis Dimension at Papillary Muscle Level. This dimen-sion is measured as the vertical distance from the septum to the posterior wall at the level of the tip of the papillary muscles (Fig. 2–84). The normal values are 4.7 cm (3.5 to 5.8 cm range) at end-diastole and 3.1 cm (2.2 to 4 cm range) at end-systole. The percentage of fractional shortening is 34 per cent (25 to 43 per cent range).

C. Apical Four-Chamber View

1. Left Ventricular Major Axis Dimension. This dimension is measured from the atrioventricular valve plane to the apical endocardium (Figs. 2–85, 2–86). The normal measurement is 8.6 cm (6.9 to 10.3 cm range) at end-diastole.

2. Left Ventricular Minor Axis Dimension. This dimension is measured at one third of the length of the major axis from the atrioventricular plane and perpendicular to the major plane (Figs. 2–85, 2–86). The normal measurements are 4.7 cm (3.5 to 6.1 range) at end-diastole and 2.8 cm (1.9 to 3.7 cm range) at end-systole.

3. Major Axis of Left Atrium. This dimension is measured from the atrioventricular plane to the atrial back wall (Figs. 2–85, 2–86). The normal measurement is 5.1 cm (4.1 to 6.2 cm range).

4. Minor Axis of Left Atrium. This dimension is measured perpendicular to and at the midpoint of the major axis (Figs. 2–85, 2–86). The normal measurement is 3.5 cm (2.8 to 4.3 cm range).

5. Right Ventricular Major Axis Dimension. This dimension is measured in a similar way to the left ventricle (Figs. 2–85, 2–86). The normal measurement is 8 cm (6.5 to 9.5 cm range).

6. Right Ventricular Minor Axis Dimension. This dimension is measured in a similar way to the left ventricle (Figs. 2–85, 2–86). The normal measurement is 3.3 cm (2.2 to 4.4 range).

7. Major Axis of Right Atrium. This dimension is measured in a similar way to the left atrium (Figs. 2–85, 2–86). The normal measurement is 4.5 cm (3.5 to 5.5 cm range).

8. Minor Axis of the Right Atrium. This dimension is measured in a similar way to the left atrium (Figs. 2–85, 2–86). The normal measurement is 3.7 cm (2.5 to 4.9 cm range).

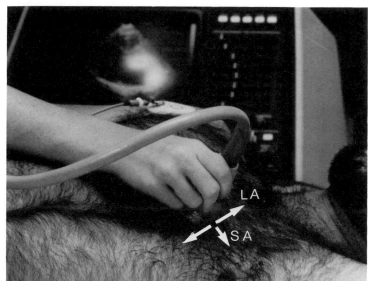

FIGURE 2–1
LEFT PARASTERNAL TRANSDUCER POSITION
The transducer is placed in the third, fourth, or fifth intercostal space in the left parasternal region and perpendicular to the chest. LA = long-axis plane; SA = short-axis plane.

(Keep probe flat on chest, not angled off of chest WALL).

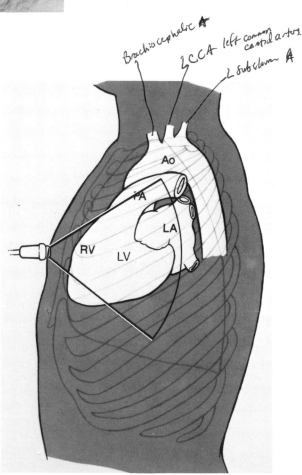

Brachiocephalic A
L CCA left common carotid artery
L subclavian A

FIGURE 2–2
LONG AXIS OF THE LEFT VENTRICLE
With the transducer in the left parasternal position, the sector image is oriented parallel to the long axis of the left ventricle, which usually moves along an imaginary line from the right sternoclavicular joint to the apex of the heart. Ao = aorta; PA = pulmonary artery; LA = left atrium; RV = right ventricle; LV = left ventricle.

iKnow

FIGURE 2–3
LONG AXIS OF THE LEFT VENTRICLE

In this view the right ventricular free wall and the right ventricular cavity (RV) are the most anterior structures. The interventricular septum (S) continues along the line of the anterior wall of the aorta (Ao) and is anterior to the left ventricular cavity (LV). The posterior wall of the left ventricle is the most posterior structure and superiorly continues along the line of the posterior wall of the left atrium (LA). The left atrium is behind the aorta and is separated from the left ventricle by the mitral valve (MV).

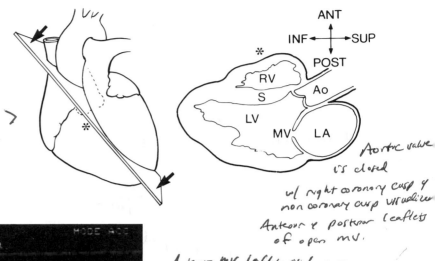

Aortic valve is closed

w/ right coronary cusp & non coronary cusp visualized

Anterior & posterior leaflets of open mv.

Anterior mv leaflet is longer

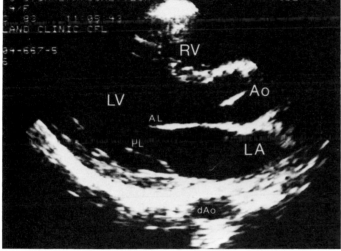

FIGURE 2–4
LONG AXIS OF THE LEFT VENTRICLE

Echocardiogram of the long axis of the left ventricle obtained from the left parasternal transducer position. RV = right ventricle; LV = left ventricle; Ao = aorta; LA = left atrium; AL = anterior mitral leaflet; PL = posterior mitral leaflet; dAo = descending aorta.

Anterior mv together comes very close to ventricular septum

FIGURE 2–5
LONG AXIS OF THE LEFT VENTRICLE, CARDIAC CYCLE

(1) Ventricular systole: the mitral valve is closed, the aortic valve is open, the cavity dimensions are small, and wall thickness is at its maximum. (2) Early diastole: the mitral valve is fully open, and the aortic valve is closed. (3) Rapid filling period: the mitral valve moves to a semiclosed position. (4) Atrial systole: the mitral valve reopens. (5) Ventricular systole: after atrial systole, the mitral valve closes again, and the aortic valve opens. RV = right ventricle; LV = left ventricle; Ao = aorta; LA = left atrium.

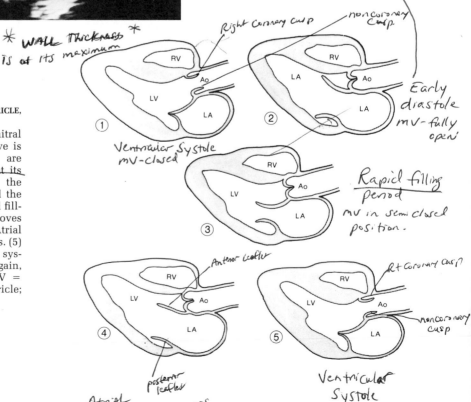

WALL Thickness is at its maximum

Right Coronary cusp   *noncoronary cusp*

Ventricular Systole mv-closed

Early diastole mv-fully open

Rapid filling period mv in semi closed position.

Anterior leaflet

posterior leaflet

Atrial Systole - mv reopens

Rt coronary cusp   *noncoronary cusp*

Ventricular Systole

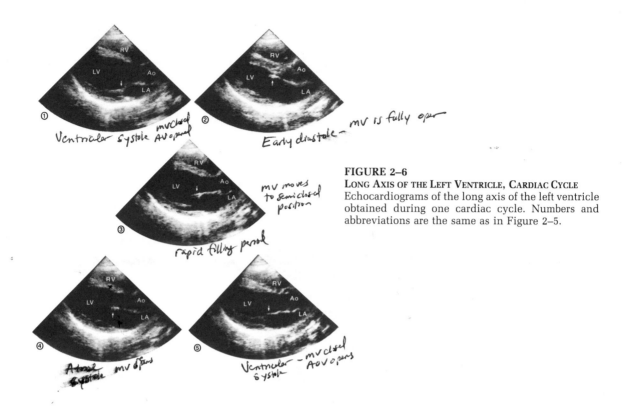

Ventricular systole mv closed AV opened

Early diastole – mv is fully open

mv moves to semiclosed position

rapid filling period

Atrial systole mv open

Ventricular systole – mv closed Aov opens

FIGURE 2–6
LONG AXIS OF THE LEFT VENTRICLE, CARDIAC CYCLE
Echocardiograms of the long axis of the left ventricle obtained during one cardiac cycle. Numbers and abbreviations are the same as in Figure 2–5.

FIGURE 2–7
LONG AXIS OF THE LEFT VENTRICLE, FORE-SHORTENED APEX
Note how the septum and the posterior wall appear to meet distal to the papillary muscles. This does not represent the true apex. In this view the true apex usually is not seen. RV = right ventricle; RA = right atrium.

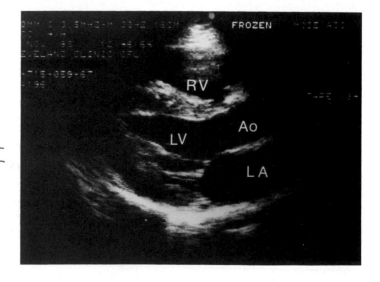

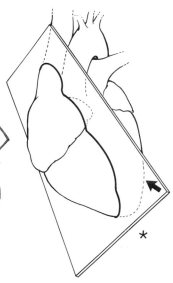

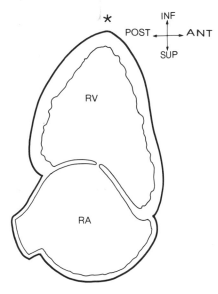

INF

POST ⟷ ANT

SUP

RV

RA

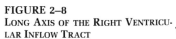

FIGURE 2–8
**LONG AXIS OF THE RIGHT VENTRICU-
LAR INFLOW TRACT**
With the transducer aligned to the
long axis of the heart, slight angulation of the sector scan toward
the right brings into the image the
inflow tract of the right ventricle
(RV). RA = right atrium.

(Pf 10.b)

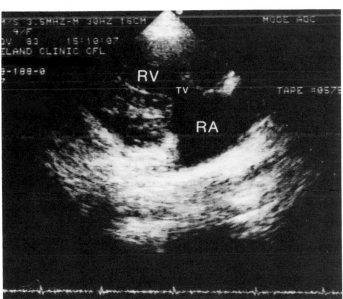

RV

TV

RA

FIGURE 2–9
**LONG AXIS OF THE RIGHT VENTRICULAR IN-
FLOW TRACT**
An echocardiogram obtained with slight
angulation to the right from the long-axis
plane of the left ventricle permits visualization of the anterior region. RV =
right ventricle; TV = tricuspid valve;
RA = right atrium.

TV
valve
is closed
in
systole

TV

FIGURE 2–10
**LONG AXIS OF THE RIGHT VENTRICULAR IN-
FLOW TRACT**
Systolic frame of the same section as in
Figure 2–9. Note the closed tricuspid
valve.

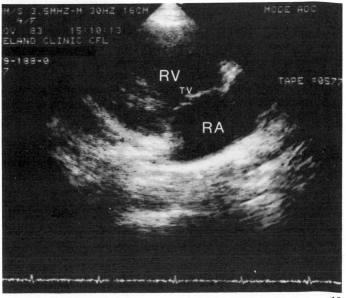

RV

TV

RA

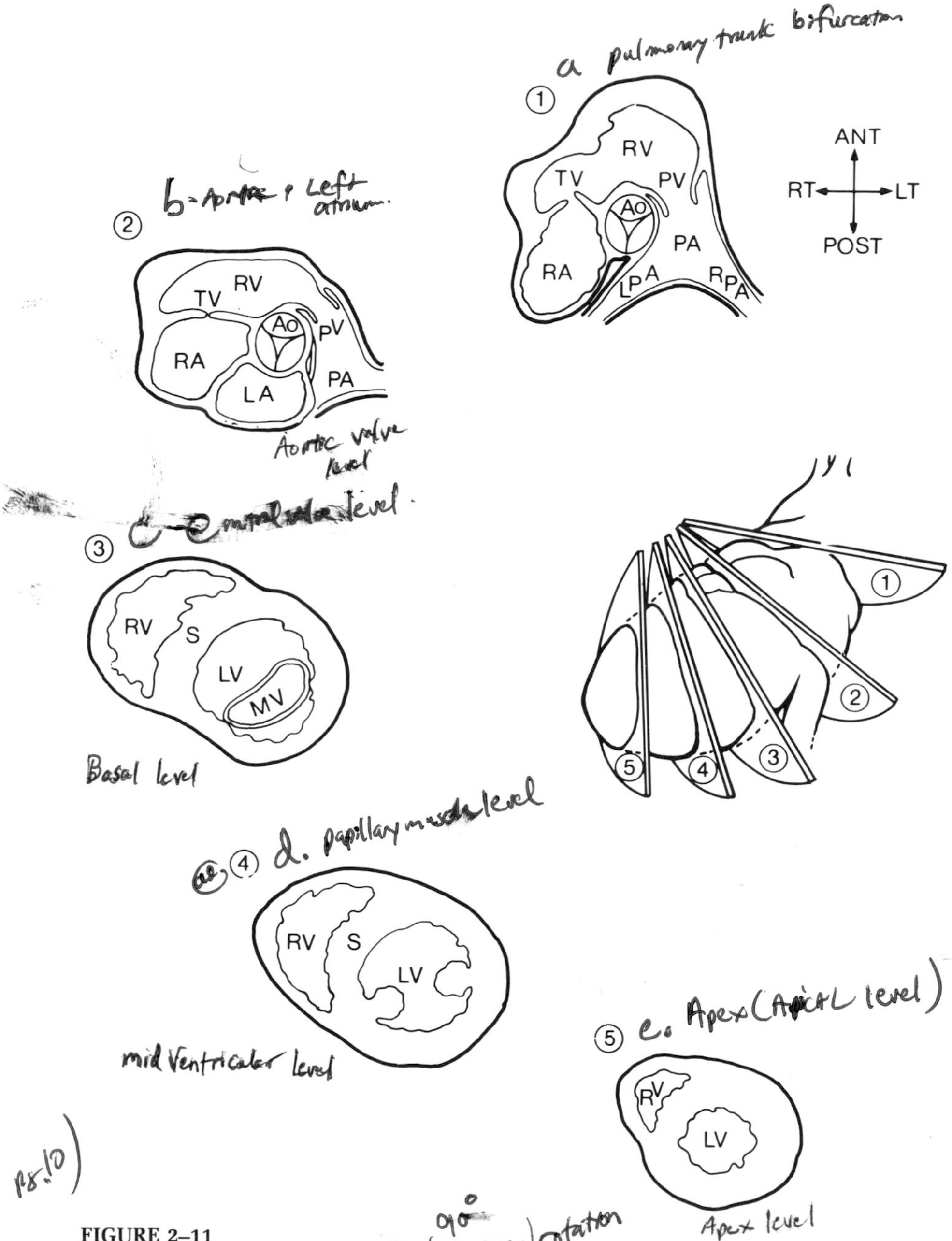

FIGURE 2–11
SHORT-AXIS VIEWS OF THE HEART
By rotating the transducer 90 degrees from the long-axis plane, short-axis views of the left ventricle are obtained. With high angulation, the sector plane is directed toward the bifurcation of the pulmonary artery (PA). Serial inferior angulation directs the sector plane through the aorta (Ao) and left atrium (LA), mitral valve (MV), papillary muscle level, and apex.

FIGURE 2–12
PULMONARY TRUNK BIFURCATION
The main pulmonary artery (PA) is seen to the left of the aorta (Ao). The right pulmonary artery (RPA) is to the left and posterior to the aorta. The left pulmonary artery (LPA) is further to the left. In front of the aorta is the right ventricular outflow tract (RVOT), and to its right is the right atrium (RA). TV = tricuspid valve; PV = pulmonic valve.

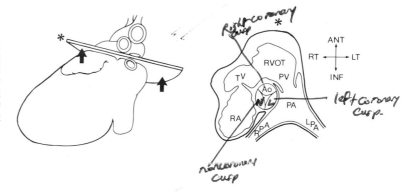

FIGURE 2–13
PULMONARY TRUNK BIFURCATION
Echocardiogram obtained at the level of the pulmonary trunk bifurcation demonstrates the aorta (Ao), the right ventricular outflow tract (RVOT), the pulmonary trunk (PA) and its bifurcation into the right pulmonary artery (RPA), and the left pulmonary artery (LPA).

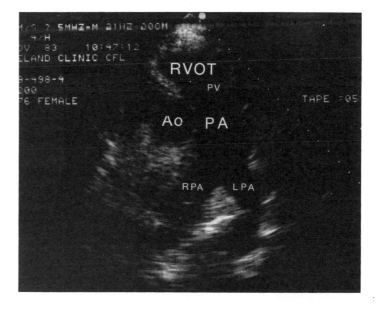

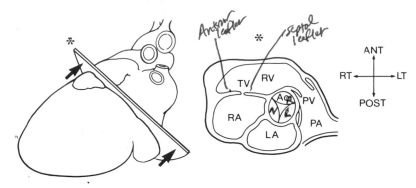

FIGURE 2–14
AORTA AND LEFT ATRIUM
At this level the sector plane is directed slightly inferiorly from the pulmonary trunk bifurcation plane. The aorta (Ao) is in the middle of the image. The outflow tract of the right ventricle (RV) is anterior to the aorta, and the left atrium (LA) is posterior to it. The right atrium (RA) and the pulmonary artery (PA) are to the sides of the aorta. TV = tricuspid valve; PV = pulmonic valve.

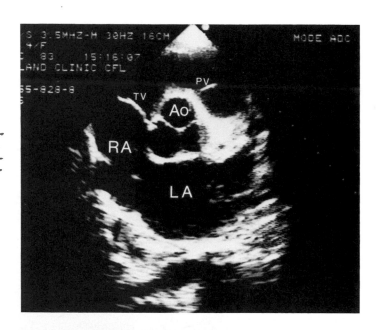

FIGURE 2–15
AORTA AND LEFT ATRIUM
Echocardiogram recorded at the level of the aortic valve in the short axis. The aortic valve is seen within the aorta (Ao) with an inverted Y configuration. The right coronary cusp is the most anterior, the noncoronary cusp is posterior and to the right, and the left coronary cusp is posterior and to the left. Behind the aorta the left atrium (LA) can be visualized. In this section it is also possible to visualize the right atrium (RA), the tricuspid valve (TV), and the pulmonic valve (PV).

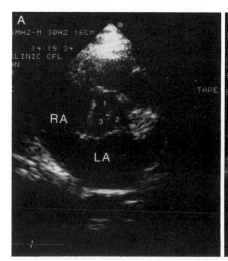
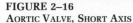

FIGURE 2–16
AORTIC VALVE, SHORT AXIS
Systolic (A) and diastolic (B) frames from a patient with a normal aortic valve. (1) Right coronary cusp; (2) left coronary cusp; (3) noncoronary cusp. During systole the three cusps move toward the aortic walls (arrows). RA = right atrium; LA = left atrium.

FIGURE 2–17
LEFT VENTRICLE AT MITRAL VALVE LEVEL
With the sector plane in the short axis and perpendicular to the chest, the left ventricle (LV) is imaged at the level of the mitral valve (MV). The left ventricle appears as a round structure, with the right ventricle (RV) anterior and to the left. The mitral valve during diastole has a "fish mouth" appearance. S = septum.

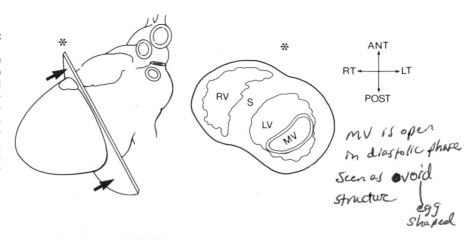

MV is open in diastolic phase seen as ovoid structure egg shaped

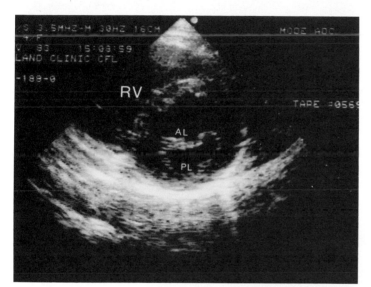

FIGURE 2–18
LEFT VENTRICLE AT MITRAL VALVE LEVEL
Short-axis echocardiogram of the left ventricle at the level of the mitral valve. The left ventricle has a doughnut-like appearance. The interventricular septum forms the anteromedial wall of the left ventricle. The right ventricle (RV) is anterior and to the right. This is a diastolic frame; the mitral valve is open and is seen as an ovoid structure within the left ventricle. AL = anterior leaflet; PL — posterior leaflet.

FIGURE 2–19
MITRAL VALVE, SHORT AXIS
Diastolic frame of the mitral valve at the base of its funnel. Note the large orifice size of the valve at this level. MVO = mitral valve orifice; RV = right ventricle; S = septum.

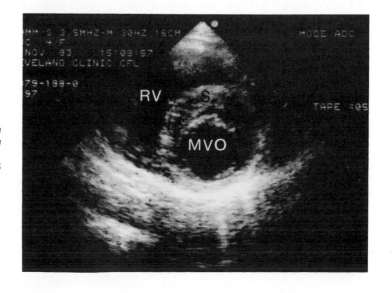

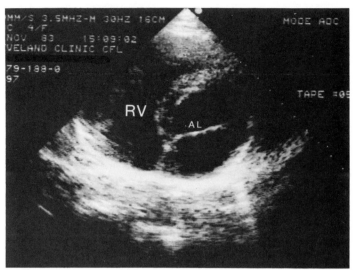

FIGURE 2–20
MITRAL VALVE, SHORT AXIS
Diastolic frame of the base of the mitral valve. Only the anterior leaflet (AL) is visualized in this area of transition between the left ventricle and the left atrium. RV = right ventricle.

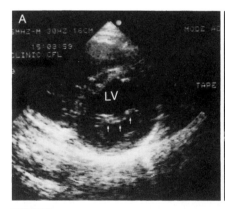
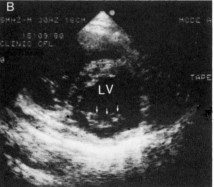

FIGURE 2–21
LEFT VENTRICLE AT MITRAL LEVEL
During diastole (A) the left ventricular circumference is larger, the walls are thinner, and the open mitral valve appears as an ovoid structure within the left ventricular circumference. During systole (B) the left ventricle is at its smallest size, the walls are thickened, and the mitral valve is closed, appearing as a diagonal linear structure. LV = left ventricle.

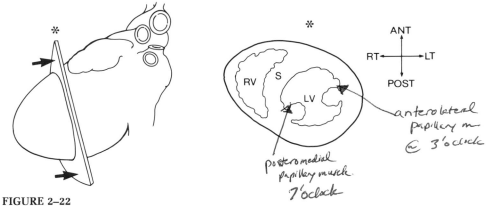

ANT

RT ←→ LT

POST

anterolateral papillary m. @ 3'oclock

posteromedial papillary muscle. 7'oclock

FIGURE 2–22
LEFT VENTRICLE AT PAPILLARY MUSCLE LEVEL
Slight inferior angulation of the sector plane from the mitral valve level brings the cross section cut to the level of the papillary muscles. The posteromedial papillary muscle is situated at about 7 o'clock and the anterolateral papillary muscle at about 3 o'clock of the left ventricular circumference. RV = right ventricle; S = septum; LV = left ventricle.

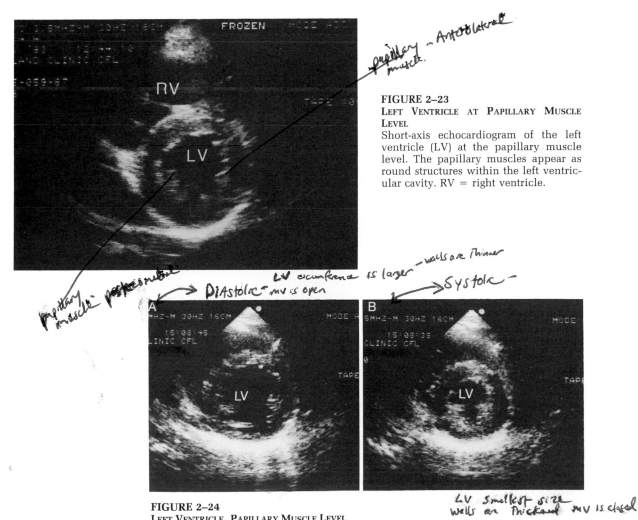

papillary muscle - Anterolateral

FIGURE 2–23
LEFT VENTRICLE AT PAPILLARY MUSCLE LEVEL
Short-axis echocardiogram of the left ventricle (LV) at the papillary muscle level. The papillary muscles appear as round structures within the left ventricular cavity. RV = right ventricle.

papillary muscle - posteromedial

LV circumference is larger - walls are Thinner

DIAStolic - MV is open

Systole -

LV smallest size walls are Thickened MV is closed

FIGURE 2–24
LEFT VENTRICLE, PAPILLARY MUSCLE LEVEL
Diastolic (A) and systolic (B) recordings of the left ventricle (LV) in the short-axis view. Note the change in internal diameter and wall thickness.

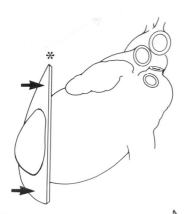

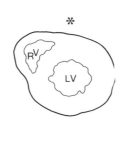

Move transducer one or two intercostal spaces below former views

FIGURE 2–25
LEFT VENTRICLE AT APICAL LEVEL

Further inferior angulation brings the sector plane to the level of the left ventricular apex. The papillary muscles are no longer visualized. The left ventricular cavity is rather small (LV). If part of the right ventricle (RV) can be visualized, it is to the right of the septum.

See pg 10 - Apical level (E)

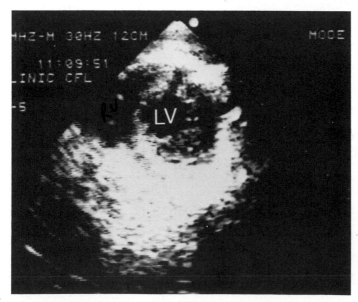

FIGURE 2–26
LEFT VENTRICLE AT APICAL LEVEL

Short-axis echocardiogram at the level of the apex. The left ventricular cavity (LV) is rather small. A small portion of the right ventricle is seen to the right of the septum.

 # dropout – absence of reflected signal from the region of fossa ovalis

Figure 2-29

trabecula(e) carneae
dis - array of thick muscular
tissue bands attached to the inner walls
of the ventricles of the heart

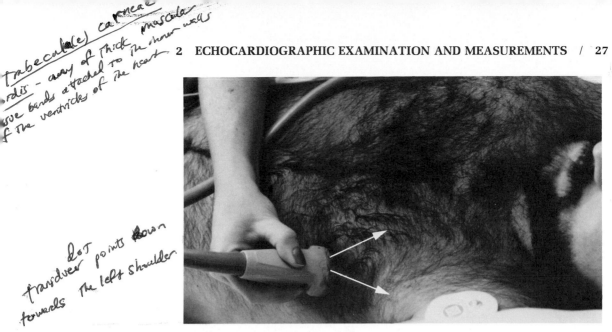

FIGURE 2–27
APICAL TRANSDUCER POSITION
With the patient in the left lateral decubitus position, the transducer is placed directly over the apical impulse of the left ventricle and is oriented parallel to the long axis of the heart.

transducer points down
towards the left shoulder

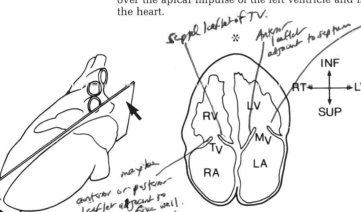

septal leaflet of TV.
Anterior leaflet adjacent to septum
Posterior mv leaflet adjacent to lateral wall.
In diastole
maybe anterior or posterior leaflet adjacent to free wall.

FIGURE 2–28
APICAL FOUR CHAMBER VIEW
With the transducer in the cardiac apex, the sector plane is oriented parallel to the long axis of the heart. This plane encompasses both ventricles (RV, LV) and both atria (RA, LA), as well as the mitral (MV) and tricuspid valves (TV).

LV w/ longer length than width
w/ a tapered but rounded apex

The anterolateral wall, apex, and inferior septum lie in this tomographic plane.
In systole.

FIGURE 2–29
APICAL FOUR-CHAMBER VIEW
Echocardiogram obtained from the cardiac apex permits imaging of the left ventricle (LV), the right ventricle (RV), the left atrium (LA), and the right atrium (RA). The interventricular septum is visualized in its entire longitude. Echo dropouts at the level of the fossa ovalis (FO) are common. The tricuspid valve (TV) is inserted in the interventricular septum at a point closer to the cardiac apex than the mitral valve (MV). MB = moderator band; PV = pulmonary vein.

View permits visualization of long axis of LV, interventricular septum, free lateral wall, & left ventricular apex.

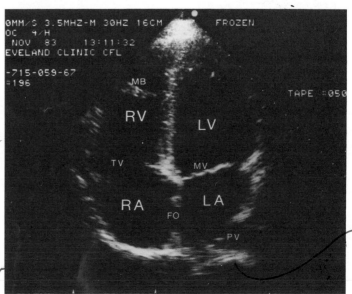

DTA lateral to LA

In systole closure plane of leaflets may appear flat - 180° closure angle.

More anterior portion of septum and lateral wall are seen

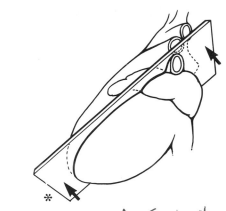

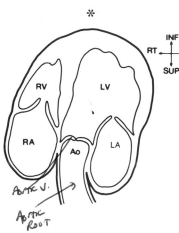

Angulating the transducer anteriorly the aortic valve and root are seen. This view "5C view"

Aortic V.
Aortic Root

FIGURE 2–30
APICAL FIVE-CHAMBER VIEW
With the transducer in a position similar to that used for obtaining the apical four-chamber view, slight anterior angulation will bring the aorta into the image. RV = right ventricle; LV = left ventricle; RA = right atrium; Ao = aorta; LA = left atrium.

FIGURE 2–31
APICAL FIVE-CHAMBER VIEW
This view is obtained from the apex with slight anterior angulation. This orientation permits visualization of the aorta (Ao), left ventricle (LV), right ventricle (RV), left atrium (LA), and right atrium (RA).

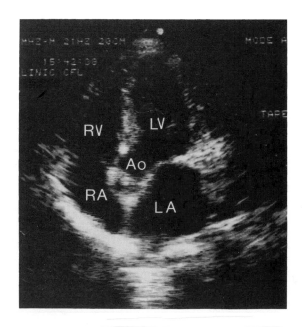

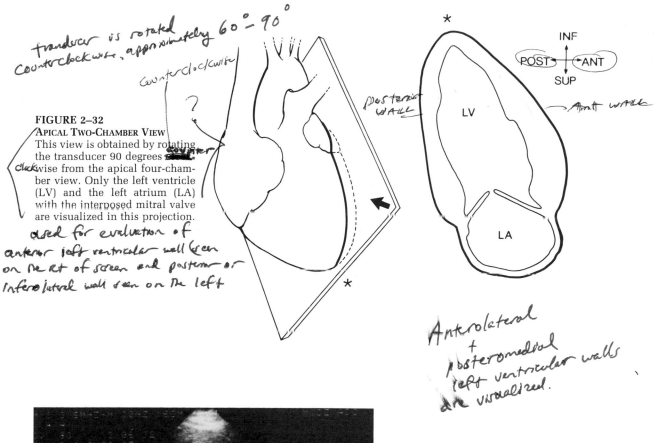

[handwritten annotations: transducer is rotated counterclockwise, approximately 60°–90°]

[handwritten: counterclockwise]

[handwritten: posterior wall]

[handwritten: Ant wall]

INF
POST — ANT
SUP

LV

LA

FIGURE 2–32
APICAL TWO-CHAMBER VIEW
This view is obtained by rotating the transducer 90 degrees *counterclockwise* from the apical four-chamber view. Only the left ventricle (LV) and the left atrium (LA) with the interposed mitral valve are visualized in this projection.

[handwritten: used for evaluation of anterior left ventricular wall (seen on the Rt of screen) and posterior or inferolateral wall seen on the left]

[handwritten: Anterolateral + posteromedial left ventricular walls are visualized.]

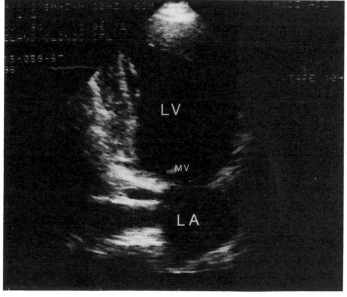

LV

MV

LA

FIGURE 2–33
APICAL TWO-CHAMBER VIEW
Echocardiogram obtained from the apical position by rotating the transducer 90 degrees from the apical four-chamber view. With this view it is possible to image the left ventricle (LV) and the left atrium (LA). No right ventricle is recorded. MV = mitral valve.

[handwritten: counter clockwise]

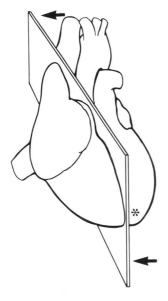

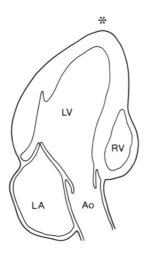

FIGURE 2–34
APICAL LONG-AXIS VIEW
This view is obtained by rotating the transducer 45 degrees clockwise from the apical four-chamber view. In addition to the true apex, this view encompasses the interventricular septum, the posterior ventricular wall, the left atrium (LA), the aortic root, and the aortic and mitral valves. LV = left ventricle; RV = right ventricle; Ao = aorta.

FIGURE 2–35
APICAL LONG-AXIS VIEW
Echocardiogram obtained from the apex after rotating the transducer 45 degrees from the apical four-chamber view. This view is similar to the left parasternal long-axis view of the left ventricle except that it includes the true apex. In addition, it permits visualization of the left ventricle (LV), left atrium (LA), aorta (Ao), and interventricular septum.

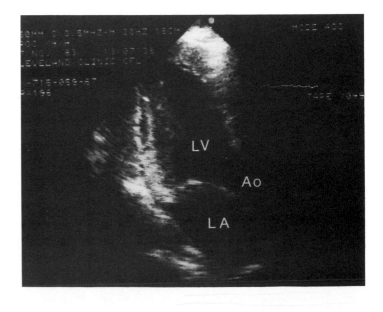

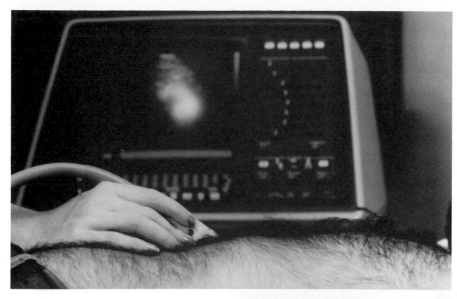

FIGURE 2–36
SUBCOSTAL TRANSDUCER
POSITION
With the patient in the
decubitus position, the
transducer is placed in
the subxiphoid region
and is directed toward
the area of interest.

FIGURE 2–37
INFERIOR VENA CAVA AND HEPATIC VEINS
Echocardiogram obtained from the subcostal region demonstrates the inferior
vena cava (IVC) in its long axis, with the
hepatic veins (HV) draining into it.
RA = right atrium; LA = left atrium.

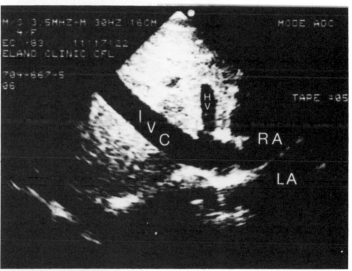

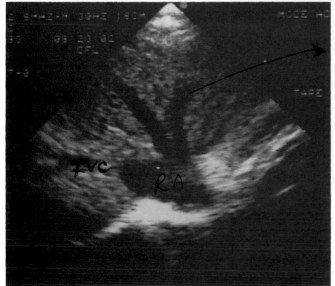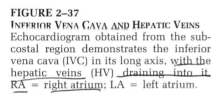

FIGURE 2–38
INFERIOR VENA CAVA AND HEPATIC VEINS
Echocardiogram obtained from the subcostal
region demonstrates the inferior vena cava
in its short axis. The hepatic veins are seen
communicating with the inferior vena cava
(note the "bunny head" appearance).

FIGURE 2-39
SUBCOSTAL FOUR-CHAMBER VIEW
With the transducer in the subcostal region, superior tilting will bring into the image the subcostal four-chamber view. RA = right atrium; LA = left atrium; RV = right ventricle; LV = left ventricle.

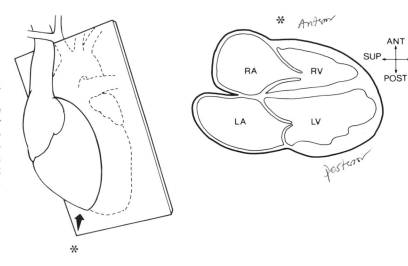

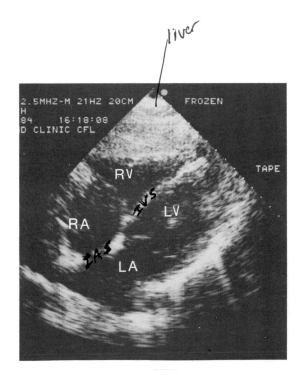

FIGURE 2-40
SUBCOSTAL FOUR-CHAMBER VIEW
Echocardiogram obtained from the subcostal region. The two atria and interatrial septum are best visualized. The tricuspid and mitral valves, as well as the right and left ventricles, are also imaged.

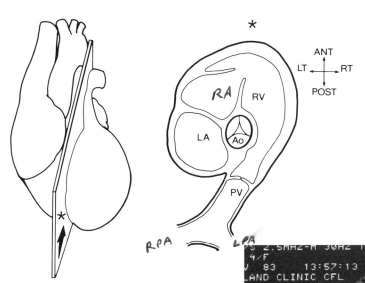

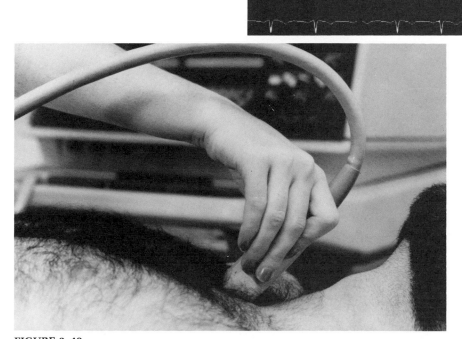

FIGURE 2–41
SUBCOSTAL RIGHT VENTRICULAR OUTFLOW TRACT
From the subcostal four-chamber view, 90 degrees of clockwise rotation and slight superior angulation bring the sector plane to the right ventricular outflow tract view. The aorta (Ao) is visualized in the short axis, and the entire right ventricular outflow tract can be viewed. RV = right ventricle; LA = left atrium; PV = pulmonic valve.

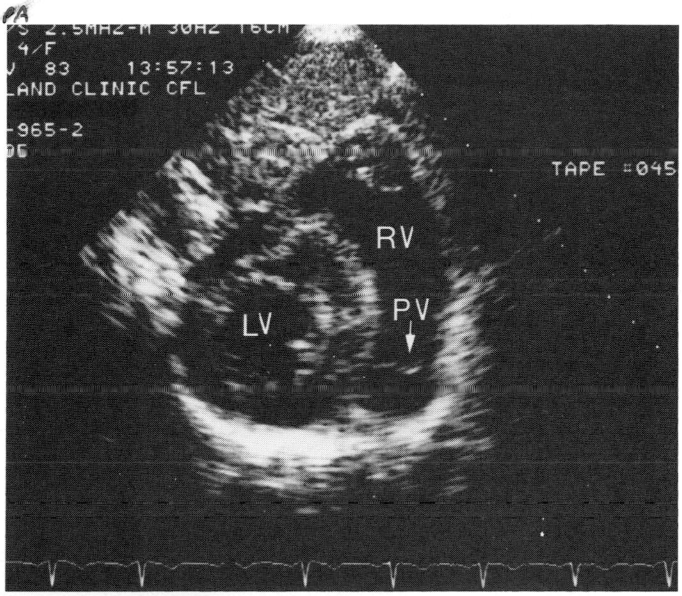

FIGURE 2–42
SUBCOSTAL RIGHT VENTRICULAR OUTFLOW TRACT
Echocardiogram obtained from the subcostal area demonstrates the left ventricle (LV) in its short axis and the entire right ventricular outflow tract (RV). PV = pulmonic valve.

FIGURE 2–43
SUPRASTERNAL TRANSDUCER POSITION
With the patient in the decubitus position with hyperextension of the neck, the transducer is placed in the suprasternal region, and the sector plane is directed to the area of interest.

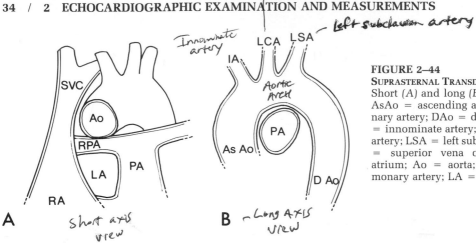

Left Common carotid artery

Innominate artery

LCA LSA — Left subclavian artery

IA

Aortic Arch

SVC

Ao

RPA

LA PA

RA

A Short axis view

As Ao

PA

D Ao

B — Long Axis view

FIGURE 2–44
SUPRASTERNAL TRANSDUCER POSITION
Short (A) and long (B) axes of the aorta. AsAo = ascending aorta; PA = pulmonary artery; DAo = descending aorta; IA = innominate artery; LCA = left carotid artery; LSA = left subclavian artery; SVC = superior vena cava; RA = right atrium; Ao = aorta; RPA = right pulmonary artery; LA = left atrium.

FIGURE 2–45
LONG AXIS OF THE AORTIC ARCH
Echocardiogram obtained from the suprasternal region demonstrates the long axis of the aortic arch. IN = innominate artery; Ao = aorta; ASC = ascending aorta; DES = descending aorta; RPA = right pulmonary artery; LA = left atrium.

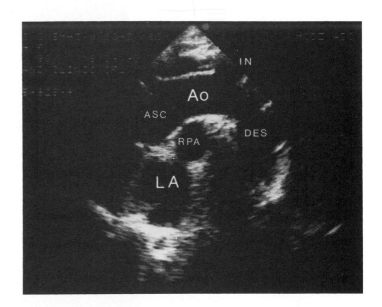

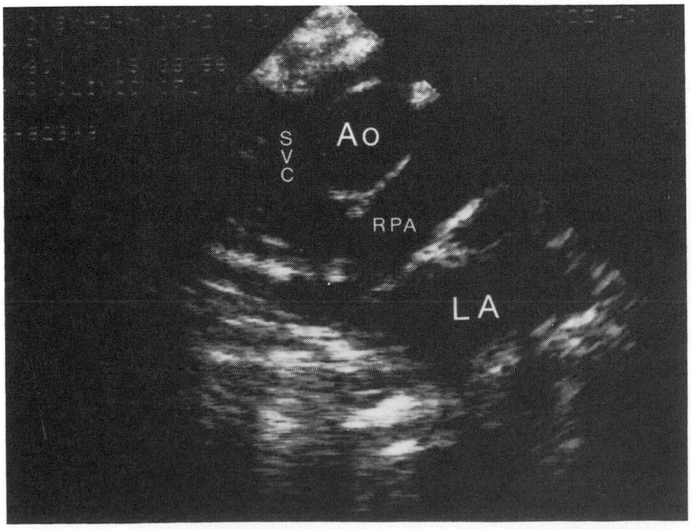

FIGURE 2–46
SHORT AXIS OF THE AORTA
Echocardiogram obtained from the suprasternal region demonstrates the short axis of the aorta. SVC = superior vena cava; RPA = right pulmonary artery; LA = left atrium; Ao = aorta.

in its Long axis

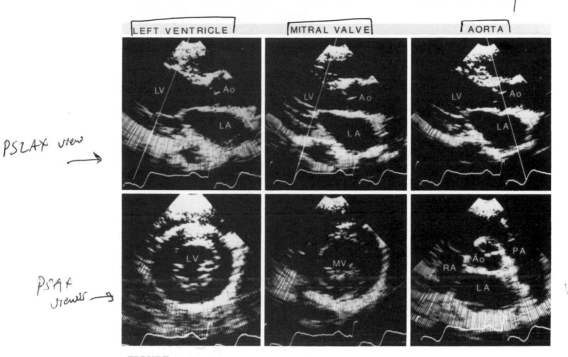

PSLAX view →

PSAX views →

FIGURE 2–47
LONG- AND SHORT-AXIS LEFT PARASTERNAL VIEWS
Long- and short-axis sections at the level of the left ventricle (LV), mitral valve (MV), and aortic valve. Ao = aorta; LA = left atrium; PA = pulmonary artery; RA = right atrium.

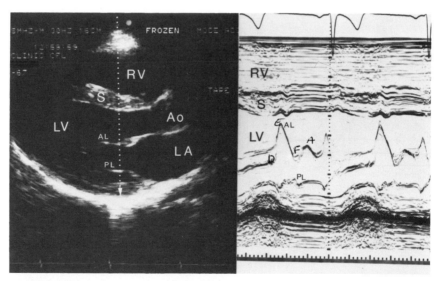

FIGURE 2–48
ECHOCARDIOGRAPHIC EXAMINATION OF THE MITRAL VALVE
The areas through which the echocardiographic beam transects the heart when the beam is directed toward the mitral valve are the anterior wall of the right ventricle, the right ventricular cavity (RV), and the interventricular septum (S). In the left ventricular cavity (LV), the beam passes through the anterior (AL) and posterior (PL) mitral valve leaflets and then exits through the posterior wall of the left ventricle. Ao = aorta; LA = left atrium.

[handwritten annotations: Atrial systole - reopened mv - Finally of beginning of ventricular systole mv moves back to a closed position ___ D line. During systole, both leaflets remain together]

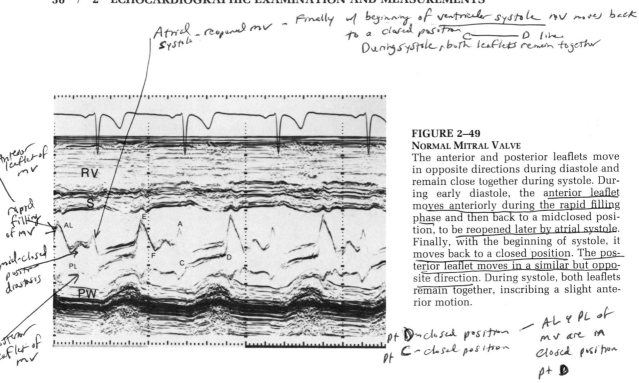

[handwritten annotations on left: Anterior leaflet of mv; rapid filling of mv; mid-closed positn diastasis; posterior leaflet of mv]

FIGURE 2–49
NORMAL MITRAL VALVE

The anterior and posterior leaflets move in opposite directions during diastole and remain close together during systole. During early diastole, the anterior leaflet moves anteriorly during the rapid filling phase and then back to a midclosed position, to be reopened later by atrial systole. Finally, with the beginning of systole, it moves back to a closed position. The posterior leaflet moves in a similar but opposite direction. During systole, both leaflets remain together, inscribing a slight anterior motion.

[handwritten annotations: pt D = closed position; pt C - closed position — AL & PL of mv are in closed position pt D]

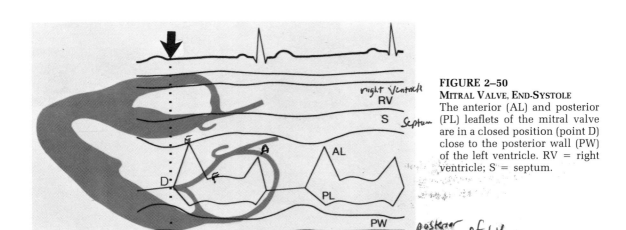

[handwritten annotations: right ventricle RV; S Septum; posterior wall of LV]

FIGURE 2–50
MITRAL VALVE, END-SYSTOLE

The anterior (AL) and posterior (PL) leaflets of the mitral valve are in a closed position (point D) close to the posterior wall (PW) of the left ventricle. RV = right ventricle; S = septum.

Early Diastole

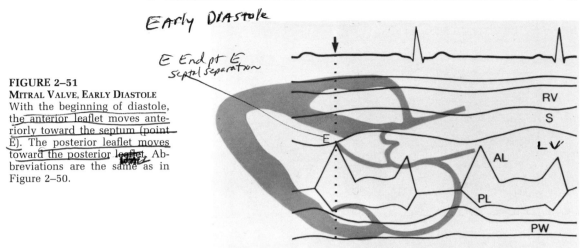

E End pt E
septal separation

FIGURE 2–51
MITRAL VALVE, EARLY DIASTOLE
With the beginning of diastole, the anterior leaflet moves anteriorly toward the septum (point E). The posterior leaflet moves toward the posterior leaflet. Abbreviations are the same as in Figure 2–50.

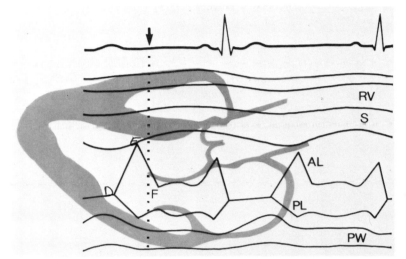

FIGURE 2–52
MITRAL VALVE, MID-DIASTOLE
As the rapid filling period of the left ventricle begins, the mitral valve moves to a semiclosed position (point F). Abbreviations are the same in Figure 2–50.

mv moves back to a
semi closed position

mv is reopened by atrial systole
and finally closes ~ w beginning
of ventricular systole.

FIGURE 2–53
MITRAL VALVE, ATRIAL SYSTOLE
With atrial systole, the mitral valve reopens from the prior semiclosed position to point A. Abbreviations are the same as in Figure 2–50.

atrial systole
mv reopens

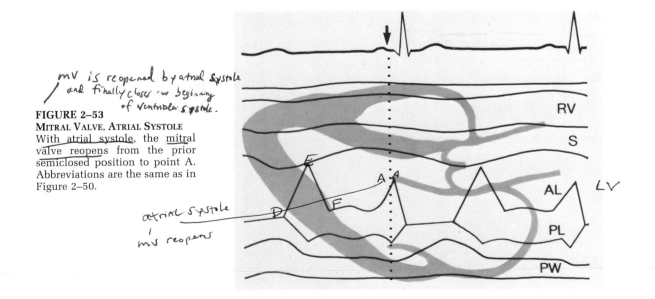

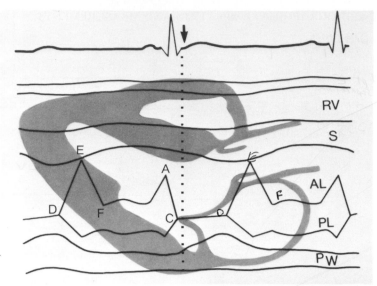

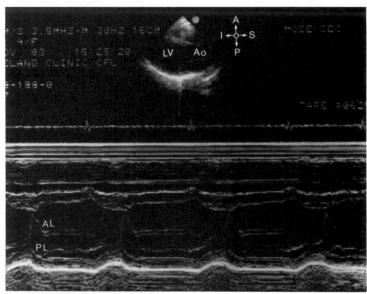

FIGURE 2–55
MITRAL VALVE, LONG AXIS
M-mode echocardiogram of the mitral valve obtained from the long-axis two-dimensional scan. AL = anterior leaflet; PL = posterior leaflet; Ao = aorta; LV = left ventricle.

FIGURE 2–56
MITRAL VALVE, SHORT AXIS
M-mode echocardiogram of the mitral valve obtained from the short-axis two-dimensional scan. Note that the M-mode echocardiogram is similar to that obtained from the long-axis scan. AL = anterior leaflet; PL = posterior leaflet; LV = left ventricle; RV = right ventricle.

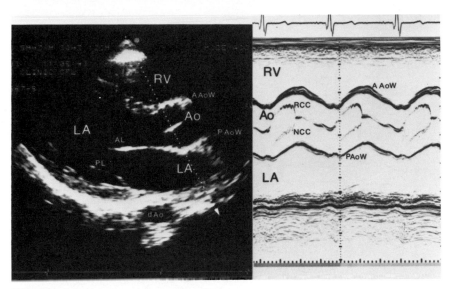

FIGURE 2–57

ECHOCARDIOGRAPHIC EXAMINATION OF THE AORTA

The areas of the heart transected by the echocardiographic beam when directed toward the aortic valve are the right ventricular outflow tract, the anterior wall of the aorta (Ao), the aortic leaflets, the posterior wall of the aorta, and the left atrium (LA). The beam exits through the posterior wall of the left atrium. RV = right ventricle; A AoW = anterior aortic wall; P AoW = posterior aortic wall; AL = anterior leaflet; PL = posterior leaflet; dAo = descending aorta; RCC = right coronary cusp; NCC = noncoronary cusp.

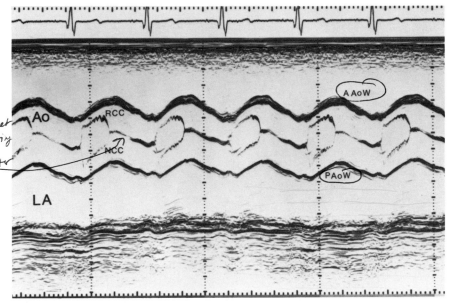

RCC & NCC close and meet at the end of ejection During diastole, The leaflets remain together at the center of the aortic root

w/ beginning of ejection (systole)

the Right coronary Cusp moves anteriorly and the Non coronary cusp moves posteriorly

FIGURE 2–58

NORMAL AORTA AND AORTIC VALVE

The anterior (A AoW) and posterior (P AoW) aortic walls move parallel throughout the cardiac cycle. They have an anterior motion during systole and a posterior motion during diastole. Within the aortic root, two of the three aortic cusps are usually recorded. With the beginning of ejection, the right coronary cusp (RCC) moves anteriorly, and the noncoronary cusp (NCC) moves posteriorly. Both remain separated and close to the aortic walls throughout systole. They close and meet at the end of ejection. During diastole, the leaflets remain together at the center of the aortic root and follow its motion. The left coronary cusp is usually not recorded. Behind the posterior wall of the aorta (Ao), the left atrium (LA) appears as an echo-free space, limited posteriorly by its posterior wall, which has only very minimal motion.

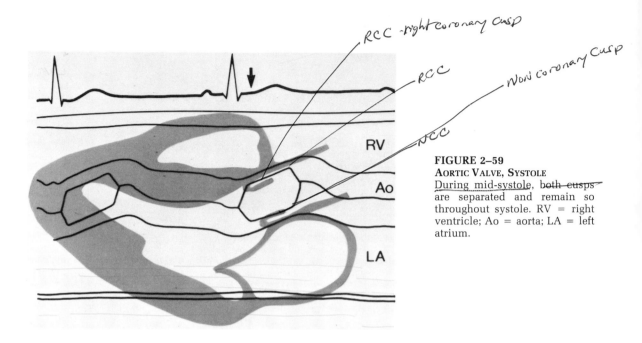

RCC - right coronary cusp

RCC

Non coronary cusp

NCC

FIGURE 2–59
AORTIC VALVE, SYSTOLE
During mid-systole, both cusps
are separated and remain so
throughout systole. RV = right
ventricle; Ao = aorta; LA = left
atrium.

END SYSTOLE
- both leaflets come
together

FIGURE 2–60
AORTIC VALVE, END-SYSTOLE
At the end of systole, both leaflets come together in the center
of the aortic root. RV = right
ventricle; Ao = aorta; LA = left
ventricle.

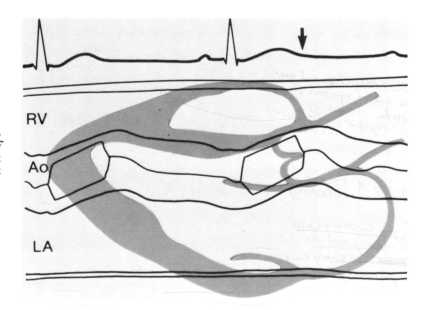

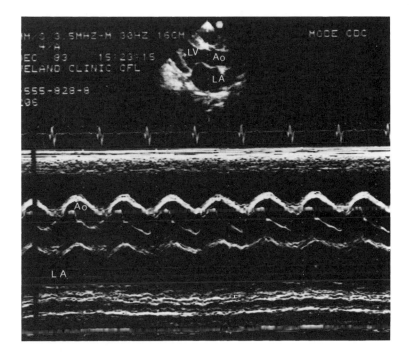

FIGURE 2–61
AORTIC VALVE, LONG AXIS
M-mode echocardiogram of the aorta obtained from the long-axis two-dimensional scan. LV = left ventricle; Ao = aorta; LA = left atrium.

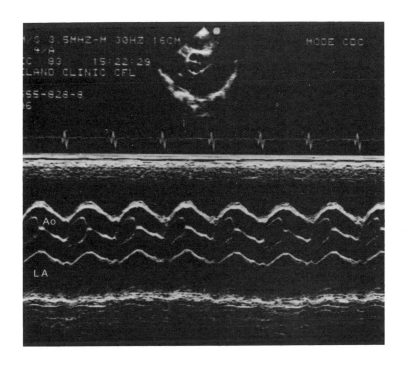

FIGURE 2–62
AORTIC VALVE, SHORT AXIS
M-mode echocardiogram of the aorta obtained from the short-axis two-dimensional scan. Note that both M-mode echocardiograms (see Fig. 2–61) appear the same.

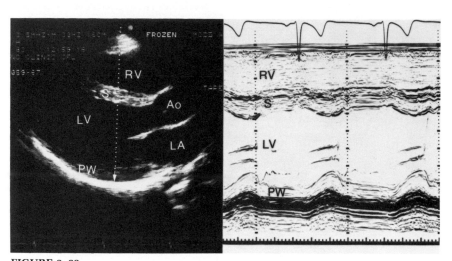

FIGURE 2–63
ECHOCARDIOGRAPHIC EXAMINATION OF THE LEFT VENTRICLE
When the echocardiographic beam is directed toward the left ventricular cavity, it transects the anterior wall of the right ventricle, the right ventricular cavity (RV), the interventricular septum (S), and the left ventricular cavity (LV). The beam exits through the posterior wall of the left ventricle (PW). Ao = aorta; LA = left atrium.

FIGURE 2–64
NORMAL LEFT VENTRICLE
Behind the stationary chest wall echoes, the right ventricular wall and the right ventricular cavity (RV) are recorded. The interventricular septum (S) moves posteriorly during systole and anteriorly during diastole. Behind the septum, the left ventricular cavity (LV) appears as an echo-free space with only very fine echoes in it. The endocardial and epicardial surfaces of the posterior wall (PW) are seen posterior to this space. They move anteriorly during systole and posteriorly during diastole.

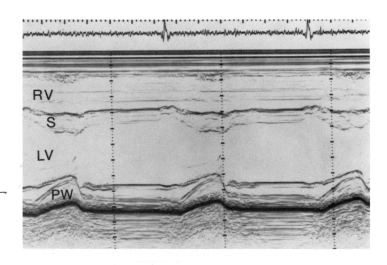

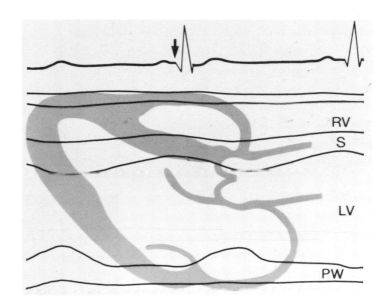

FIGURE 2–65
LEFT VENTRICLE, DIASTOLE
The interventricular septum (S) and the posterior wall of the left ventricle (PW) are at their maximal separation and the wall thickness is the smallest during diastole. RV = right ventricle; LV = left ventricle.

RV wall and IVS move anteriorly
PW moves posteriorly

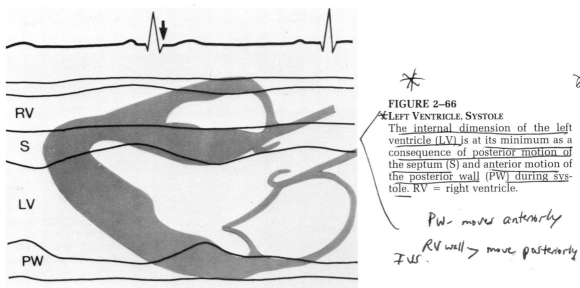

FIGURE 2–66
LEFT VENTRICLE, SYSTOLE
The internal dimension of the left ventricle (LV) is at its minimum as a consequence of posterior motion of the septum (S) and anterior motion of the posterior wall (PW) during systole. RV = right ventricle.

PW- moves anteriorly
IVS. RV wall > move posteriorly

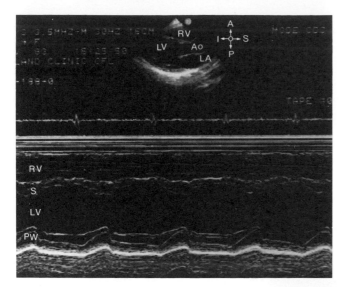

FIGURE 2–67

LEFT VENTRICLE, M-MODE FROM LONG AXIS
The M-mode echocardiographic tracing of
the left ventricle is obtained by selecting the
M-mode line. This transects the left ventricle at the chordae tendineae level, proximal
to the tip of the papillary muscles. RV =
right ventricle; Ao = aorta; LV = left ventricle; S = septum; PW = posterior wall.

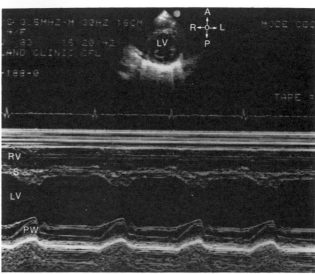

FIGURE 2–68

LEFT VENTRICLE, M-MODE FROM SHORT AXIS
A similar M-mode echocardiogram of the
left ventricle can be obtained from the short-
axis sector scan by directing the M-mode
line between the papillary muscles. RV =
right ventricles; S = septum; LV = left
ventricle; PW = posterior wall.

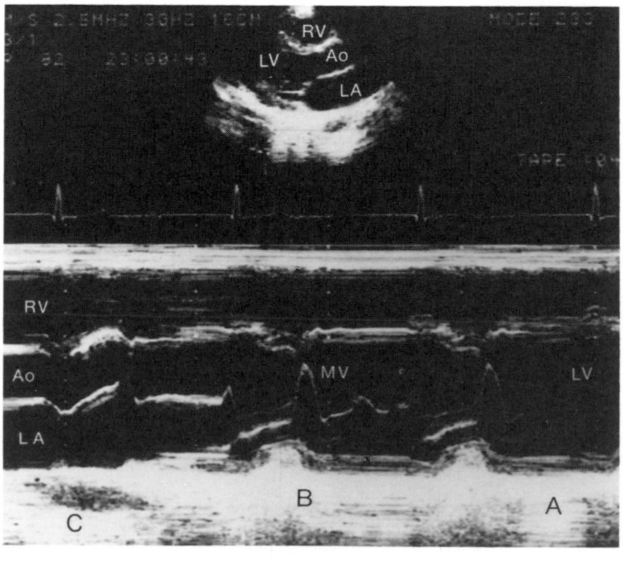

FIGURE 2–69

ECHOCARDIOGRAPHIC SCAN
Echocardiographic scan demonstrates the
left ventricular cavity (LV) at level A, the
mitral valve (MV) at level B, and the aorta
(Ao) at level C. RV = right ventricle; LA =
left atrium.

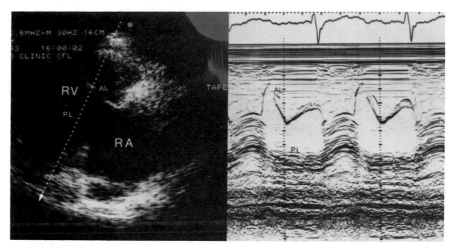

FIGURE 2–70

EXAMINATION OF THE TRICUSPID VALVE

For examination of the tricuspid valve, the transducer is oriented to the inflow tract of the right ventricle (RV). The echocardiographic motion of the tricuspid valve is very similar to that of the mitral valve. The anterior leaflet (AL) moves anteriorly during diastole and to a midclosed position after the rapid filling. It reopens with the atrial kick and is closed with the beginning of systole. A posterior leaflet (PL) moves in the opposite direction. This posterior leaflet usually has more excursion than does the posterior leaflet of the mitral valve. In front of the tricuspid valve, the right ventricular wall is recorded.

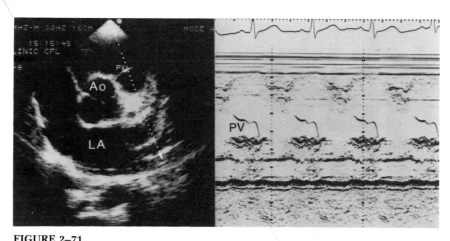

FIGURE 2–71

EXAMINATION OF THE PULMONIC VALVE

To examine the pulmonic valve (PV), the transducer is oriented to the short axis of the great vessels, and the M-mode line is directed to the pulmonary artery. Usually only one of the pulmonic leaflets is recorded. The cycle of pulmonic valve motion starts with a posterior deflection produced by atrial systole; then the leaflet moves back, at which time ejection starts. Finally, the leaflet moves posteriorly to a fully open position. It remains open throughout systole and then returns to a closed position. During diastole, a mild posterior displacement of the leaflet is noted. The size of the a wave varies, with respiration becoming larger in full inspiration. Ao = aorta; LA = left atrium.

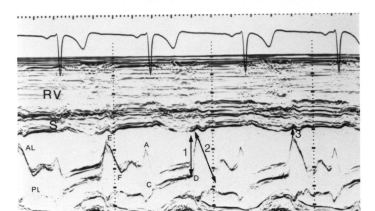

FIGURE 2–72

NORMAL MITRAL VALVE MEASUREMENTS
Echocardiogram of a normal mitral valve with good visualization of the anterior leaflet (AL) and the posterior leaflet (PL). Routine echocardiographic measurements include valve excursion (1), E to F slope (2), and septal-mitral valve distance (3). See text for definitions and normal values. Points E, F, A, C, and D are conventionally used to define the mitral valve motion during the cardiac cycle. RV = right ventricle; PW = posterior wall.

FIGURE 2–73

AORTA AND AORTIC VALVE MEASUREMENTS
This echocardiogram demonstrates a normal aorta (Ao) and aortic valve. The routine measurements obtained from this recording are (1) aortic valve leaflet separation, (2) left ventricular ejection time, and (3) aortic root dimension. LA = left atrium.

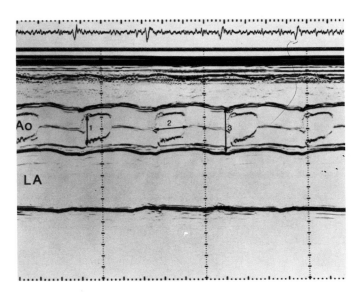

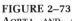

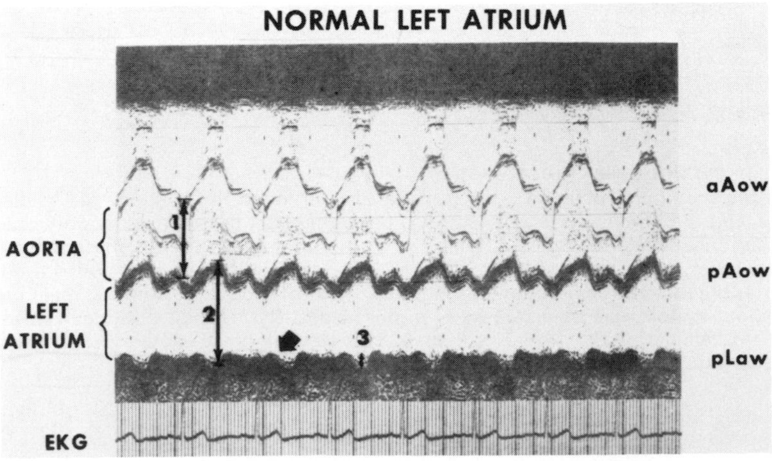

FIGURE 2–74

NORMAL LEFT ATRIUM
This echocardiogram illustrates the normal aortic and left atrial measurements: (1) aortic root diameter, (2) left atrial diameter, and (3) posterior wall motion. The arrow points to the posterior systolic motion of the left atrial wall. See text for definitions and normal values. aAow = anterior aortic wall; pAow = posterior aortic wall; pLaw = posterolateral aortic wall.

See Pg 14   Text

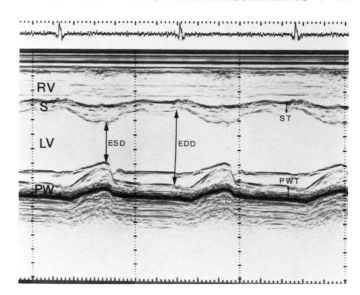

FIGURE 2–75
VENTRICULAR DIMENSIONS
The routine echocardiographic dimensions that are measured at the level of the left ventricle include (1) end-diastolic diameter (EDD), (2) end-systolic diameter (ESD), (3) end-diastolic septal thickness (ST), and (4) end-diastolic posterior wall thickness (PWT). See text for definitions and normal values. RV = right ventricle; S = septum; LV = left ventricle; PW = posterior wall.

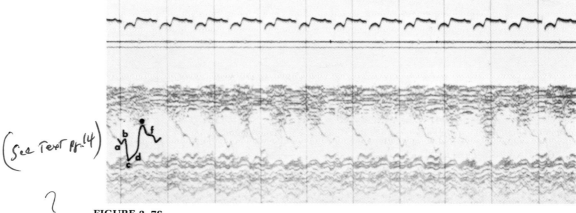

(See Text pg. 14)

FIGURE 2–76
NORMAL PULMONIC VALVE
The normal pulmonic valve measurements are illustrated. These include (1) E to F slope, (2) a wave amplitude, (3) amplitude of opening, and (4) opening velocity. See text for definitions and normal values.

BC-Slope - slope of pulmonic valve opening in early systole.
amplitude of normal value is 2 mm
amplitude is ↑ in pulmonary hyper-

RIGHT VENTRICLE - MEASUREMENTS

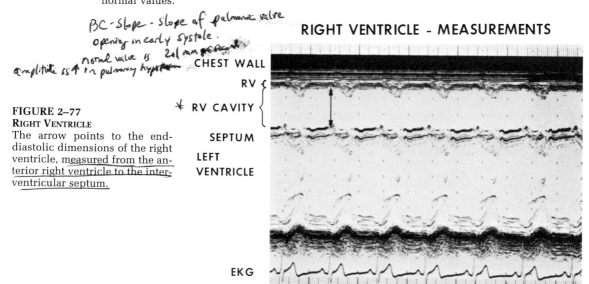

FIGURE 2–77
RIGHT VENTRICLE
The arrow points to the end-diastolic dimensions of the right ventricle, measured from the anterior right ventricle to the interventricular septum.

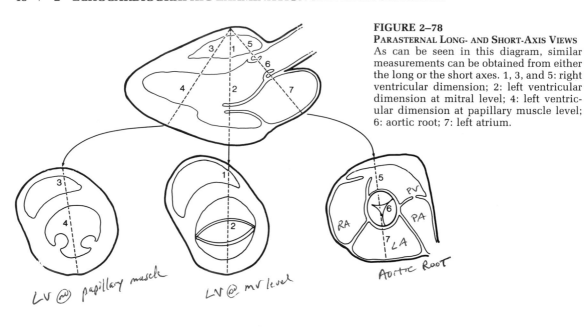

FIGURE 2–78
PARASTERNAL LONG- AND SHORT-AXIS VIEWS
As can be seen in this diagram, similar measurements can be obtained from either the long or the short axes. 1, 3, and 5: right ventricular dimension; 2: left ventricular dimension at mitral level; 4: left ventricular dimension at papillary muscle level; 6: aortic root; 7: left atrium.

FIGURE 2–79
PARASTERNAL LONG AXIS
This view allows for measuring the aorta (Ao), left atrium (LA), right ventricle (RV), septum (S), left ventricular dimension (LVD), and posterior wall thickness (PW).

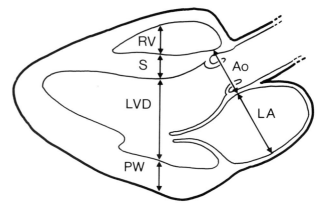

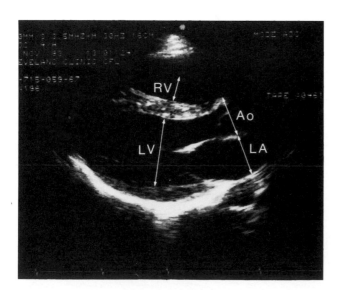

FIGURE 2–80
PARASTERNAL LONG AXIS
Two-dimensional echocardiogram demonstrates the routine dimensions that can be measured from the long axis in the left parasternal view. RV = right ventricle; LV = left ventricle; Ao = aorta; LA = left atrium.

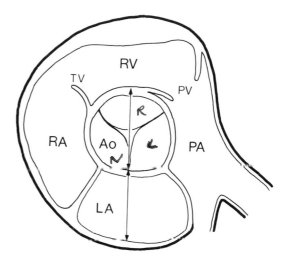

FIGURE 2–81
PARASTERNAL SHORT AXIS, AORTA, AND LEFT ATRIUM
The anteroposterior dimensions of the aorta (Ao) and left atrium (LA) are measured from this view. RA = right atrium; TV = tricuspid valve; RV = right ventricle; PV = pulmonic valve; PA = pulmonary artery.

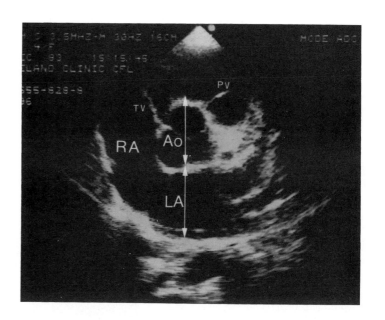

FIGURE 2–82
PARASTERNAL SHORT AXIS, AORTA, AND LEFT ATRIUM
This echocardiogram demonstrates the routine measurements to be obtained at this level. Ao = aorta; LA = left atrium; RA = right atrium; TV = tricuspid valve; PV = pulmonic valve.

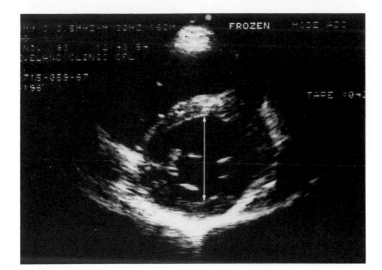

FIGURE 2–83
SHORT-AXIS, MITRAL LEVEL
At this level the minor anteroposterior diameter is measured as the ventrical distance from the septum to the posterior left ventricular wall.

FIGURE 2–84
SHORT-AXIS, MITRAL, AND PAPILLARY MUSCLE LEVELS
These minor anteroposterior diameters are measured in a similar way as described in Figure 2–83.

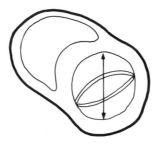 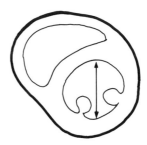

MITRAL LEVEL   PAPILLARY MUSCLE LEVEL

FIGURE 2–85
APICAL FOUR-CHAMBER VIEW
From this view these measurements are made: (1) long axis of the left ventricle; (2) short axis of the left ventricle; (3) major axis of the left atrium; (4) minor axis of the left atrium; (5) long axis of the right ventricle; (6) short axis of the right ventricle; (7) major axis of the right atrium; (8) minor axis of the right atrium. RV = right ventricle; LV = left ventricle; RA = right atrium; LA = left atrium.

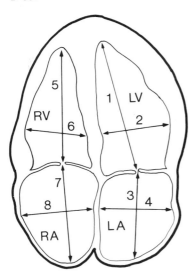

FIGURE 2–86
APICAL FOUR-CHAMBER VIEW
Two-dimensional echocardiogram with the routine measurements. The numbers are shown in Figure 2–85. Abbreviations are the same as for Figure 2–85.

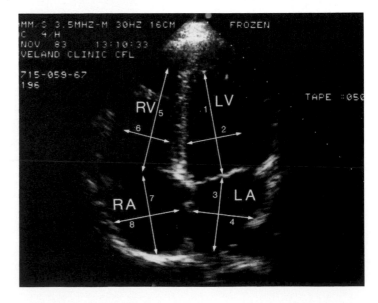

3 ECHOPHONOCARDIOGRAPHY AND ECHOCARDIOGRAPHIC FINDINGS WITH ALTERED ELECTRICAL ACTIVATION

3.1 ECHOPHONOCARDIOGRAPHY

The echocardiogram can serve as a reference recording for the evaluation of heart sounds and murmurs.[1-5] Figure 3-1 illustrates the correlations between the electrocardiogram, the carotid pulse tracing, the apexcardiogram phonocardiogram, and the motion of the valves seen by echocardiography. The aortic and pulmonic valves can be used as references for ejection clicks, evaluation of the second heart sound, and measurement of ejection time.

A. First Heart Sound

Four components of the first heart sound have been identified (Fig. 3-2). The initial low-frequency component occurs at the beginning of mechanical systole and precedes the actual closure of the mitral valve. The second component coincides with mitral valve closure, and the third and fourth components are related to the beginning of ejection and acceleration of flow into the great vessels.

Patients with complete heart block present an opportunity to evaluate the relation of mitral valve closure to the first heart sound (Figs. 3-3 to 3-5). A short PR interval is related to a loud first heart sound because both atrial and ventricular systoles find the mitral valve in a fully open position, which by an additive effect produces a forceful valve closure. With a long PR interval, the mitral valve may actually close by the atrial systole, producing an atrial sound. At the beginning of ventricular systole, the mitral valve is closed, causing the first heart sound to be soft. With a longer PR interval, the mitral valve may reopen, and its closure with the beginning of ventricular systole produces a loud or normal first heart sound.

B. Second Heart Sound

Although mean intervals of 12 and 60 msec, respectively, have been found between aortic closure and A_2 and pulmonic closure and P_2, the early components of A_2 and P_2 do correspond to the coaptation of the aortic (Fig. 3–6) and pulmonic valves (Fig. 3–7). The echocardiographic record of the semilunar valves may be used for identifying A_2 and P_2 when these are buried in a holosystolic or continuous murmur or when there is paradoxic splitting of the second heart sound.

C. Third Heart Sound

A third heart sound occurs at the time of rapid ventricular filling. This can be precisely identified by the F waves of the apexcardiogram or the initial down slope of the E to F slope of the mitral valve echogram (Figs. 3–8, 3–9).

D. Fourth Heart Sound

A fourth heart sound occurs during atrial systole. It can be identified by the a wave of the apexcardiogram (Fig. 3–10) or by the a wave of the mitral valve echogram (Fig. 3–11). In some patients, both a third and a fourth sound can be registered (Fig. 3–12).

The echophonocardiographic findings in specific cardiac abnormalities are discussed under the given chapters.

3.2 SYSTOLIC TIME INTERVALS

The left ventricular ejection time measured from the opening to the closing of the aortic valve correlates well with that obtained by the carotid pulse recording. The total electromechanical time $(Q S_2)$ can be measured from the Q wave of the electrocardiogram to the closure of the aortic valve. The pre-ejection period (PEP) is obtained indirectly, by subtracting the left ventricular ejection time (LVET) from the total electromechanical time[6] (Fig. 3–13).

For the calculation of right-side systolic time intervals, the echocardiographic recording of the pulmonic valve is used. The right ventricular ejection time is measured from the opening to the closing motion of the pulmonic valve. The total electromechanical time is measured from the Q wave of the electrocardiogram to the closure of the pulmonic valve. The pre-ejection period is determined indirectly by subtracting the right ventricular ejection time from the pre-ejection period (Fig. 3–14).

3.3 ALTERED ELECTRICAL ACTIVATION

Alterations in the motion of the atrioventricular and semilunar valves, as well as of ventricular and atrial walls, can be seen in several forms of arrhythmias: sinus arrhythmia (Fig. 3–15); sinus tachycardia (Fig. 3–16); premature ventricular contraction (Figs. 3–17, 3–18); atrial fibrillation (Figs. 3–19, 3–20); atrial flutter[7] (Fig. 3–21); ventricular tachycardia (Fig. 3–22); first-degree atrioventricular block (Fig. 3–23); and complete heart block (Figs. 3–3 to 3–5).

Alterations in cardiac motion can be demonstrated in the following conditions with abnormal ventricular depolarization:

1. Left bundle branch block (Fig. 3–24)
   a. Brief downward dip of the septum toward the left ventricle shortly after the mitral valve opening.
   b. Systolic anterior motion of the septum.
2. Ventricular pacing (Fig. 3–25)
   When the right ventricle is paced from the apex, septal motion abnormalities similar to those seen in left bundle branch block are present.
3. Right bundle branch block
   a. Normal septal motion.
   b. Delayed pulmonic valve opening.
   c. Delayed tricuspid valve closure.
4. Wolff-Parkinson-White syndrome (Fig. 3–26)
   Type A: abnormal motion of the posterior wall consisting of a brief anterior displacement following the beginning of electrical depolarization.
   Type B: abnormal septal motion similar to that of left bundle branch block.

Left ventricular ejection time (LVET) – from aortic valve opening (AVO) to closure (AVC)

ECHO-PHONO-GRAPHICS CORRELATIONS

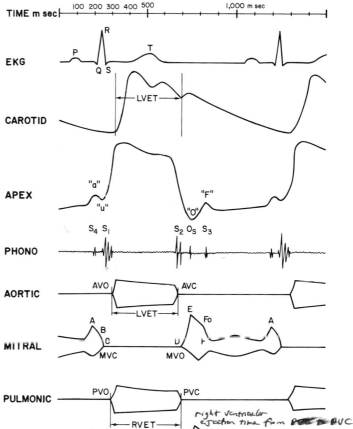

FIGURE 3–1
ECHOCARDIOGRAPHIC, PHONOCARDIOGRAPHIC, AND GRAPHIC RECORDING CORRELATIONS

This illustration correlates the motion of the aortic, mitral, pulmonary, and tricuspid valves with the electrocardiogram, carotid pulse, apexcardiogram, and phonocardiogram. Note the relation of mitral valve closure (MVC) and tricuspid valve closure (TVC) to the first heart sound. Aortic valve closure (AVC) and pulmonary valve closure (PVC) coincide with the two components of the second heart sound. The mitral valve opening (MVO) and the tricuspid valve opening (TVO) can be used as reference points for identification of opening snaps (OS). Left ventricular ejection time (LVET) can be recorded from the carotid pulse or from the aortic valve echo from valve opening (AVO) to closure (AVC). Right ventricular ejection time (RVET) can be measured from pulmonary valve opening (PVO) to pulmonary valve closure (PVC). Note the relation of S_4 and S_3 to the mitral valve motion.

MVC, TVC – to first heart sound S_1
Aortic AVC, PVC – coincide w/ S_2 heart sound – MVO & TVO can be used as reference pts for identification of opening snaps (OS)

FIRST HEART SOUND

FIGURE 3–2
FIRST HEART SOUND

This echocardiogram of the mitral valve illustrates the coincidence of mitral valve closure with the first high-frequency component of the first heart sound. Note that this first component is preceded by a low-frequency sound and is followed by a high-frequency component and a low-frequency component.

PHONO
APEX

EKG

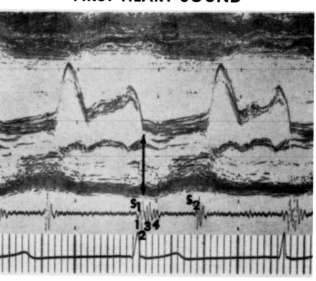

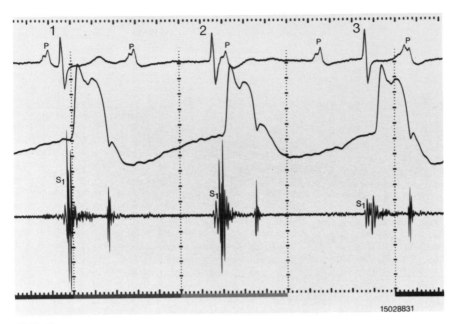

FIGURE 3–3
COMPLETE HEART BLOCK
Electrocardiogram, carotid pulse tracing, and phonocardiogram at the apex in a patient with complete heart block. With a short PR interval (1) the first heart sound is very loud and with a long PR interval (2) S_1 is also very loud, but with a moderately large PR interval (3) the first heart sound is soft.

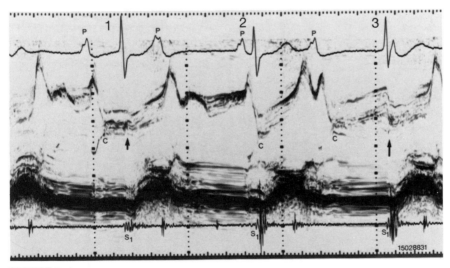

FIGURE 3–4
COMPLETE HEART BLOCK
Echocardiogram of the mitral valve in the same patient as in Figure 3–3. With a long PR interval (1) ventricular systole finds the mitral valve closed; hence S_1 is soft. With a short PR interval (2), the mitral valve is closed by the combined atrial and ventricular systoles, resulting in a loud S_1. With a very long PR interval (3), the mitral valve reopens, and with ventricular systole it closes, producing a loud S_1.

FIGURE 3–5
COMPLETE HEART BLOCK
The alterations on the intensity of the first heart sound present with complete heart block are illustrated in this echocardiogram. The first PR interval lasts only 60 milliseconds, and the intensity of the first heart sound is increased during this beat. Note that the mitral valve closes as a result of both atrial and ventricular systole. The second PR interval is 400 milliseconds. The mitral valve in this instance closes as a result of atrial systole alone; an atrial sound (AS) is recorded at this point. Later, with the beginning of ventricular systole, a soft first heart sound is recorded. On the third beat the PR interval lasts 1400 milliseconds. The mitral valve closes after atrial systole but later reopens. In ventricular systole the mitral valve is open, and the intensity of this first heart sound is increased.

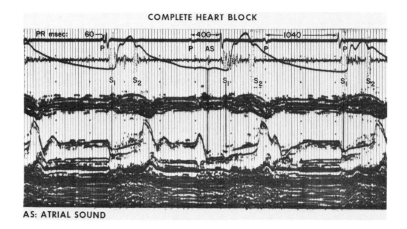

SECOND HEART SOUND

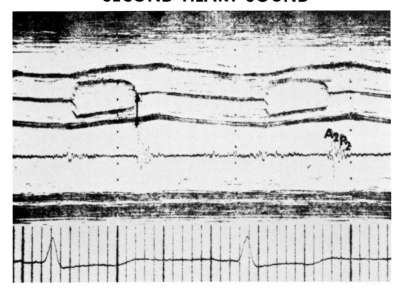

FIGURE 3–6
SECOND HEART SOUND
An echocardiogram of the aortic valve illustrates the correlation between aortic valve closure and the first component of the second heart sound.

FIGURE 3–7
SECOND HEART SOUND
A simultaneously recorded echocardiogram of the pulmonic valve and a phonocardiogram recorded in the second intercostal space illustrate the correlation between pulmonic valve closure and the second component of the second heart sound.

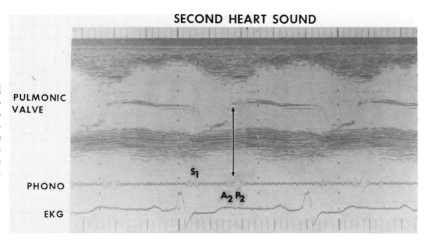

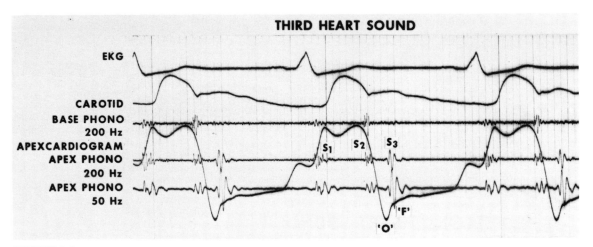

FIGURE 3–8
THIRD HEART SOUND
A simultaneous recording of the electrocardiogram, carotid pulse, apexcardiogram, and phonocardiogram shows a loud third heart sound (S₃) coinciding with the F point of the apexcardiogram.

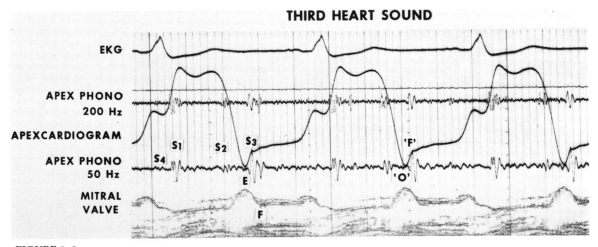

FIGURE 3–9
THIRD HEART SOUND
An echocardiogram of the mitral valve recorded simultaneously with the phonocardiogram and an apexcardiogram illustrate the relation of mitral valve motion with the apexcardiogram and the third heart sound. The F point of the apexcardiogram coincides with the third heart sound and with the initial down slope of the E to F slope of the mitral echocardiogram. A soft fourth heart sound (S₄) is also recorded.

FOURTH HEART SOUND

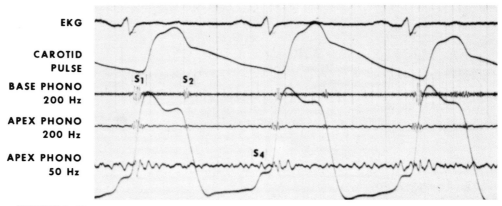

FIGURE 3–10
FOURTH HEART SOUND
A fourth heart sound (s_4), recorded in the phonocardiogram at the apex, coincides with the a wave of the apexcardiogram.

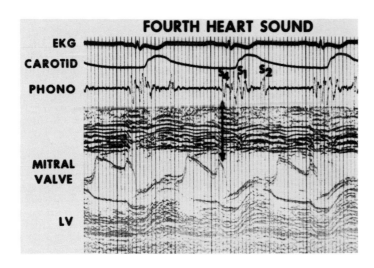

FIGURE 3–11
FOURTH HEART SOUND
A phonocardiogram and a mitral valve echocardiogram were recorded simultaneously in a patient with a loud fourth heart sound. The a wave in the mitral valve can be used as a reference for the identification of a fourth heart sound. LV = left ventricle.

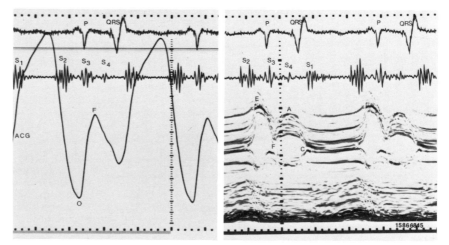

FIGURE 3–12
THIRD AND FOURTH HEART SOUNDS
A third heart sound (S_3) is seen to coincide with the early phase of the E to F slope of the mitral valve. A fourth heart sound (S_4) coincides with the closure motion of the mitral valve after atrial systole. ACG = apexcardiogram.

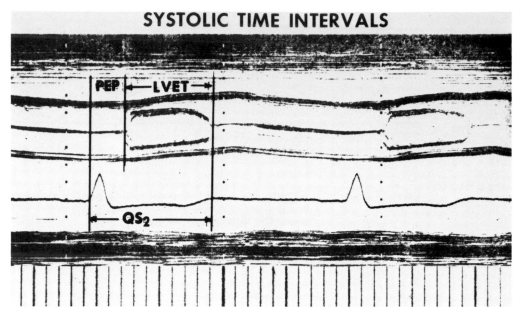

FIGURE 3–13
SYSTOLIC TIME INTERVALS
Simultaneous recording of an electrocardiogram and an aortic valve echocardiogram allows measurement of the systolic time intervals. PEP = pre-ejection period; LVET = left ventricular ejection time; QS_2 = total electromechanical systole.

FIGURE 3–14
RIGHT-SIDED SYSTOLIC TIME INTERVALS
A simultaneous recording of an electrocardiogram and an echocardiogram of the pulmonic valve allows measurement of right-sided systolic time intervals. QP_2 = total right electromechanical systole; RVET = right ventricular ejection time; PEP = pre-ejection period.

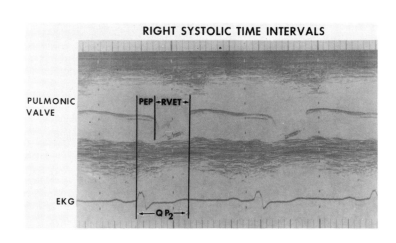

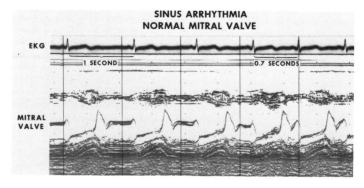

FIGURE 3–15
SINUS ARRHYTHMIA
The effects of sinus arrhythmia in a normal mitral valve are demonstrated. With shorter RR intervals, the a wave moves closer to the F point of the anterior leaflet. When the RR intervals are long, there is a pause between the F point and the a wave, with the mitral valve remaining in the semiclosed position.

SINUS TACHYCARDIA

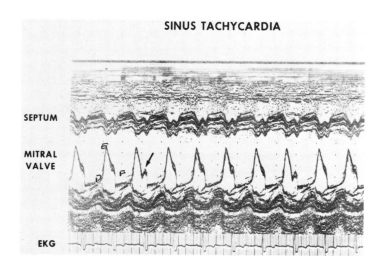

FIGURE 3–16
SINUS TACHYCARDIA
Alteration of the heart rate produces changes in the echocardiographic appearance of the mitral valve. With sinus tachycardia, the atrial kick merges into the E to F slope and changes the M-shape of the mitral valve to a triangular shape. This patient had sinus tachycardia with mild respiratory sinus arrhythmia, which made the atrial kick emerge from some of the beats, as shown by the arrow.

PREMATURE VENTRICULAR CONTRACTION

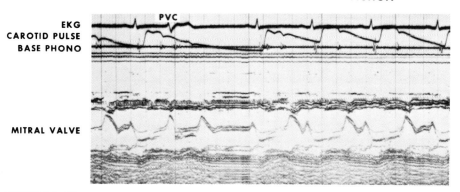

FIGURE 3–17
PREMATURE VENTRICULAR CONTRACTION
A premature ventricular contraction (PVC) moves the mitral valve to a closed position before atrial systole can occur, so that no a wave is seen during this beat. The beat that follows has a long diastolic filling period, with the mitral valve remaining stationary in a midopen position until the next atrial contraction, which reopens the valve.

VENTRICULAR BIGEMINY

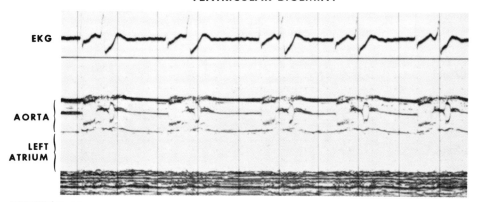

FIGURE 3–18
VENTRICULAR BIGEMINY
Decreased stroke volume influences the normal aortic valve motion. The aortic valve excursion is decreased in every other beat in this patient with ventricular bigeminy. The duration of systole and the velocity of opening of the leaflets are also decreased. There are fine systolic vibrations in the noncoronary cusps of the valve in the normally conducted beats. This is a normal finding that represents normal flow through a normal pliable valve.

ATRIAL FIBRILLATION

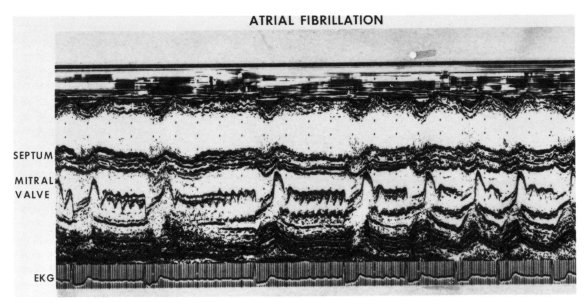

FIGURE 3–19
ATRIAL FIBRILLATION
Coarse vibratory waves are seen during diastole in both the anterior and the posterior mitral valve leaflets of this patient with coronary artery disease and a normal mitral valve. This pattern is frequently seen in patients who have atrial fibrillation with slow ventricular response and otherwise normal and pliable mitral valve leaflets. These wave patterns should not be confused with the fine vibrations seen in aortic insufficiency or ruptured chordae tendineae.

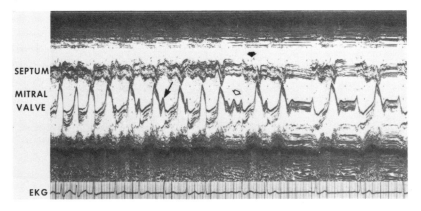

FIGURE 3–20
ATRIAL FIBRILLATION, NORMAL SINUS RHYTHM
This echocardiogram was recorded in a patient whose condition spontaneously converted from atrial fibrillation to normal sinus rhythm (short black arrow). Note the variable appearance of the anterior leaflet of the mitral valve during atrial fibrillation. Black and white arrows point to fibrillatory waves. During sinus rhythm, valve motion is normal.

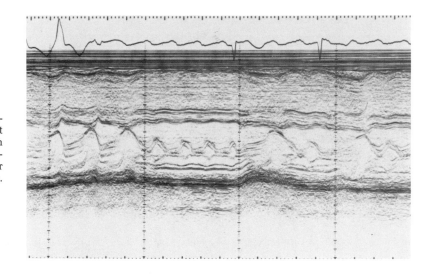

FIGURE 3–21
ATRIAL FLUTTER
The diastolic motion of the mitral valve is characteristic of that seen in atrial flutter, in which the leaflet opens and closes synchronously with the flutter waves on the electrocardiogram.

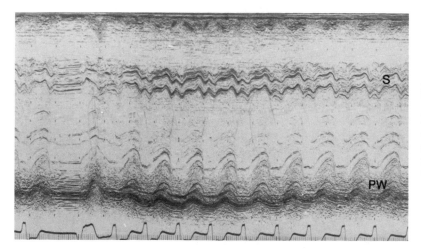

FIGURE 3–22
VENTRICULAR TACHYCARDIA
Echocardiogram of the left ventricle in a patient with sustained ventricular tachycardia. The only abnormality demonstrated is paradoxic septal motion. S = septum; PW = posterior wall.

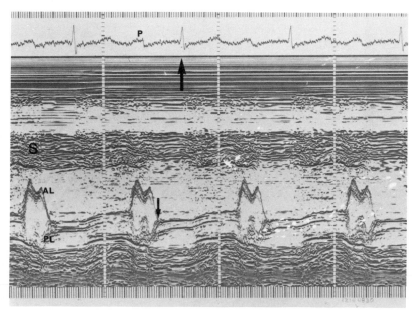

FIGURE 3–23
FIRST-DEGREE BLOCK
In patients with first-degree atrioventricular block, the *a* wave of the mitral valve echogram occurs earlier. Often it is very close to the F point, and occasionally it may be buried on the E to F slope. Note there is prematue closure of the mitral valve.

LEFT BUNDLE BRANCH BLOCK

Brief downward dip of the septum toward the LV shortly after MV opening —

← IVS

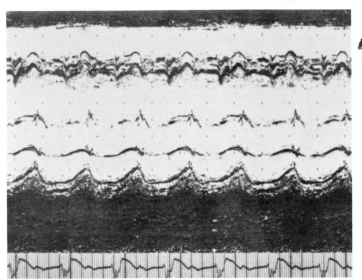

FIGURE 3–24
LEFT BUNDLE BRANCH BLOCK (LBBB)
Paradoxic septal motion is shown in a patient with LBBB. A sharp posterior displacement of the septum occurs during early systole, followed by systolic anterior motion during ventricular ejection.

FIGURE 3–25
PACEMAKER RHYTHM
Type B paradoxic septal motion is demonstrated in a patient with pacemaker rhythm. The mitral valve and the posterior wall of the left ventricle (LV) are normal. Note the normal septal motion during normal sinus rhythm. S = septum; RV = right ventricle.

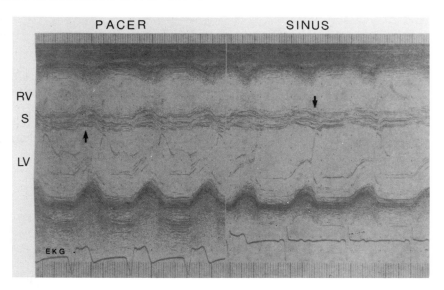

FIGURE 3–26
TYPE B WOLFF-PARKINSON-WHITE SYNDROME (WPW)
After the inscription of the delta wave in the electrocardiogram, there is a rapid posterior motion of the septum(s) followed by anterior systolic motion. PW = posterior wall.

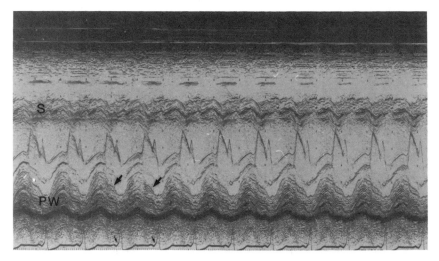

4 MITRAL VALVE DISEASE

4.1 MITRAL STENOSIS

Mitral stenosis, with very few exceptions (congenital malformations and calcified mitral annulus), is the result of rheumatic carditis.[1] There is thickening of both leaflets, preferentially toward their free edges; fusion of the commissures, with more severe and earlier compromise of the medial commissure; and fibrosis and shortening of the chordae tendineae. The mitral valve acquires a funnel shape, with the narrow orifice facing toward the apex. The base of this funnel, the mitral annulus, is usually not affected. As the mitral valve orifice area narrows from the normal range of 4 to 6 sq cm to 2 sq cm or less, the mitral valve flow decreases and the pressure in the left atrium increases and stays high throughout diastole. This increased pressure is transmitted to the capillary wedge and the pulmonary artery, producing pulmonary hypertension and increased right ventricular pressure.

Echocardiographic Findings

A number of echocardiographic findings can be observed in patients with mitral stenosis.

1. Thickened Mitral Leaflets. With M-mode echocardiography, it is possible to determine the degree of thickening of the mitral leaflets (Fig. 4–1). M-mode echocardiography can differentiate mild from mod-

erate and severe degrees of thickening. The leaflets are more thickened toward their free edges and close to the commissures. Two-dimensional echocardiography permits this characterization better than does the M-mode study (Fig. 4–2).

2. Decreased E to F Slope. The persistently high pressure in the left atrium throughout diastole maintains the mitral leaflets in an open position so that the mid-diastolic semiclosure (E to F slope) is reduced or absent (Fig. 4–3). With progressive decrease in the E to F slope, there is a parallel decrease in the size of the a wave.

3. Diastolic Anterior Motion of the Posterior Leaflet. Both mitral leaflets move anteriorly during diastole. This motion is caused by diastolic anterior pulling of the posterior leaflet by the larger and more mobile anterior leaflet.[2] This process can be observed by the two echocardiographic techniques but is better characterized by M-mode echocardiography.

4. Diastolic Doming of the Mitral Leaflets. Leaflet doming is one characteristic common to all stenotic valves. In mitral stenosis, such doming can be viewed best by two-dimensional echocardiography in the long-axis parasternal view (Fig. 4–4). At the beginning of diastole the anterior leaflet arcs into the left ventricle with its tip pointing to a mirror-image posterior leaflet.

5. Commissure Fusion. This can be studied best in the short-axis left parasternal view. There is increased echo density and decreased leaflet motion at the level of one or both commissures. In some patients, there may be marked fusion and calcification of the medial commissure, while the lateral commissure is nearly normal. This condition can create totally different M-mode recordings in two different areas. Two-dimensional echocardiography serves to clarify these findings (Fig. 4–5).

6. Decreased Mitral Orifice Size. The end result of commissure fusion is narrowing of the mitral valve orifice area. Two-dimensional echocardiography is probably the best method available to measure this area. The mitral valve orifice is best visualized in the parasternal short-axis view, with the scan plane passing directly through the tip of the mitral valve funnel (Fig. 4–6). The smallest orifice is found by angling the scan plane in a superior-inferior arc from the level of the papillary muscles to the base of the left ventricle until the smallest orifice is found (Figs. 4–7, 4–8).

In the M-mode echocardiogram this narrowing is seen as decreased diastolic separation of the leaflets (Fig. 4–9). The single-plane image of the M-mode technique has obvious limitations in this respect.

7. Shortening and Fibrosis of Chordae Tendineae. The same thickening and fibrosis that affects the mitral leaflets extends into the chordae tendineae, producing short and dense chordae. If there is a significant degree of fibrosis and fusion, a true subvalvular stenosis may occur. This condition can be observed best by two-dimensional echocardiography in the four-chamber apical view (Fig. 4–10). With M-mode echocardiography the dense chordae appear at the left ventricular level as dense linear echoes behind the mitral valve.

8. Abnormal Septal Motion. In patients with significant mitral stenosis, an early diastolic dip of the interventricular septum may be seen (Fig. 4–11). This phenomenon appears to be related to a more rapid filling of the right ventricle, which pushes the interventricular septum toward the left ventricular cavity.[3]

In the presence of pulmonary hypertension, flattening of the interventricular septum may be evident with two-dimensional echocardiography.

9. Left Atrial Enlargement. Variable degrees of left atrial dilatation are usually present. Occasionally, aneurysmal left atrial dilatation may be seen (Figs. 4–12, 4–13).

10. Left Atrial Thrombus. Only rarely is a left atrial thrombus detected. Thrombi usually are found in the left atrial appendage, an area difficult to visualize with echocardiography.

11. Right Ventricular Dilatation. This condition is commonly seen in the presence of pulmonary hypertension.

12. Pulmonary Hypertension. In patients with severe mitral stenosis, echocardiographic findings of pulmonary hypertension are frequently seen. Abnormalities of septal motion related to this pulmonary hypertension already have been mentioned.

13. Small Left Ventricle. This is a common finding in patients with isolated mitral stenosis.

Severity of Mitral Stenosis

For the estimation of the severity of mitral stenosis, five parameters have been used.

1. E to F Slope. This measurement has not proved helpful in predicting the degree of mitral stenosis in large numbers of patients.[4] Patients with a mitral E to F slope of less than 15 mm per second usually have valve areas of less than 1.3 sq cm, and patients with an E to F slope of more than 35 mm per second have valve areas greater than 1.8 sq cm, but there are significant overlaps.[5]

The E to F slope can be used only as a crude index in the estimation of severity; it has more value in following a given patient's condition.

2. Mitral Valve Closure Index. This parameter is based on the rate of diastolic apposition of the anterior and posterior mitral leaflet echoes. It excludes movements extraneous to the mitral apparatus and hence is considered to be more specific than the E to F slope for the assessment of the severity of mitral stenosis.[6, 7] This index is not widely used.

3. Left Atrial Emptying Index. This parameter is defined as the fraction of passive posterior aortic wall motion occurring in the first third of diastole. It has been found to be related to the mitral valve area index,[8] but it can be affected by changes in the elasticity of the aortic root and left ventricular compliance.

4. Left Ventricular Posterior Wall Velocity. This measurement is determined by calculating the slope of the posterior left ventricular wall endocardial motion in diastole.[9] This index has not been widely accepted because it may also be affected by factors other than the mitral valve orifice size, such as decreased left ventricular compliance. There is a report suggesting its use to determine the presence of mitral prosthetic stenosis.[9]

5. Measurement of Mitral Valve Orifice Area. A very useful parameter that can be obtained with two-dimensional echocardiography is the measurement of the mitral valve orifice area.[10-13] Several reports have confirmed its accuracy when compared with cardiac catheterization measurements. It is reproducible to 0.3 sq cm of measurements obtained by catheterization or surgery, and it is not affected by the presence of mitral insufficiency. It can certainly differentiate a normal orifice area from one with severe narrowing (Fig. 4–14) (less than 1 sq cm) or mild narrowing (Fig. 4–15) (less than 2 sq cm). For this measurement to be valid, care must be taken to: (a) record the true valve orifice location (Figs. 4–16 to 19); (b) measure the valve orifice when the leaflet is fully open; and (c) have an adequate reciber gain setting. Once the proper frame has been selected, the orifice size can be measured using planimetry.

Cross-sectional echocardiographic measurement of the mitral area also correlates well with catheterization measurements in patients with associated mitral regurgitation.[12]

In patients that have a severely calcified and narrowed mitral valve orifice, because of the high echo reflectivity in that area, it may not be possible to measure the mitral valve orifice area (Fig. 4–20).

Surgical Considerations

Patients with significant mitral stenosis that will benefit from commissurotomy,[14, 15] rather than valve replacement, usually have pliable valves, absence of calcium, and absence of mitral regurgitation.

1. PLIABLE VALVES. These are recognized as having only a mild increase in thickness and normal excursion (Fig. 4–21). There is more than 20 mm of aperture motion (DE excursion). The maximal excursion should be measured with M-mode echocardiography at the base of the heart, at which point the motion of the leaflets is more pronounced. Conversely, a nonpliable valve has significant reduction in its excursion even at the base of the leaflets (Fig. 4–22).

2. ABSENCE OF CALCIUM. Valvular calcium is seen in echocardiography as areas of high

reflectivity, thick conglomerate, and "fuzzy" or "shaggy" echo recordings observed in the mitral valve in diastole (Fig. 4–20). Care must be taken to adjust the gain controls appropriately.

3. NO MITRAL REGURGITATION. This is a clinical or angiographic diagnosis, but a small left ventricle and absence of left ventricular volume overload suggest the absence of significant mitral insufficiency.

Echocardiography has also been used to study patients after commissurotomy to evaluate the immediate results of the operation and for long-term follow-up to evaluate the presence of restenosis. A successful commissurotomy significantly increases the E to F slope of the mitral valve and may restore to normal the motion of the posterior leaflet (Figs. 4–23, 4–24). Diastolic flutter of the mitral valve is occasionally seen in patients after commissurotomy (Fig. 4–25). On two-dimensional echocardiography, the mitral valve orifice is increased and usually is in the range of 2.7 to 2.9 sq cm.[16]

Mitral valve replacement should be considered for symptomatic patients, for whom commissurotomy is not suitable and who have severely stenotic valves as determined by two-dimensional echocardiography.

Patients who are found to have small left ventricles and particularly narrow left ventricular outflow tracts on echocardiography are better candidates for low-profile prostheses.[17]

Differential Diagnosis

Several conditions should be considered in the differential diagnosis of mitral stenosis.

1. Pseudomitral Stenosis. This condition is evidenced by decreased E to F slope but normal leaflet thickness and normal motion of the posterior leaflet.[18] Pseudomitral stenosis is seen in conditions of decreased left ventricular compliance.

2. Normal Motion of the Posterior Leaflet. This may be seen in about 10 per cent of patients with mitral stenosis. The posterior mitral leaflet moves posteriorly (Fig. 4–26)—in an opposite direction from the anterior leaflet. Occasionally, both normal and diastolic anterior motion of the posterior mitral leaflet may be observed.[19, 20]

3. Rheumatic Mitral Insufficiency. The echocardiogram of patients with rheumatic mitral insufficiency may be indistinguishable from that in mitral stenosis, but often there is a "ski-slope" E to F slope and evidence of left ventricular volume overload.

4. Left Atrial Myxoma. The E to F slope can be flat, but usually a mass of echo recordings is seen behind the mitral valve and in the left atrium.

5. Calcified Mitral Annulus. Dense echoes are recorded at the level of the mitral ring. The leaflets are usually thick and move normally.

6. Low Cardiac Output. Conditions with decreased cardiac output may have an apparent small mitral valve orifice area.

7. Aortic Insufficiency. The diagnosis of aortic insufficiency associated with mitral stenosis may be difficult to make because the dense and fibrotic mitral leaflets tend not to show the characteristic diastolic fluttering. The diastolic vibrations induced by aortic insufficiency may have to be sought in the interventricular septum (Fig. 4–27). Only rarely can they be seen in a thickened and stenotic mitral valve (Fig. 4–28). Conversely, a patient with aortic insufficiency may have echocardiographic findings of pseudomitral stenosis (Fig. 4–29).

8. Left Atrial Thrombus. Echocardiography has not proved to be very useful in detecting left atrial thrombus in patients with mitral stenosis. The thrombi are usually located in the atrial appendage, which cannot be imaged well by echocardiography.

Echophonocardiography

The auscultatory and phonocardiographic findings of mitral stenosis include: (1) loud first heart sound; (2) opening snap; (3) diastolic rumble; and (4) presystolic murmur. The apexcardiogram shows a small a wave and a slow or absent rapid filling wave (Fig. 4–30).

An M-mode echocardiogram can be recorded simultaneously to serve as a reference for timing of the abnormal heart sound and murmurs. The E point of the anterior mitral leaflet coincides with the opening snap and the O point of the apexcardiogram. The diastolic rumble occurs during the E to F slope, the presystolic murmur occurs at the time of mitral closure (AC interval), and the loud S_1 coincides with leaflet coaptation (Fig. 4–31).

4.2 MITRAL INSUFFICIENCY

In contrast to mitral stenosis, which essentially has only one cause (rheumatic), there

are many causes of mitral insufficiency.[21] Mitral regurgitation can occur not only with dysfunction of the mitral leaflets, but with abnormalities of the mitral ring, chordae tendineae, papillary muscles, and left ventricular wall.[22, 23]

In chronic mitral insufficiency, there is enlargement of the left ventricle and the left atrium. In acute mitral regurgitation the chamber size may be normal.

Secondary Echocardiographic Abnormalities

Although there are no definite echocardiographic findings to make the diagnosis of mitral insufficiency or to estimate its severity, there are several secondary echocardiographic abnormalities that support the diagnosis of mitral regurgitation. These include:

1. Left Ventricular Volume Overload. This consists of normal size or enlarged left ventricle with increased septal and posterior wall motion, (Fig. 4–32).

2. Increased E to F Slope. Together with excessive mitral valve motion, this is related to increased mitral valve flow (Fig. 4–33).

3. Early Closure of the Aortic Valve. The aortic valve is fully open only at the beginning of systole. It then gradually moves back to a semiclosed position. The left ventricular stroke volume is partially lost to the left atrium (Fig. 4–34).

4. Pulsations of Left Atrial Walls. Excessive motion of the posterior left atrial wall (greater than 1 cm) can be seen with M-mode echocardiography.[24] This, in the author's experience, has not been easy to document and is not a very sensitive sign. The initial velocity of the posterior motion of the left atrial wall may be increased.

5. Abnormal Interatrial Septal Motion. In acute mitral insufficiency, the interatrial septum has been shown to bow toward the right atrium during systole.[25] This has been demonstrated with two-dimensional subxiphoid echocardiography. On M-mode echocardiography, the interatrial septum amplitude is increased (12.4 ± 1.9 mm). Systolic flutter of the interatrial septum has also been demonstrated.

6. Left Atrial Enlargement. In chronic mitral insufficiency this is a common and prognostic finding (Fig. 4–33).

7. Left Atrial Volume Overload. The patient with severe mitral regurgitation may have systolic expansion of the left atrium and an increased left atrial ejection fraction.[26]

Echocardiography has been most helpful in determining the causes of mitral insufficiency in a number of conditions.[27] These include (1) rheumatic mitral insufficiency; (2) mitral valve prolapse; (3) ruptured chordae tendineae; (4) papillary muscle dysfunction; (5) mitral annulus calcification; (6) endocarditis; and (7) cleft mitral valve.

4.3 RHEUMATIC MITRAL INSUFFICIENCY

The M-mode echocardiogram (Figs. 4–35, 4–36) of a patient with pure rheumatic mitral insufficiency may be indistinguishable from that of a patient with mitral stenosis. The E to F slope is mildly decreased and may show a biphasic or "ski slope" pattern. The posterior mitral leaflet may have normal or abnormal motion during diastole, and the diastolic separation between the leaflets is usually not significantly reduced. Enlargement of the left atrium and left ventricular volume overload are usually seen. With two-dimensional echocardiography (Fig. 4–37), the fibrotic and thickened leaflets produce increased echo density, especially at the leaflet tips. With pure mitral regurgitation, there is no commissure fusion or doming of the leaflets during diastole. The mitral valve orifice size is normal or minimally reduced. Occasionally the pattern of mitral valve prolapse may be seen (Fig. 4–38).

Incomplete systolic leaflet coaptation has been noted on short-axis views at the level of the mitral valve orifice.[28]

4.4 MITRAL VALVE PROLAPSE

Echocardiographic Abnormalities

Many echocardiographic abnormalities have been described in patients with mitral valve prolapse. These include:

1. Systolic Bowing of the Mitral Valve Toward the Left Atrium. This is characterized by M-mode echocardiography[29–34] as a late (Figs. 4–39 to 4–41) or holosystolic motion (Figs. 4–42, 4–43) of one or both mitral leaflets toward the posterior left atrial wall. The maximal degree of prolapse is usually seen at the level of the atrioventricular groove (Fig. 4–44).

With two-dimensional echocardiography[35, 36] this abnormal motion is seen as arching of one or both leaflets superiorly toward the left atrium so that part of the valve moves beyond the mitral ring during systole (Figs. 4–45, 4–46). This abnormal motion can be seen on the long-axis parasternal view or in the apical views (Fig. 4–47). The apical four-chamber view (Fig. 4–48) is considered by some authors as the "gold standard" for the diagnosis of mitral valve prolapse.[37]

2. Thickened and Redundant Leaflets. The mitral valve leaflets of patients with mitral valve prolapse appear thickened, redundant, and as having excessive motion. Areas of localized thickness may have the appearance of a mass attached to the leaflet (Figs. 4–49, 4–50). This localized increase in leaflet thickness makes the diagnosis of infective endocarditis difficult in patients with mitral valve prolapse.[38] Leaflet redundancy is possibly the cause of the systolic anterior motion of the mitral valve that is seen occasionally in patients with mitral valve prolapse. In the short axis parasternal view, the redundant leaflets give a scalloped appearance to the mitral valve (Fig. 4–51).

3. Hyperactive Atrioventricular Groove. Not uncommonly, the atrioventricular groove of patients with mitral valve prolapse has an exaggerated motion. With M-mode echocardiography, this may produce a cloud of echoes behind the posterior leaflet of the mitral valve and give the appearance of a left atrial mass (Figs. 4–52, 4–53).

4. Large Mitral Annulus. The mitral annulus size in patients with mitral valve prolapse ranges from normal (4.2 ± 0.5 sq cm per square millimeter) to markedly dilated.[39]

Maneuvers to Enhance Diagnostic Accuracy

In the author's experience, provocative maneuvers have not been very useful in demonstrating mitral valve prolapse. Nevertheless, several maneuvers have been described as possibly enhancing the accuracy of echocardiography for the diagnosis of mitral valve prolapse.

1. Valsalva Maneuver. Adequate and reproducible echocardiograms are difficult to obtain after the Valsalva maneuver or with the patient standing up. Occasionally, a mitral valve prolapse can be seen only after the Valsalva maneuver.

2. The Inhalation of Amyl Nitrate. Inhalation of amyl nitrate makes a systolic pro-lapse become holosystolic but apparently does not bring on a prolapse that is not seen in the resting state[40] (Fig. 4–54).

Conditions Obscuring Diagnosis

Conditions that may create confusion in the echocardiographic diagnosis of mitral valve prolapse include transducer place-ment in the chest, pseudo prolapse caused by pericardial effusion, systolic anterior mi-tral valve motion, and pseudo vegetations.

1. Transducer Placement in the Chest. High chest positioning of the M-mode trans-ducer may give the false appearance of a holosystolic prolapse in a normal individ-ual.[41] Proper transducer placement can be recognized by recording the left atrial wall of the atrioventricular groove behind the posterior mitral leaflet. The appearance of a holosystolic prolapse should be questioned if the left ventricular wall is seen well be-hind the mitral valve; this probably means that the transducer was placed too high in the chest.

Conversely, a very low transducer place-ment may not permit identification of a true prolapse (Fig. 4–55).

2. Pseudo Prolapse Caused by Pericar-dial Effusion. A large pericardial effusion may produce swinging of the heart in which systolic posterior displacement of the entire heart produces motion of the mitral valve similar to that seen in mitral valve prolapse (Fig. 4–56). Mitral valve prolapse should be diagnosed in the presence of pericardial ef-fusion only if the effusion is small and the mitral valve motion does not follow that of the heart walls.

3. Systolic Anterior Motion of the Mitral Valve. Mild systolic anterior motion occa-sionally can be seen in patients with mitral valve prolapse (Fig. 4–57).[42, 43] Normal septal thickness and normal left ventricular size differentiate this condition from idiopathic hypertrophic subaortic stenosis.

4. Pseudo Vegetations. Localized thick-ening of the mitral valve may give the ap-pearance of a vegetation (Fig. 4–58).

Secondary Mitral Valve Prolapse

Secondary causes of mitral valve prolapse include (1) papillary muscle dysfunction, (2) ruptured chordae tendineae, (3) rheumatic mitral insufficiency, (4) primary pulmonary hypertension, and (5) ostium secundum atrial septal defect.[44]

4.5 RUPTURED CHORDAE TENDINEAE

The most common causes of ruptured chordae tendineae include (1) idiopathic causes: affect mainly the posterior leaflet; (2) myxomatous degeneration: usually associ-ated with mitral valve prolapse; (3) infective endocarditis; (4) rheumatic carditis; (5) con-nective tissue disorders; and (6) trauma.

Echocardiographic Abnormalities

Several echocardiographic abnormalities have been described in patients with rup-tured chordae tendineae. These include vis-ualization of the flail chordae, flail leaflet, mitral valve prolapse, and systolic mitral valve flutter.

1. Visualization of the Flail Chordae. With two-dimensional echocardiography, the actual ruptured chordae can be seen (Figs. 4–59 to 4–61).[45, 46] With M-mode ech-ocardiography, fine lines with systolic vibra-tions in the left atrium are commonly seen (Figs. 4–62, 4–63).

2. Flail Leaflet. If a significant portion of the valve does not have adequate support, it flails. With M-mode echocardiography, coarse flutter and disorganized motion of the affected leaflet is seen (Fig. 4–64). Marked variation of the diastolic pattern of the mo-tion from beat to beat is frequently present (Fig. 4–65). Exaggerated leaflet motion is common, and the leaflets may become close together during diastole (Fig. 4–66). The parts of the valve that have normal support may appear normal, so that a complete scan of the mitral valve is needed to exclude the diagnosis. With two-dimensional echocar-diography, an exaggerated motion in which the leaflets inscribe a very large angle of motion can be viewed. The top of the af-fected leaflet loses its point of coaptation and moves into the left atrium, with its tip pointing superiorly into the left atrial cav-ity.[47]

3. Mitral Valve Prolapse. Mitral valve prolapse is usually seen.[48] One pattern is indistinguishable from mitral valve prolapse without ruptured chordae tendineae (Fig. 4–67). With two-dimensional echocardiog-raphy, the tip of the mitral valve points toward the left ventricle, whereas in rup-tured chordae it points to the left atrium (Fig. 4–68).

4. Systolic Flutter of the Mitral Valve. Fine systolic flutter of the mitral valve is characteristic of ruptured chordae tendineae.[49] Although this finding is probably not very sensitive, it is quite specific (Figs. 4–69, 4–70).

Echophonocardiography

Echophonocardiography may assist in the evaluation of patients with ruptured chordae. In addition to the holosystolic murmur and a third heart sound characteristic of most forms of mitral insufficiency, patients with ruptured chordae tendineae frequently have an associated fourth heart sound that is related to a noncompliant left atrium (Figs. 4–71 to 4–73).

4.6 PAPILLARY MUSCLE DYSFUNCTION

The posteromedial papillary muscle receives its blood supply from the posterior descending branch of the right coronary artery and becomes ischemic and infarcted more frequently than does the anterolateral papillary muscle, which receives its blood supply from the left anterior descending and circumflex arteries.

Mitral insufficiency can occur not only by direct ischemic involvement of the papillary muscles but by scarring of the left ventricular wall adjacent to the papillary muscles or by dilatation of the left ventricle. Left ventricular dilatation can alter the spatial relationship between the papillary muscles and the chordae and result in ischemia.

The echocardiographic diagnosis of papillary muscle dysfunction is often made indirectly. In the presence of mitral insufficiency the demonstration of segmental left ventricular dysfunction without other abnormalities of the mitral valve apparatus supports the diagnosis of papillary muscle dysfunction. The echocardiographic abnormalities that have been reported in this disorder include:[50–52]

1. Failure of one or both mitral leaflets to reach the normal peak systolic position relative to the mitral ring. This has been best characterized with two-dimensional echocardiography from the two- or four-chamber apical views (Fig. 4–74).

2. Mitral valve prolapse.

3. Fibrosis or calcification of the papillary muscles.

4. Segmental left ventricular dysfunction.

5. Secondary findings of mitral insufficiency.

4.7 MITRAL ANNULUS CALCIFICATION

The mitral annulus is part of the fibrous skeleton of the heart and serves to anchor the mitral valve. Anteriorly it joins the aortic ring, and posteriorly it is at the level of the atrioventricular ring.

The mitral annulus starts to develop fibrosis and deposits of calcium at age 65 years. This process starts in the posterior aspect of the atrioventricular ring and progresses laterally, occasionally involving the whole circumference.[53] As the deposits of calcium increase, they are not confined to the annulus itself but grow into the left ventricular cavity, particularly in the subvalvular space behind the posterior mitral leaflet. Calcification of the aortic valve is a common association.

Calcification of the mitral annulus appears in the echocardiogram as a mass of dense and highly reflective echo recordings in any point along the circumference of the mitral ring.[54–60] In the short axis (Fig. 4–75), this mass of echoes is initially seen in the posterior aspect of the ring. As the calcification becomes more severe, it involves its medial aspect and eventually the whole circumstance. In the long-axis left parasternal view (Fig. 4–76), the dense band of echoes is seen at the level of the atrioventricular groove, often extending into the left ventricular cavity behind the posterior mitral leaflet.

With M-mode echocardiography, a dense band of echoes is seen behind the posterior mitral leaflet and in front of the posterior wall endocardium (Fig. 4–77). An echocardiographic scan permits examination of how far into the ventricle the band extends (Fig. 4–78).

When the calcification extends to the anterior ring, a band of echoes is seen anterior to the mitral valve (Fig. 4–79). The thickness of the annular calcification varies from very mild in which only a line is seen, to very severe in which the thickness may be 10 mm or more (Fig. 4–80).

A very severely calcified mitral annulus can make the visualization of the leaflets difficult and can eventually restrict their motion to produce the appearance of mitral stenosis.

There appears to be a higher association of mitral annulus calcification with idiophathic hypertrophic subaortic stenosis.

M.S.

mild   moderate   severe

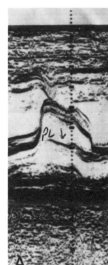
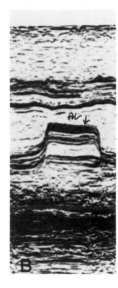
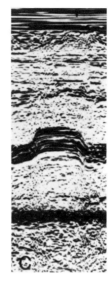

"m-mode"

FIGURE 4–1
MITRAL STENOSIS, THICKENED LEAFLETS
Thickening of both anterior and posterior mitral leaflets is characteristic of mitral stenosis. The degree of thickening is variable, and M-mode echocardiography permits differentiation of (A) mild from (B) moderate and (C) severe leaflet thickening. The other characteristic findings of mitral stenosis—decreased E to F slope and abnormal motion of the posterior leaflet—are also evident in these patients.

↓ Drastic anterior motion (pulling) of the posterior leaflet by the larger, anterior leaflet. more mobile.

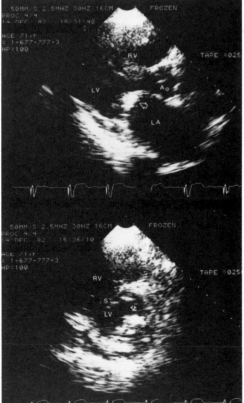

← PSLAX view
Leaflet thickening at the tips.
Doming of AL
LA is enlarged

"2-D" → shows thickened MV leaflets better than m-mode.

FIGURE 4–2
MITRAL STENOSIS, TWO-DIMENSIONAL ECHOCARDIOGRAPHY
Left parasternal long- and short-axis echocardiograms demonstrate the typical leaflet thickening at their tips (arrows). Doming of the anterior leaflet is also apparent. The left atrium (LA) is enlarged. The aorta (Ao) and right ventricle (RV) are normal. LV = left ventricle; S = septum.

PSAX view

M.S. — Decreased E to F slope.

mildly reduced   severely reduced   absent

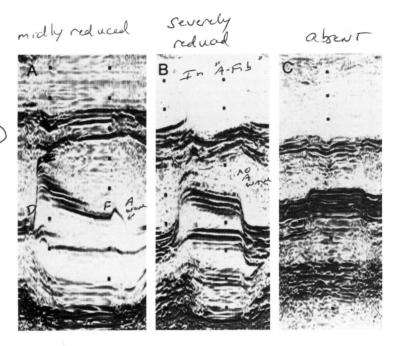

In "A-Fib"

No A wave

FIGURE 4–3
MITRAL STENOSIS, DECREASED E to F SLOPE
The persistently high pressure in the left atrium throughout diastole maintains the mitral leaflets in an open position so that the E to F slope is (A) mildly reduced, (B) severely reduced, or (C) absent. There is only a gross correlation between this finding and the severity of mitral stenosis.

MV area narrows to 2 sq cm² or less from normal of (4–6 sq cm²) valve

LA is enlarged + pressure overload throughout diastole.

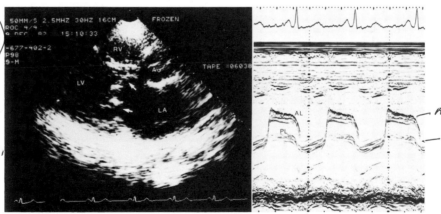

AL
PL

FIGURE 4–4
MITRAL STENOSIS, DOMING OF THE ANTERIOR LEAFLET
The long-axis parasternal view permits observation of diastolic doming of the anterior mitral leaflet, a characteristic finding of mitral stenosis. The posterior leaflet (PL) is pulled anteriorly by the larger anterior leaflet. The M-mode echocardiogram from the same patient shows the decreased E to F slope of the anterior leaflet (AL) and the diastolic anterior motion of the posterior leaflet. RV = right ventricle; LV = left ventricle; Ao = aorta.

PSLAX view shows — diastolic doming of mitral leaflets common to all stenotic valves. — Best viewed in 2D-PSLAX view

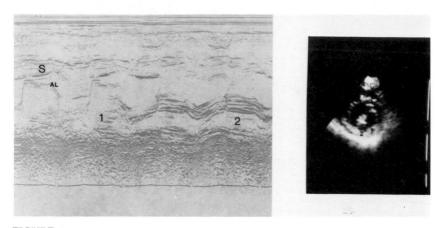

FIGURE 4–5

MITRAL STENOSIS, COMMISSURE FUSION

M-mode and two-dimensional echocardiograms. The M-mode echocardiogram shows marked difference in leaflet thickness in areas 1 and 2. The anterior leaflet (AL) has normal excursion in area 1, whereas it hardly moves in area 2. The cross-sectional echocardiogram shows that this difference is caused by fusion of the medial commissure (2) with little involvement of the lateral commissure (1). S = septum.

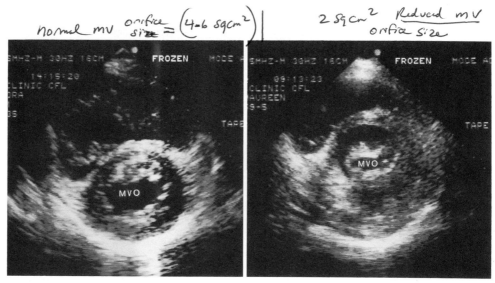

FIGURE 4–6

MITRAL STENOSIS, DECREASED ORIFICE SIZE

Short-axis left parasternal view of (A) normal mitral orifice size as compared with a reduced mitral valve area in a patient with mitral stenosis (B).

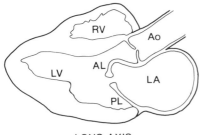

LONG-AXIS
PARASTERNAL VIEW

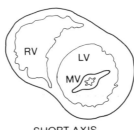

SHORT-AXIS
PARASTERNAL VIEW

FIGURE 4–7

MITRAL STENOSIS, DECREASED ORIFICE SIZE

The long-axis parasternal view shows the typical doming of the anterior leaflet (AL) and the posterior leaflet (PL) being pulled forward to cause decreased leaflet separation at their tips. The short-axis parasternal view shows decreased orifice size of the mitral valve (MV). RV = right ventricle; LV = left ventricle; Ao = aorta; LA = left atrium.

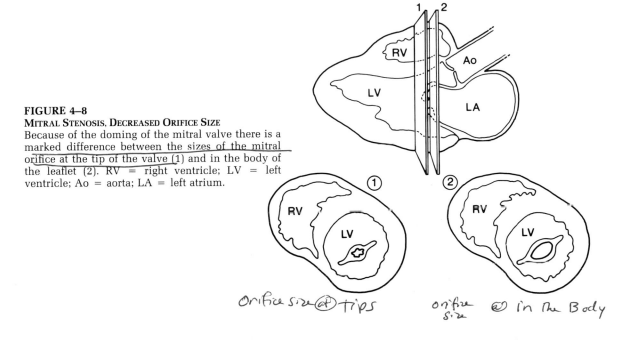

FIGURE 4–8
MITRAL STENOSIS, DECREASED ORIFICE SIZE
Because of the doming of the mitral valve there is a
marked difference between the sizes of the mitral
orifice at the tip of the valve (1) and in the body of
the leaflet (2). RV = right ventricle; LV = left
ventricle; Ao = aorta; LA = left atrium.

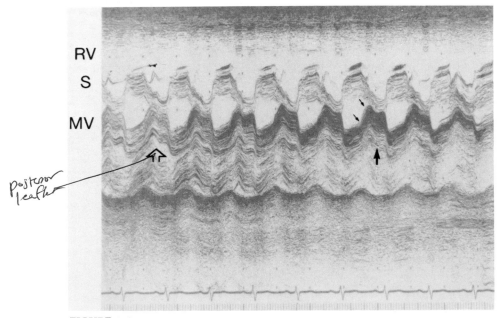

FIGURE 4–9
MITRAL STENOSIS, DECREASED LEAFLET SEPARATION
M-mode echocardiogram of a patient with severe mitral stenosis with markedly
thickened leaflets. The separation between the anterior leaflet (small arrows) and the
posterior leaflet (open arrow) is markedly reduced and not even apparent in one area
(black arrow). This area is the M-mode equivalent of a reduced mitral leaflet orifice
size. RV = right ventricle; S = septum; MV = mitral valve.

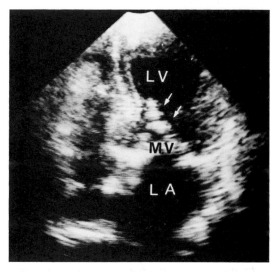

FIGURE 4–10
MITRAL STENOSIS, THICKENED CHORDAE TENDINEAE
Apical four-chamber view in a patient with mitral stenosis
and marked thickening of the chordae tendineae *(arrows)*,
producing obstruction into the left ventricle (LV). The left
atrium (LA) is enlarged. MV = mitral valve.

normal LA < 4.0 cm²

Mitral Stenosis — Abnormal Septal motion

frequent finding in patients w/ severe m.s.

IVS early diastolic dip

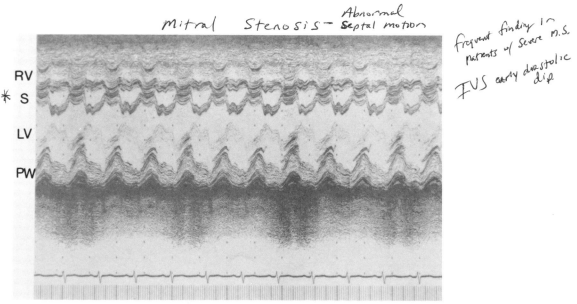

FIGURE 4–11
MITRAL STENOSIS, ABNORMAL SEPTAL MOTION
M-mode echocardiogram shows an early diastolic dip of the interventricular septum
(S), a frequent finding in patients with severe mitral stenosis. RV = right ventricle; LV
= left ventricle; PW = posterior wall.

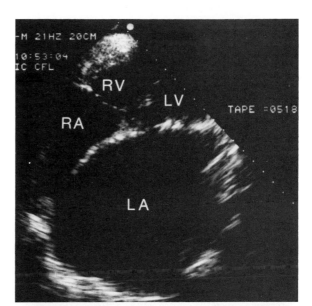

FIGURE 4–12
MITRAL STENOSIS, ANEURYSMAL DILATATION OF THE LEFT ATRIUM
Apical four-chamber section in a patient with severe pure mitral stenosis. Aneurysmal dilatation of the left atrium (LA) is present. RV = right ventricle; LV = left ventricle; RA = right atrium.

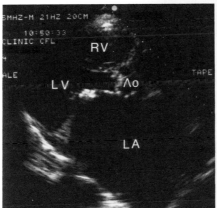

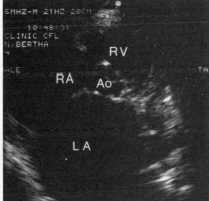

FIGURE 4–13
MITRAL STENOSIS, ANEURYSMAL DILATATION OF THE LEFT ATRIUM
Left parasternal short- and long-axis views from the same patient as in Figure 4–12. The anteroposterior diameter of the left atrium (LA) is 10 cm. RV = right ventricle; LV = left ventricle; Ao = aorta; RA = right atrium.

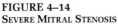

FIGURE 4–14
SEVERE MITRAL STENOSIS
Short-axis left parasternal view from a patient with severe mitral stenosis with a calculated mitral valve area of 0.7 sq cm.

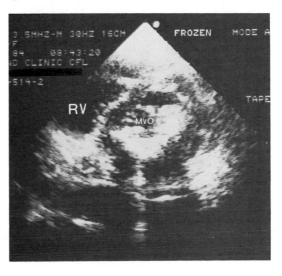

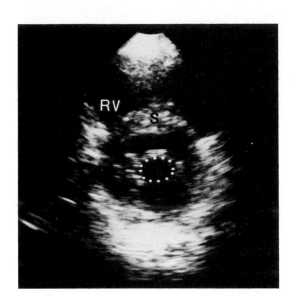

FIGURE 4–15
MILD MITRAL STENOSIS
Short-axis parasternal view in a patient with mitral
stenosis with a calculated valve area of 2 sq cm. Cardiac
catheterization showed normal pulmonary pressure and
a 6 mm Hg gradient across the mitral valve. RV = right
ventricle; S = septum.

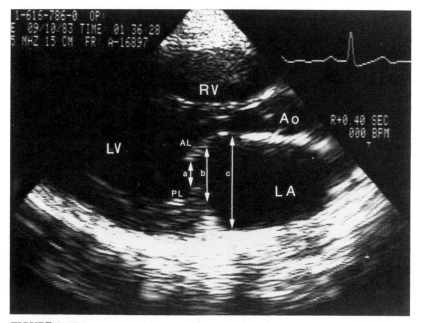

FIGURE 4–16
MITRAL STENOSIS, VALVE ORIFICE SIZE
Long-axis parasternal views in a patient with mitral stenosis. There are significant
differences in the distances from the anterior (AL) to the posterior (PL) leaflets at
the tip of the valve (a), at the body (b), and at the base (c). RV = right ventricle;
LV = left ventricle; Ao = aorta; LA = left atrium.

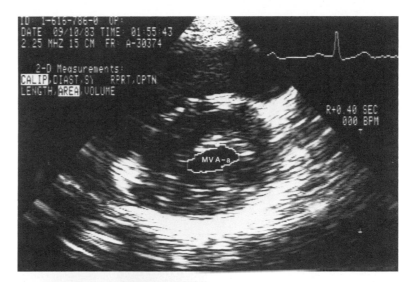

FIGURE 4–17
MITRAL STENOSIS, VALVE ORIFICE SIZE
Short-axis left parasternal view at level a of Figure 4–16. This represents the true mitral orifice size. MVA = mitral valve area.

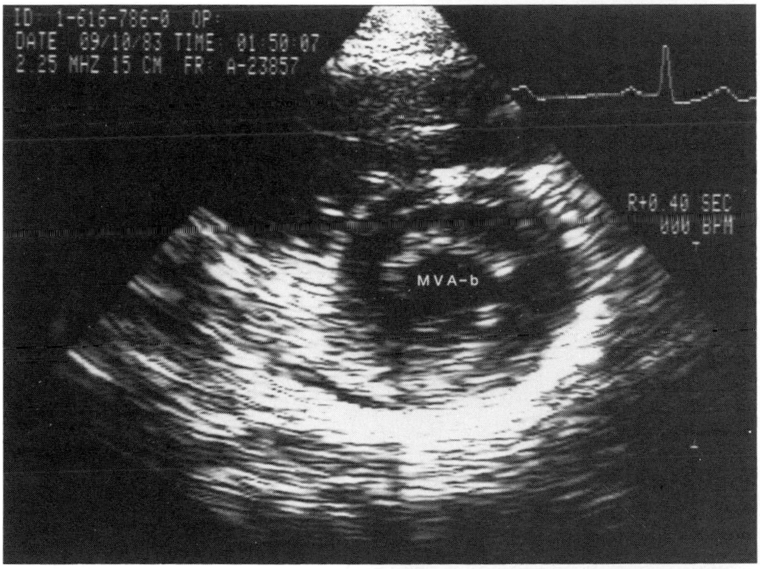

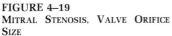

FIGURE 4–18
MITRAL STENOSIS, VALVE ORIFICE SIZE
Short-axis section at level b of Figure 4–16. Note that this area is somewhat larger than that shown in Figure 4–17. MVA = mitral valve area.

FIGURE 4–19
MITRAL STENOSIS, VALVE ORIFICE SIZE
Short-axis section of level c of Figure 4–16. This area is close to the mitral annulus, and there is no apparent narrowing of the orifice size.

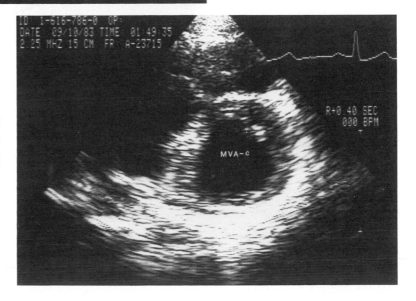

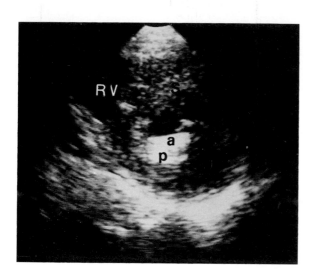

FIGURE 4–20
MITRAL STENOSIS, CALCIFIED LEAFLETS
Short-axis parasternal view in a patient with severe mitral stenosis with calcification of the leaflets (a = anterior; p = posterior). The high echo reflectivity in that area does not permit visualization of the true valve orifice, so that the valve area cannot be measured echocardiographically. RV = right ventricle.

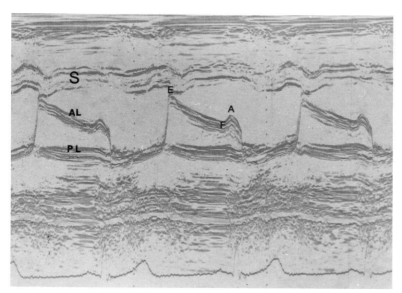

FIGURE 4–21
MITRAL STENOSIS, PLIABLE VALVE
M-mode echocardiogram from a 33-year-old patient with severe mitral stenosis (24 mm Hg gradient) and a pliable valve. The patient underwent successful commissurotomy the day after this echocardiogram was recorded. Note the normal leaflet excursion and the absence of thick shaggy echoes to suggest calcium. The absence of left ventricular volume overload does not suggest mitral regurgitation. S = septum; AL = anterior leaflet; PL = posterior leaflet.

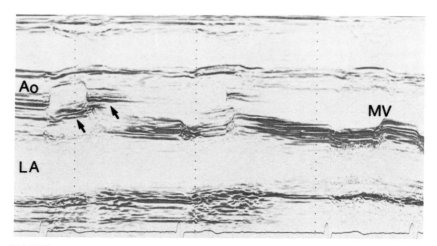

FIGURE 4–22
MITRAL STENOSIS, NONPLIABLE VALVE
M-mode echocardiographic scan from the aorta (Ao) to the mitral valve (MV) in a patient with severe (26 mm Hg gradient) mitral stenosis. The leaflets are quite thickened and the valve excursion is markedly reduced, even at the base of the leaflets. This patient also had mild aortic stenosis with a 30 mm Hg gradient. The arrows point to a thickened aortic valve. LA = left atrium.

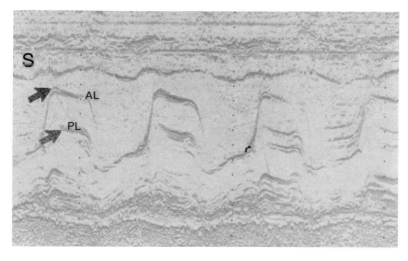

FIGURE 4–23
MITRAL STENOSIS, BEFORE COMMISSUROTOMY
Preoperative echocardiograms in a patient who underwent a successful commissurotomy. There is significant reduction of the E to F slope of the anterior leaflet (AL). The posterior leaflet (PL) moves anteriorly during diastole. The patient had a 23 mm Hg gradient across the mitral valve. S = septum.

FIGURE 4–24
MITRAL STENOSIS, AFTER COMMISSUROTOMY
Echocardiogram obtained seven days after successful commissurotomy in the same patient as in Figure 4–23. Notice the normalization of the E to F slope and the nearly normal motion of the posterior mitral leaflet. S = septum; AL = anterior leaflet; PL = posterior leaflet.

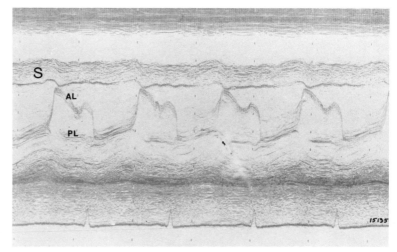

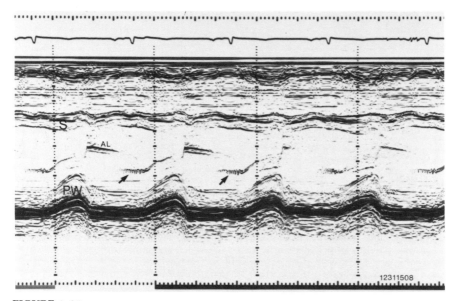

FIGURE 4–25
MITRAL STENOSIS, AFTER COMMISSUROTOMY
Late diastolic flutter of the posterior mitral leaflet is apparent in this patient with mitral stenosis after commissurotomy. S = septum; AL = anterior leaflet; PW = posterior wall.

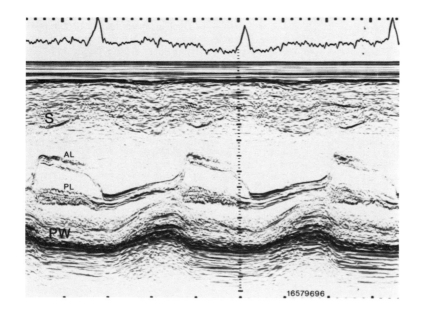

FIGURE 4–26
MITRAL STENOSIS, NORMAL POSTERIOR LEAFLET MOTION
M-mode echocardiogram from a 23-year-old patient with aortic insufficiency and mild mitral stenosis (5 mm Hg gradient). There is decreased E to F slope and increased leaflet thickening. The posterior leaflet (PL) moves normally (in the direction opposite to the anterior leaflet). The left ventricle is dilated as a result of aortic insufficiency. Fine fluttering of the posterior leaflet secondary to aortic insufficiency is seen in the first beat. S = septum; AL = anterior leaflet; PW = posterior wall.

FIGURE 4–27
MITRAL STENOSIS, AORTIC INSUFFICIENCY

The echocardiographic diagnosis of associated aortic insufficiency in patients with mitral stenosis may be difficult. The mitral valve, because of increased thickness, usually does not show the fine diastolic vibrations characteristic of aortic insufficiency. Septal vibrations as shown by the open arrow may be the only clue for the echocardiographic diagnosis of aortic insufficiency in the presence of mitral stenosis.

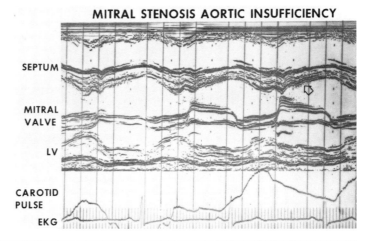

MITRAL STENOSIS AORTIC INSUFFICIENCY

SEPTUM

MITRAL VALVE

LV

CAROTID PULSE

EKG

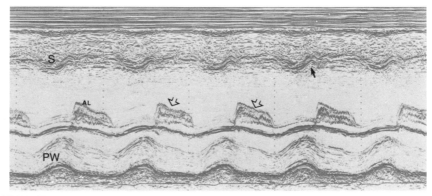

FIGURE 4–28
MITRAL STENOSIS, AORTIC INSUFFICIENCY

Echocardiogram from a 67-year-old patient with severe mitral stenosis (22 mm Hg gradient), aortic stenosis (74 mm Hg gradient), and aortic insufficiency. The fine diastolic flutter of the mitral valve characteristic of aortic insufficiency was only evident at the tip of the leaflets (arrows). At the level of the body of the anterior (AL) and posterior leaflets (PL) the vibrations are not seen. S = septum; PW = posterior wall.

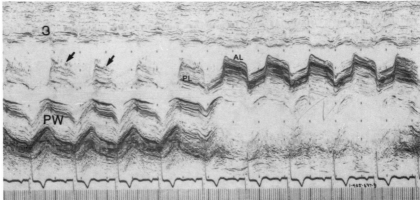

FIGURE 4–29
AORTIC INSUFFICIENCY, PSEUDO MITRAL STENOSIS

Echocardiogram from a 50-year-old patient with 4+ aortic insufficiency and no gradient across the mitral valve. The anterior leaflet (AL) has decreased E to F slope caused by decreased left ventricular compliance. The leaflet appears thickened, but in reality this is related to diastolic flutter (open arrows). A calcified mitral ring obscures the posterior mitral leaflet and gives the appearance of diastolic anterior motion of the posterior leaflet. The left ventricle is dilated. The black arrow points to a septal notch frequently seen in severe aortic insufficiency. S = septum; PW = posterior wall.

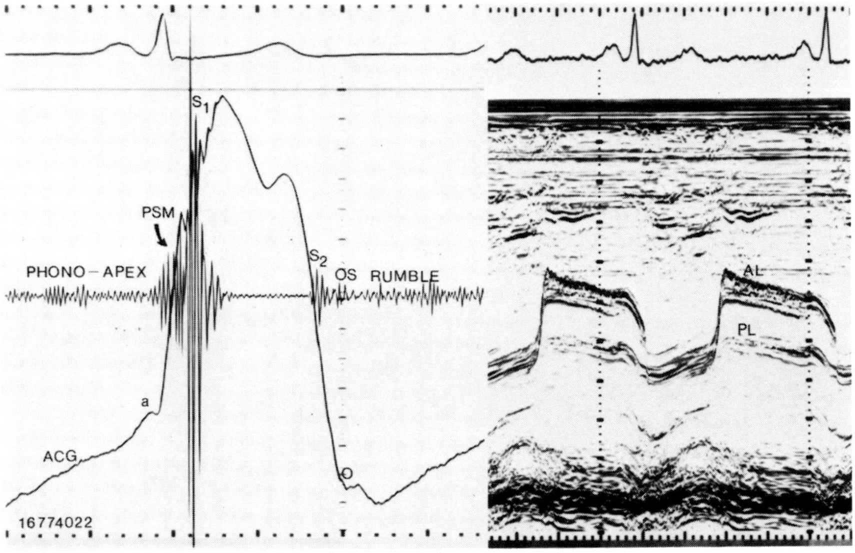

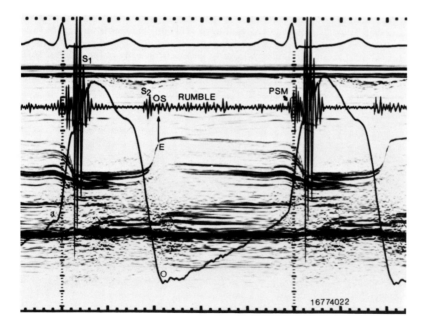

FIGURE 4–30
MITRAL STENOSIS, GRAPHICS
Phonocardiogram recorded at the apex in a patient with mitral stenosis. A presystolic murmur (PSM) precedes a very loud first heart sound (S_1). An opening snap (OS) is recorded 50 msec after the second heart sound (S_2) and is followed by a diastolic rumble. The apexcardiogram (ACG) shows a decreased a wave, an o point that coincides with the opening snap, and an absent rapid filling wave.

FIGURE 4–31
MITRAL STENOSIS, ECHOPHONOCARDIOGRAPHY
Simultaneous recording of phonocardiogram at the apex, apexcardiogram, and M-mode echocardiogram. Note that point E of the mitral valve coincides with the opening snap and the o point of the apexcardiogram. The diastolic rumble occurs during the E to F slope; the presystolic murmur (PSM) occurs during the closure of the mitral valve (AC interval), and the loud S_1 coincides with leaflet coaptation.

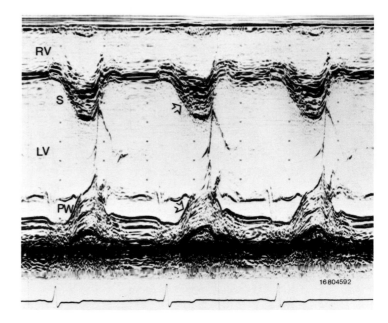

FIGURE 4–32
MITRAL INSUFFICIENCY, LEFT VENTRICULAR VOLUME OVERLOAD
Echocardiogram from a patient with severe mitral insufficiency demonstrates increased septal and posterior wall (PW) motion and a dilated left ventricle (LV). These findings are characteristic of left ventricular volume overload. RV = right ventricle; S = septum.

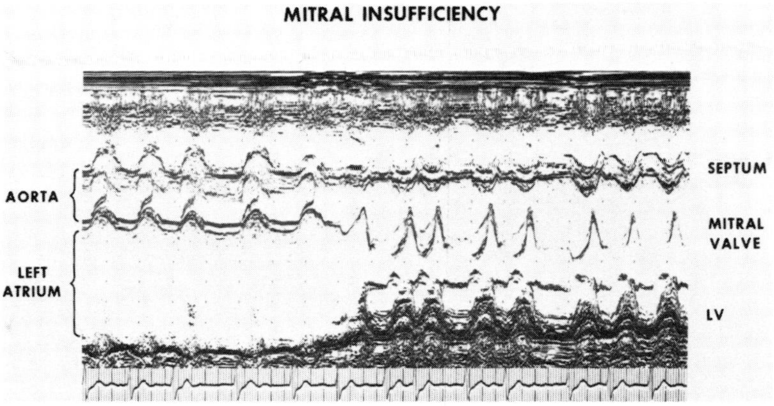

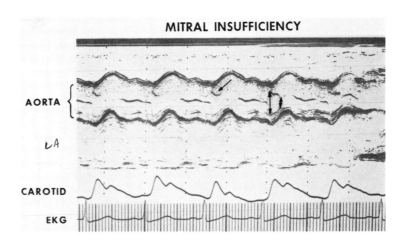

FIGURE 4–33
MITRAL INSUFFICIENCY
Echocardiogram from a patient with severe long-term nonrheumatic mitral insufficiency. Most of the secondary echo findings of mitral insufficiency are apparent in this study. The pattern of left ventricular (LV) volume overload, increased E to F slope of the mitral valve, and dilated left atrium is apparent.

FIGURE 4–34
MITRAL INSUFFICIENCY, EARLY AORTIC VALVE CLOSURE
With mitral insufficiency, the left ventricular stroke volume is partially lost to the left atrium, and as a result the aortic valve is fully open only at the beginning of systole. Note the difference in lengths of the arrows at the origin of systole as compared with the end of systole. The oblique arrow points to semiclosure of the aortic valve, which is a frequent finding in severe mitral insufficiency.

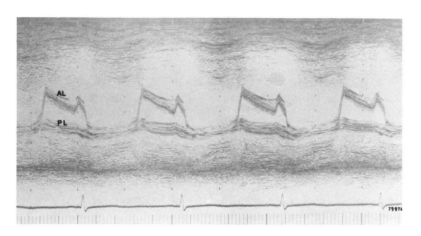

FIGURE 4–35
RHEUMATIC MITRAL INSUFFICIENCY
M-mode echocardiogram in a 47-year-old patient with mild mitral regurgitation and no gradient across the mitral valve. The diagnosis of rheumatic mitral valve disease can be made in this case on the basis of the increased thickness of the leaflets, the decreased E to F slope, and the abnormal motion of the posterior leaflet (PL). The prominent *a* wave suggests no gradient across the mitral valve, and the dilated ventricle is consistent with left ventricular volume overload secondary to mitral regurgitation. AL = anterior leaflet.

FIGURE 4–36
RHEUMATIC MITRAL INSUFFICIENCY
M-mode echocardiogram from a 23-year-old patient with pure rheumatic mitral insufficiency of moderate degree. Note the thickened leaflets, decreased E to F slope *(black arrow)*, diastolic anterior motion of the posterior leaflet *(open arrow)*, and increased septal motion with a dilated left ventricle (LV) suggestive of left ventricular volume overload. S = septum; PW = posterior wall.

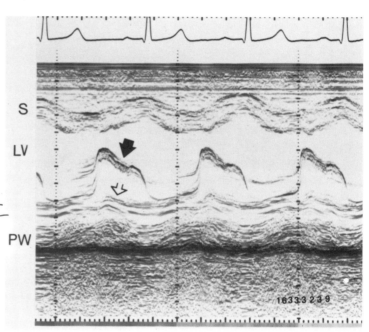

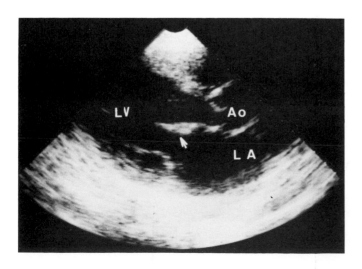

FIGURE 4–37
RHEUMATIC MITRAL INSUFFICIENCY
Long-axis parasternal view of the same patient as in Figure 4–36 shows increased leaflet thickening, relatively unrestricted leaflet aperture, and absence of diastolic doming—all characteristics of rheumatic mitral insufficiency. LV = left ventricle; Ao = aorta; LA = left atrium.

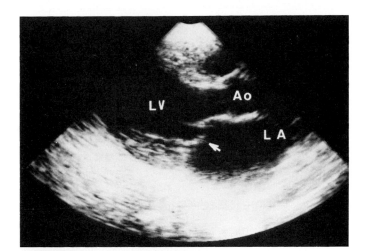

FIGURE 4–38
RHEUMATIC MITRAL INSUFFICIENCY
Long-axis parasternal view from the same patient as in Figures 4–36, 4–37. This recording, made during systole, demonstrates mitral valve prolapse (arrow), a finding occasionally seen in patients with rheumatic mitral insufficiency. LV = left ventricle; Ao = aorta; LA = left atrium.

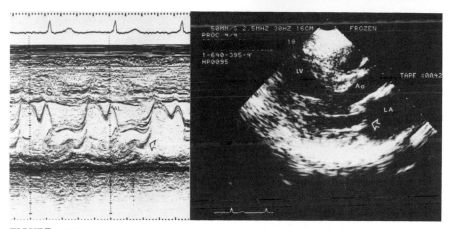

FIGURE 4–39
MITRAL VALVE PROLAPSE
M-mode and two-dimensional echocardiograms from a patient with mitral valve prolapse. The arrow in the M-mode echocardiogram points to the late systolic motion of the mitral valve toward the left atrium (LA). In the two-dimensional echocardiogram, the arrow points to the arcing of both leaflets toward the left atrium. S = septum; AL = anterior leaflet; LV = left ventricle; Ao = aorta.

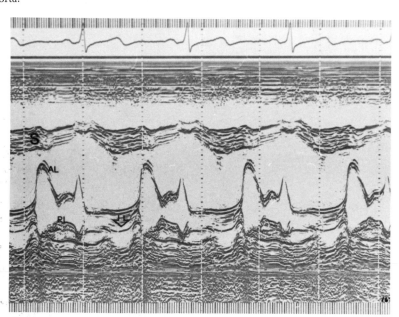
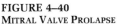

FIGURE 4–40
MITRAL VALVE PROLAPSE
Mild late systolic prolapse (arrow) in a 48-year-old woman who has had a known heart murmur since age 8 and a loud midsystolic click. The posterior leaflet (PL) is mildly thickened. S = septum; AL = anterior leaflet.

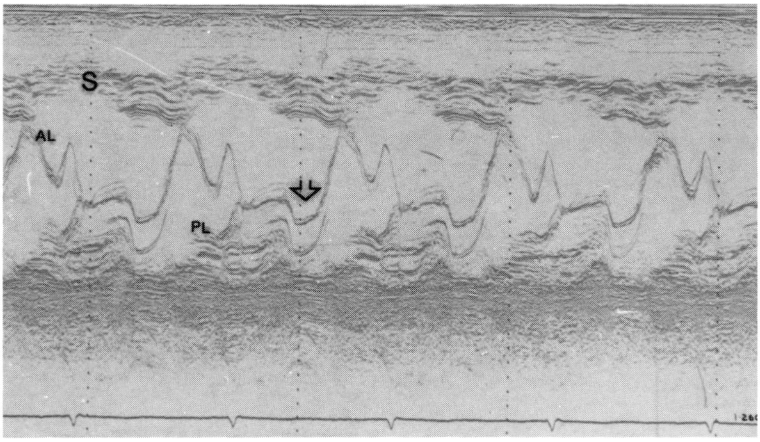

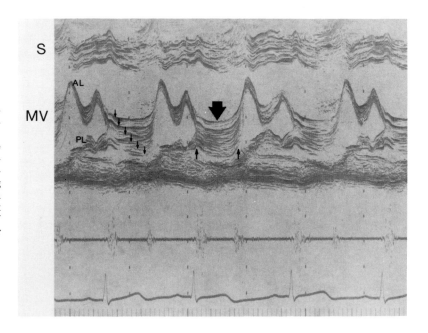

FIGURE 4–41
MITRAL VALVE PROLAPSE
M-mode echocardiogram demonstrates late systolic prolapse of both leaflets *(arrow)* in a 25-year-old woman with a mid-systolic click and late systolic murmur. Preceding the prolapse there is slight systolic anterior motion. The anterior (AL) and posterior (PL) leaflets appear normal during diastole. S = septum.

FIGURE 4–42
MITRAL VALVE PROLAPSE
Holosystolic mitral valve prolapse *(large arrow)* in a 13-year-old boy with Marfan's syndrome. Hammocking throughout systole is apparent *(small upright arrows)*. leaflet redundancy produces systolic multilayering *(small arrows)* as the echo beam transects the thickened leaflet at several points. S = septum; MV = mitral valve; AL = anterior leaflet; PL = posterior leaflet.

FIGURE 4–43

MITRAL VALVE PROLAPSE

Pansystolic mitral valve prolapse in a 16-year-old boy with
Marfan's syndrome. A simultaneous phonocardiogram demonstrates a loud first heart sound
(S_1), and a mid late systolic click
(x) followed by a late systolic
murmur. Marked thickening of
the posterior leaflet is apparent.
RV = right ventricle; S = septum; AL = anterior leaflet.

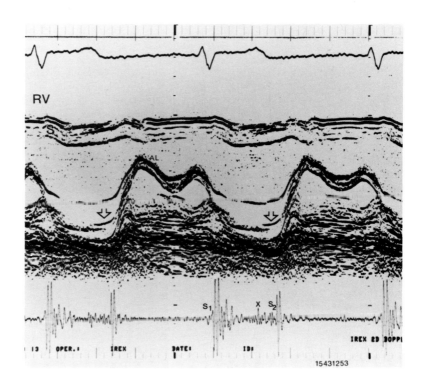

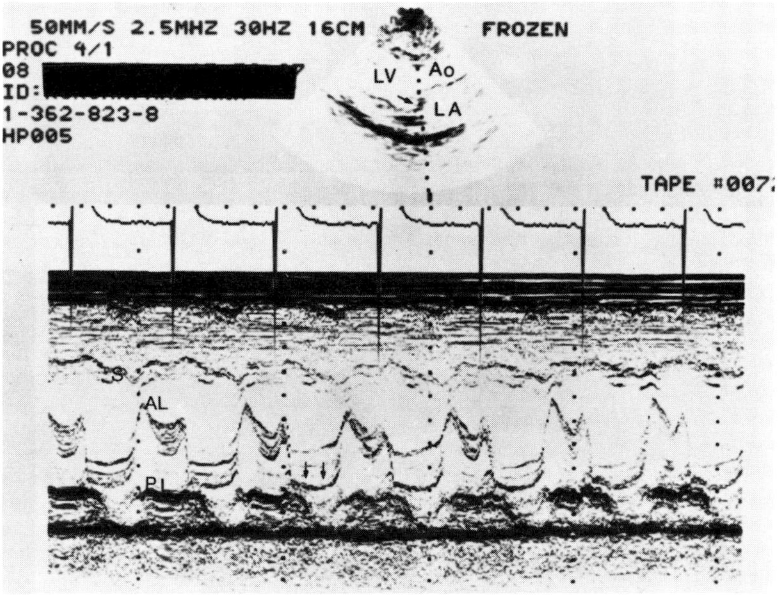

FIGURE 4–44

MITRAL VALVE PROLAPSE

Pansystolic mitral valve prolapse (*small arrows*) was demonstrated in this 37-year-old
woman with mild mitral regurgitation shown at the time of
cardiac catheterization. The M-
mode tracing was selected from
a two-dimensional long-axis
view sector scan with the M-
mode line transecting the heart
at the level of the atrioventricular groove. This is the zone in
which mitral valve prolapse is
most evident on M-mode echocardiography. LV = left ventricle; Ao = aorta; LA = left
atrium; AL = anterior leaflet; PL
= posterior leaflet.

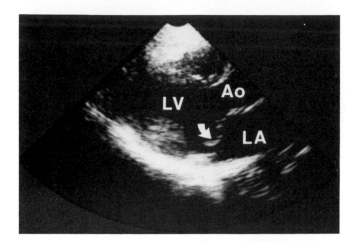

FIGURE 4–45
MITRAL VALVE PROLAPSE
Long-axis parasternal view in a patient with mitral valve prolapse demonstrates the typical arcing of the anterior leaflet toward the left atrium (LA) *(arrow)* so that part of the valve moves beyond the mitral ring during systole. LV = left ventricle; Ao = aorta.

FIGURE 4–46
MITRAL VALVE PROLAPSE
Long-axis parasternal view in a 65-year-old woman with moderate aortic and mitral insufficiency. The arrow points to the anterior mitral leaflet, which is prolapsing into the left atrium (LA). There is also mild dilatation of the aorta (Ao) and the left atrium (LA). The patient underwent mitral and aortic valve replacement and was found to have myxomatous degeneration of both valves.

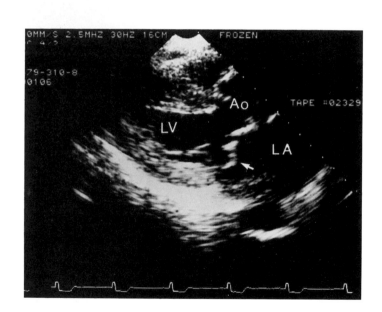

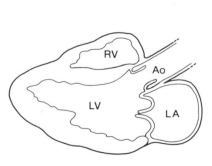

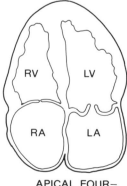

LONG-AXIS
PARASTERNAL VIEW

APICAL FOUR–
CHAMBER VIEW

FIGURE 4–47
MITRAL VALVE PROLAPSE
Long-axis parasternal and apical four-chamber views illustrate the arcing of the mitral valve leaflets that is typical of mitral valve prolapse. RV = right ventricle; LV = left ventricle; Ao = aorta; LA = left atrium; RA = right atrium.

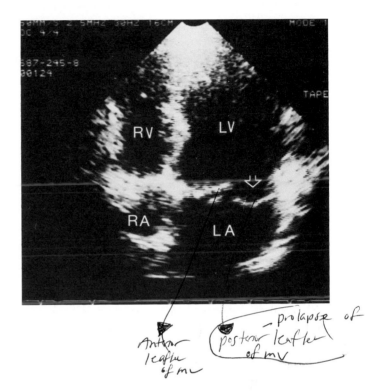

FIGURE 4–48
MITRAL VALVE PROLAPSE, APICAL VIEW
Apical four-chamber view in a patient who had
a 3/6 holosystolic murmur at the apex. The
arrow points to prolapse of the posterior mitral
valve into the left atrium (LA). RV = right
ventricle; LV = left ventricle; RA = right
ventricle.

Antior leaflet of mv

prolapse of posterior leaflet of mv

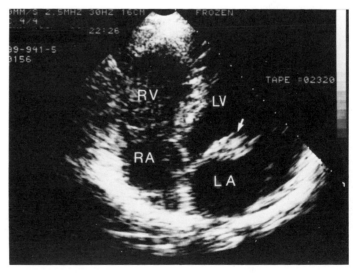

FIGURE 4–49
MITRAL VALVE PROLAPSE
Echocardiogram from a 55-year-old patient with mitral valve prolapse and severe mitral regurgitation. The arrow
points to a mass of echoes at the level of
the anterior leaflet that is suggestive of a
vegetation. The patient underwent mitral
valve replacement, and no vegetations
were found at the time of surgery. Such
a cloud of echoes is frequently seen in
patients with mitral valve prolapse with
redundant leaflet. RV = right ventricle;
LV = left ventricle; RA = right atrium;
LA = left atrium.

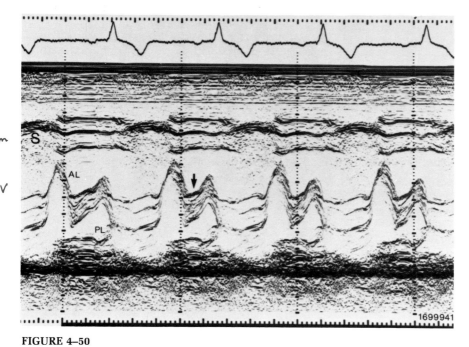

Septum

LV

FIGURE 4–50
MITRAL VALVE PROLAPSE, THICKENED LEAFLETS
M-mode echocardiogram from the same patient as in Figure 4–49. Note the marked thickening (*arrow*) of the anterior leaflet (AL). The posterior leaflet (PL) is normal. S = septum.

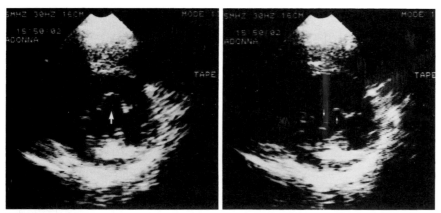

FIGURE 4–51
MITRAL VALVE PROLAPSE
Short-axis parasternal views in a patient with mitral valve prolapse show undulations (*arrows*) of the anterior leaflet. This is characteristic of a redundant and elongated valve.

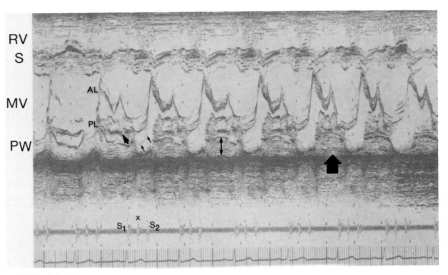

FIGURE 4–52
MITRAL VALVE PROLAPSE
Echocardiogram of a patient with mitral valve (MV) prolapse and hyperactive atrioventricular groove. The posterior leaflet (PL) is markedly thickened (*arrowhead*). The small arrows point to the prolapse. The double-headed arrow demarcates the excessive atrioventricular groove motion. The large black arrow shows the thickened posterior leaflet, which by being in contact with the atrioventricular groove gives the appearance of a mass in the inflow tract of the left ventricle. RV = right ventricle; S = septum; PW = posterior wall; AL = anterior leaflet.

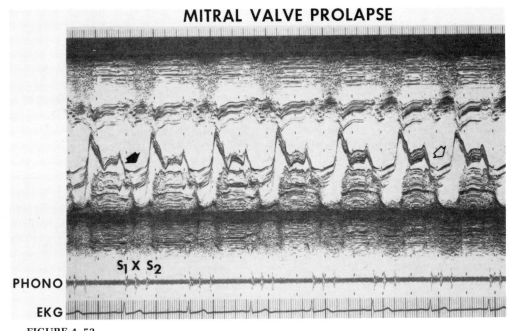

FIGURE 4–53
MITRAL VALVE PROLAPSE
Echocardiogram from the same patient as in Figure 4–52 shows the "pseudo mass" behind the mitral valve. At the level of the black arrow the prolapse is evident, whereas at the level of the white arrow it is not.

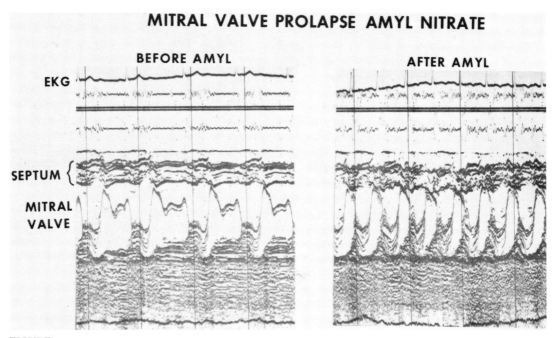

FIGURE 4–54
MITRAL VALVE PROLAPSE AND AMYL NITRATE INHALATION
Echocardiograms from a patient with mitral valve prolapse before and after the inhalation of amyl nitrate. The late systolic prolapse becomes holosystolic after the inhalation of amyl nitrate.

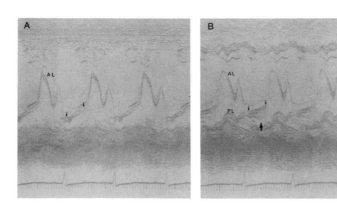

FIGURE 4–55
MITRAL VALVE PROLAPSE
These echocardiograms illustrate that a low transducer position (A) may not demonstrate a prolapse. The systolic mitral motion between the arrows in panel A is apparently normal. With proper transducer placement (B), the prolapse is evident (*black arrow*). AL = anterior leaflet; PL = posterior leaflet.

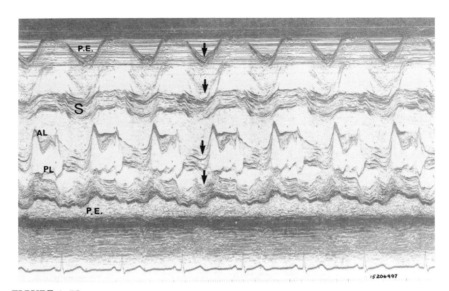

FIGURE 4–56
PSEUDO MITRAL VALVE PROLAPSE, PERICARDIAL EFFUSION
Echocardiogram from a 48-year-old patient with recurrent pericarditis and a large pericardial effusion. The mitral valve appears to have a late systolic prolapse, but on closer inspection it can be seen that the entire heart is moving backward during systole (*arrows*). P.E. = pericardial effusion; S = septum; AL = anterior leaflet; PL = posterior leaflet.

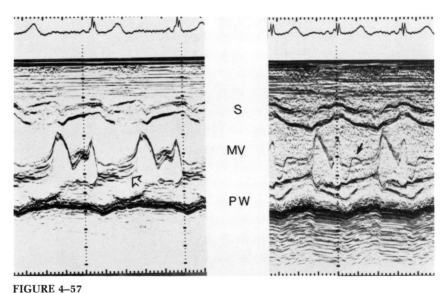

FIGURE 4–57
MITRAL VALVE PROLAPSE, SYSTOLIC ANTERIOR MOTION
In some patients with mitral valve prolapse, systolic anterior motion is present. In this case, with inferior angulation of the transducer the systolic anterior motion was evident (*black arrow*). The open arrow points to the prolapse, which was visualized at higher levels. In most patients, this abnormality is related to redundant leaflets. In this particular case it is probably related to excessive motion of the chordae tendineae. S = septum; MV = mitral valve; PW = posterior wall.

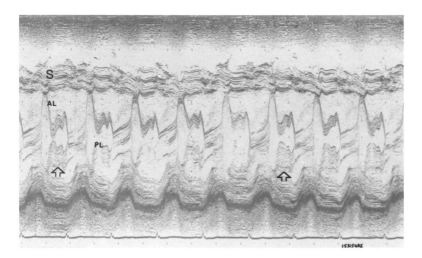

FIGURE 4–58

MITRAL VALVE PROLAPSE, PSEUDO-
VEGETATIONS

M-mode echocardiogram from a
patient with mitral valve prolapse and thickened posterior
leaflet (PL). The patient did not
have bacterial endocarditis. S =
septum; AL = anterior leaflet.

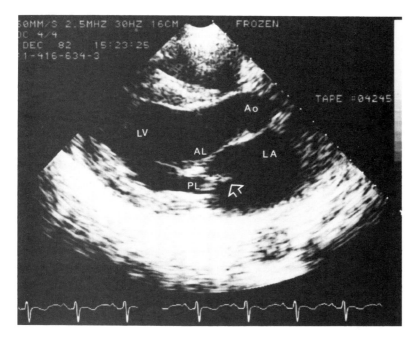

FIGURE 4–59

RUPTURED CHORDAE TENDINEAE

Long-axis parasternal view in a
21-year-old patient with Whipple's disease and acute mitral
regurgitation. The arrow points
to a flail chordae attached to the
posterior mitral valve (PL) and
prolapsing into the left atrium
(LA). At the time of cardiac surgery, ruptured chordae tendineae to the posterior leaflet were
found. Mitral valve repair was
performed. LV = left ventricle;
Ao = aorta; AL = anterior leaflet.

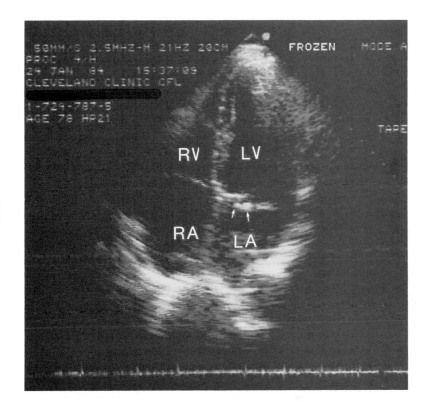

FIGURE 4–60
Ruptured Chordae Tendineae
Apical four-chamber view shows the ruptured chordae tendineae in the left atrium.

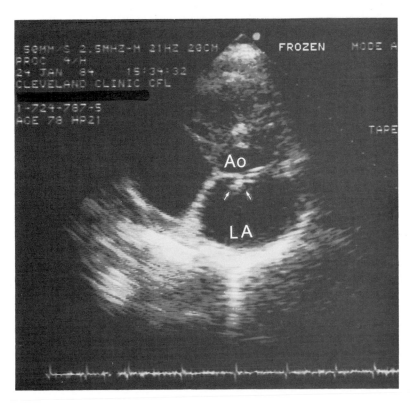

FIGURE 4–61
Ruptured Chordae Tendineae
Short-axis parasternal view shows the ruptured chordae tendineae at the level of the left atrium.

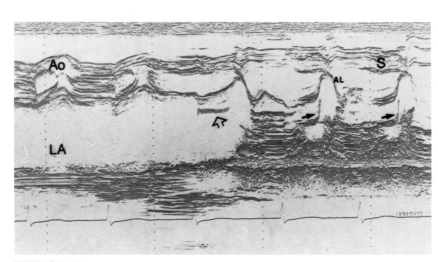

FIGURE 4–62
RUPTURED CHORDAE TENDINEAE
M-mode echocardiographic scan from the aorta to the left ventricle in a 61-year-old patient with severe mitral insufficiency. The left atrium (LA) is enlarged and contains parts of the mitral valve and chordae (*open arrow*), which are prolapsing and show fine systolic vibrations. Ao = aorta; AL = anterior leaflet; S = septum.

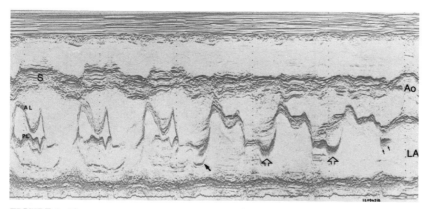

FIGURE 4–63
RUPTURED CHORDAE TENDINEAE
M-mode echocardiographic scan from the mitral valve to the aorta shows part of the mitral valve prolapsing into the left atrium (LA) (*small arrows*). Fine late systolic vibrations are indicated by the open arrows. The posterior leaflet (PL) is thickened and meets the anterior leaflet (AL) is mid-diastole. S = septum; Ao = aorta.

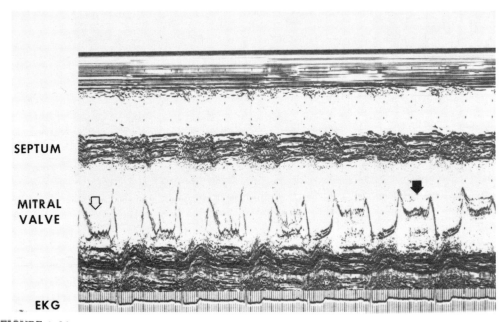

FIGURE 4–64
RUPTURED CHORDAE TENDINEAE
Diastolic abnormalities of mitral valve motion are seen in this patient with ruptured chordae tendineae to the anterior leaflet. There is variation of the diastolic pattern of motion from beat to beat. Fine and coarse flutter of the anterior leaflet is apparent during the first few beats. Toward the end of the tracing (*black arrow*), the motion of the valve is normal, probably because that part of the valve had adequate chordal support.

FIGURE 4–65
RUPTURED CHORDAE TENDINEAE
Marked variation of the diastolic pattern of motion is demonstrated in the anterior leaflet of the mitral valve in a patient with ruptured chordae tendineae to the anterior mitral valve. Despite regular sinus rhythm, no two beats have similar diastolic appearances.

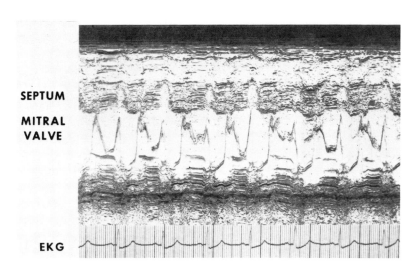

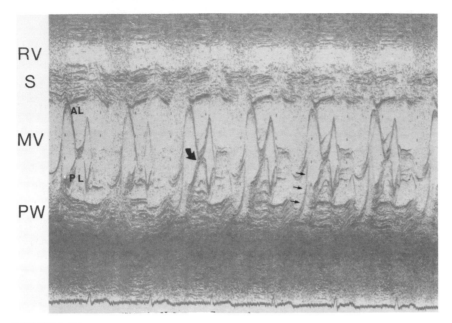

FIGURE 4–66
RUPTURED CHORDAE TENDINEAE
Mid-diastolic contact of both leaflets (*large arrow*) is apparent in this 51-year-old patient with severe mitral regurgitation. The small arrows point to the mitral valve (MV) returning from its prolapsed position. At the time of cardiac surgery, several ruptured chordae were found along the central aspect of the posterior leaflet (PL). RV = right ventricle; S = septum, PW = posterior wall; AL = anterior leaflet.

FIGURE 4–67
RUPTURED CHORDAE TENDINEAE
Apical four-chamber view during diastole in a patient with ruptured chordae tendineae. This condition appears indistinguishable from severe mitral valve prolapse. RV = right ventricle; LV = left ventricle; RA = right atrium; LA = left atrium.

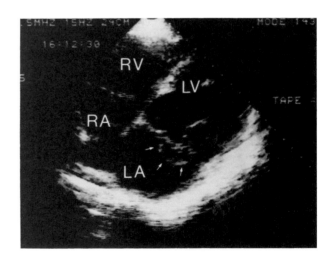

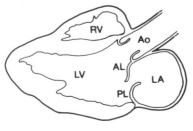

FIGURE 4–68
MITRAL VALVE PROLAPSE COMPARED WITH RUPTURED CHORDAE TENDINEAE
In the long-axis parasternal view, the tip of a prolapsing mitral valve points toward the left ventricle (LV) during systole, whereas with ruptured chordae tendineae, it points toward the left atrium (LA). RV = right ventricle; Ao = aorta; AL = anterior leaflet; PL = posterior leaflet.

FIGURE 4–69
RUPTURED CHORDAE TENDINEAE, SYSTOLIC FLUTTER
M-mode echocardiogram from a 76-year-old patient with severe mitral insufficiency, congestive heart failure, and negative blood cultures. The mitral valve (MV) is somewhat thickened and shows evidence of mitral valve prolapse (*small arrows*) and systolic vibrations (*black arrow*) consistent with the diagnosis of ruptured chordae tendineae. RV = right ventricle; S = septum.

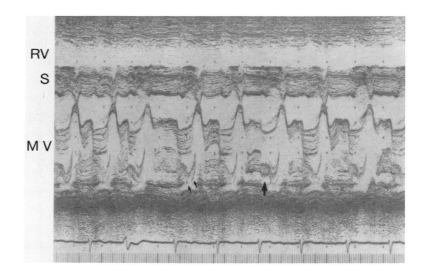

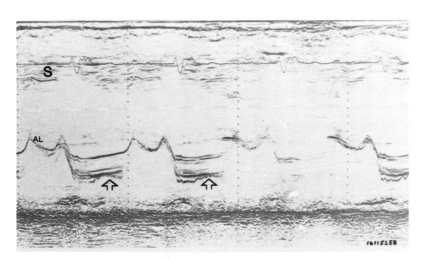

FIGURE 4–70
RUPTURED CHORDAE TENDINEAE
M-mode echocardiogram from a 68-year-old man with a history of endocarditis at age 63. The arrows point to fine systolic fluttering of the mitral valve. Ruptured chordae tendineae were evident at the time of surgery. S = septum; AL = anterior leaflet.

FIGURE 4–71
RUPTURED CHORDAE TENDINEAE
Long-axis left parasternal view in a patient with ruptured chordae tendineae and acute mitral regurgitation. The posterior leaflet is seen to prolapse into the left atrium (LA) (*arrow*). The left atrium is not significantly dilated. LV = left ventricle; Ao = aorta; AL = anterior leaflet.

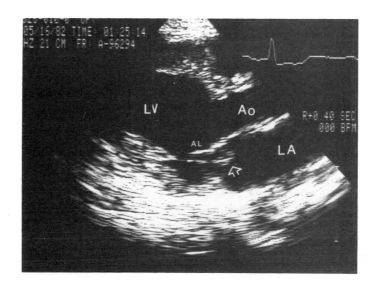

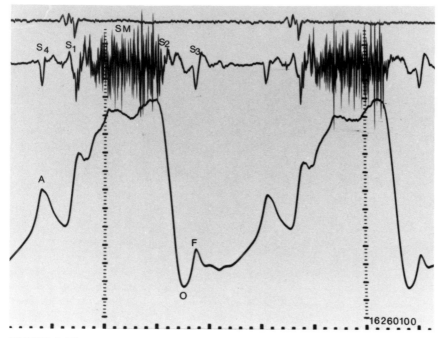

FIGURE 4–72
RUPTURED CHORDAE TENDINEAE
Apexcardiogram and phonocardiogram recorded at the apex in the same patient as in Figure 4–71. The large α wave on the apexcardiogram coincides with a fourth heart sound. A rapid filling wave (F) coincides with a third heart sound. The phonocardiogram also registers a holosystolic high-frequency murmur.

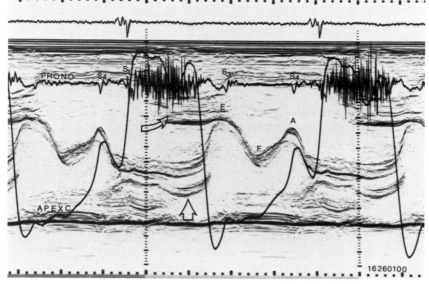

FIGURE 4–73
RUPTURED CHORDAE TENDINEAE
Simultaneous mitral valve echocardiogram, apexcardiogram, and phonocardiogram recorded at the apex in the same patient as in Figure 4–72. The large arrow points to the prolapsing mitral valve. The small arrow points to the holosystolic murmur. A fourth heart sound coincides with an α wave of the mitral valve and of the apexcardiogram. A third heart sound coincides with the E point of the mitral valve and the F point of the apexcardiogram.

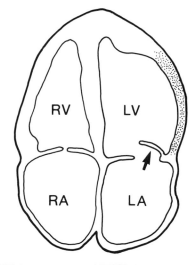

FIGURE 4–74
PAPILLARY MUSCLE DYSFUNCTION
Apical four-chamber view in a patient with a lateral wall myocardial infarction and papillary muscle dysfunction. There is failure of the posterior leaflet to reach the normal peak systolic position relative to the mitral ring. RV = right ventricle; LV = left ventricle; RA = right atrium; LA = left atrium.

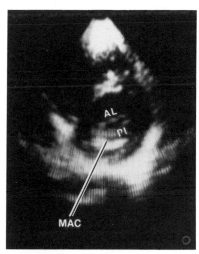
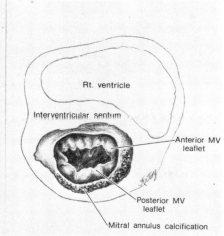

FIGURE 4–75
MITRAL ANNULUS CALCIFICATION
Short-axis left parasternal view in a patient with mitral annulus calcification (MAC), which appears as a dense mass of echoes behind the posterior mitral valve (PL). AL = anterior leaflet; MV = mitral valve.

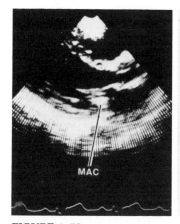
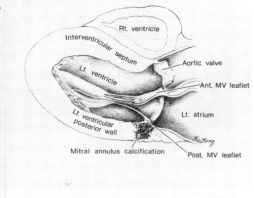

FIGURE 4–76
MITRAL ANNULUS CALCIFICATION
Long-axis left parasternal view in a patient with mitral annulus calcification (MAC), which is seen to protrude into the left ventricular cavity behind the posterior leaflet.

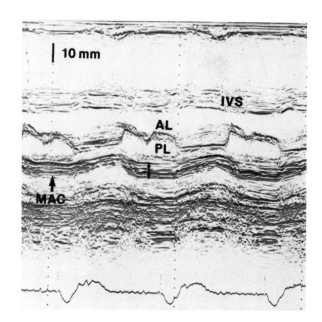

FIGURE 4–77
MITRAL ANNULUS CALCIFICATION
A dense band of echoes (MAC) is seen behind the posterior mitral leaflet (PL) in this patient with a densely calcified mitral annulus (MAC). The MAC thickness (*two-headed arrow*) is approximately 10 mm. AL = anterior leaflet; IVS = interventricular septum.

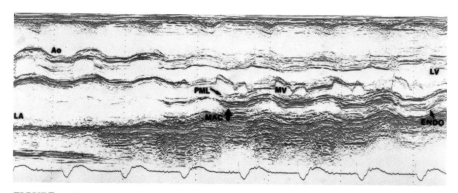

FIGURE 4–78
MITRAL ANNULUS CALCIFICATION
Echocardiographic scan from the aorta (Ao) to the left ventricle (LV) demonstrates mitral annulus calcification (MAC) behind the posterior leaflet of the mitral valve (PML) and in front of the posterior wall endocardium (endo). LA = left atrium; MV = mitral valve.

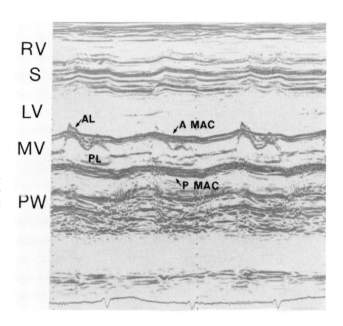

FIGURE 4–79
MITRAL ANNULUS CALCIFICATION
Anterior and posterior mitral annulus calcification (A MAC and P MAC) are demonstrated. The mitral valve (MV) is seen within the two parallel lines that are part of the anterior and and posterior mitral ring. RV = right ventricle; S = septum; LV = left ventricle; PW = posterior wall; AL = anterior leaflet; PL = posterior leaflet.

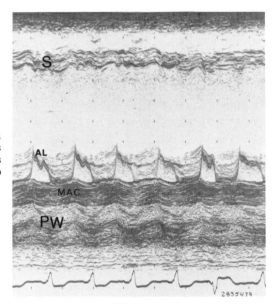

FIGURE 4–80
MITRAL ANNULUS CALCIFICATION
M-mode echocardiogram from a 78-year-old woman with congestive heart failure, chronic renal failure, and sick sinus syndrome. A markedly thickened mitral annulus (MAC) is seen posterior to the mitral valve. The left ventricle is also markedly dilated. S = septum; AL = anterior leaflet; PW = posterior wall.

5 AORTIC VALVE DISEASE

5.1 VALVULAR AORTIC STENOSIS

There are three important causes of valvular aortic stenosis in the adult.

1. Rheumatic Aortic Stenosis. This condition is usually accompanied by rheumatic mitral valve disease. There is fusion of the commissures with calcification of the valve and scarring of the leaflet edges.

2. Fibrocalcific Senile Aortic Stenosis. This form of stenosis is produced by degenerative valvular changes in the form of destruction of collagen and accumulation of calcific deposits. These processes begin at the sinuses of Valsalva and progress medially until they compromise a significant portion of the valve to obstruct normal flow.

3. Congenital Aortic Stenosis. This form is provoked by fibrocalcific degeneration in a congenitally deformed aortic valve.

The end result of all three processes is the same—that is, commissure fusion with narrowing of the aortic valve orifice. When the degeneration and calcification are severe, it may be impossible to determine which of the three forms of aortic stenosis is present.

Another common finding in patients with severe aortic stenosis is concentric left ventricular hypertrophy with thickened left ventricular walls but typically with a chamber of normal or near normal size.

Echocardiographic Findings in Calcific Aortic Stenosis

In this section the echocardiographic findings of the adult patient with calcific aortic stenosis are discussed. A description of the congenitally deformed aortic valve can be found in Chapter 16.

The echocardiographic findings in adult calcific aortic stenosis include thickened aortic leaflet, restricted leaflet motion, and a narrow aortic orifice.

1. Thickened Aortic Leaflets. With M-mode echocardiography this is seen as multiple and dense echoes coming from one leaflet during both systole and diastole (Fig. 5–1). The degree of echo return has some correlation with the degree of fibrosis of the leaflets. Occasionally the thickening is localized to one leaflet so that the increased echo density is seen in a localized area (Fig. 5–2).

Two-dimensional echocardiography permits a better evaluation of the degree and location of the leaflet thickness.[1] The fibrotic leaflets are more reflective and allow better leaflet visualization (Fig. 5–3). In contrast to the aortic leaflets of normal individuals, which are not well visualized during diastole in the long-axis view, in patients with aortic stenosis the leaflets are clearly seen throughout the cardiac cycle. In the short-axis view, the calcification typically begins at the base of the involved leaflet. The right coronary cusp is affected most commonly and the left coronary cusp least commonly (Fig. 5–4).

2. Restricted Leaflet Motion. The systolic separation between the anterior (right coronary cusp) and posterior (noncoronary cusp) leaflets is reduced to below 1.5 cm in adults (Fig. 5–5).

All or portions of the leaflets become fixed. The bases of the leaflets usually are more restricted, but in some patients the entire valve is fixed. In the long-axis left parasternal view, this restriction is manifested as diminished leaflet separation (Figs. 5–6 to 5–8).

In the presence of multiple systolic echoes, it may be difficult to clearly identify the leaflets.

3. Narrow Aortic Orifice. Commissure fusion and restricted motion reduce the aortic valve area. With two-dimensional echocardiography it is possible to estimate the aortic valve orifice area, but this value is not as reliable as with the measurement of the mitral valve area.

Other echocardiographic findings frequently seen in aortic stenosis[2] include (1) left ventricular hypertrophy, (2) decreased left ventricle compliance evidenced by decreased mitral E to F slope, (3) dilated aortic root, (4) left ventricular dilatation and dysfunction, and (5) left atrial enlargement.

Severity of Aortic Stenosis

The severity of aortic stenosis can be estimated by examining leaflet motion restriction, left ventricular hypertrophy, and aortic valve area.

1. Degree of Leaflet Motion Restriction. There is some relationship between the degree of leaflet motion restriction as seen by M-mode echocardiography[3] and the severity of aortic stenosis.

By using two-dimensional echocardiography, a relationship has been established between the maximal aortic cusp separation as seen in the long-axis parasternal view and the severity of aortic stenosis. Maximal cusp separation of less than 8 mm usually means that there is severe aortic stenosis, whereas separation of 12 mm or more usually means that if there is stenosis it is mild.[4, 5]

Another practical way to estimate the severity of aortic stenosis is by observing individual leaflet motion. If any leaflet opens completely (Fig. 5–9), there can be only mild to moderate aortic stenosis. If no leaflet motion is seen, the stenosis is probably severe.

2. Degree of Left Ventricular Hypertrophy. Most patients with significant aortic stenosis have some degree of left ventricular hypertrophy.[6–11] Several investigators have tried to correlate the degree of hypertrophy in patients with aortic stenosis with the

aortic valve area or the gradient or with both parameters. Left ventricular pressure can be estimated according to the constant wall stress hypothesis by the following formula:

$$\text{left ventricular systolic pressure} = \frac{225 \times \text{LVWTs}}{\text{LVEDS}}$$

where 225 is a stress constant, LVWTs is the systolic left ventricular wall thickness, and LVEDS is the end-systolic diameter of the left ventricle.

From this calculation the systolic pressure obtained by a sphygmomanometer can be subtracted to obtain an approximation of the aortic gradient. This formula has been validated mainly for young patients without left ventricular dysfunction. In studies of adults, this approach has not proved helpful.[12]

3. Aortic Valve Area. With two-dimensional echocardiography it is possible to visualize and measure the size of the aortic valve orifice.[13] Unfortunately, this method has not been as useful clinically as it has been in studying the mitral valve. Measuring the aortic valve orifice is much more difficult. There is more dropout of echoes, so that the borders of the image are not as clear. The recording is thus clinically unreliable because very small changes in orifice size make a significant difference in the pressure gradient, which is the parameter that has greater clinical relevance.

Conditions Complicating the Diagnosis

A number of conditions can make the diagnosis of aortic stenosis difficult:

1. Aortic Sclerosis. In this condition the aortic leaflets are thickened, but their motion is not restricted (Fig. 5–10).

2. Aortic Root Fibrosis and Calcification. This condition may make the visualization of the aortic leaflet difficult or impossible to evaluate (Fig. 5–11).

3. Decreased Cardiac Output. This condition may produce decreased leaflet excursion. If the leaflets are sclerotic, the condition may be indistinguishable from aortic stenosis.

4. Congenital Aortic Stenosis. Leaflet doming produces apparently normal leaflet separation in the presence of severe stenosis.

Echophonocardiography

Phonocardiography and pulse recordings are quite helpful in the evaluation of patients with aortic stenosis. Patients with aortic stenosis usually have a *delayed carotid upstroke* with a U time of more than 120 msec.[14] Patients with critical aortic stenosis with gradients of more than 70 mm Hg usually have U times of 200 msec or longer (Fig. 5–12). The time interval between the Q wave on the electrocardiogram and the *peak of the murmur* has been used to assess the severity of aortic stenosis. A time interval from Q to peak of the murmur of more than 240 msec has been found in patients with gradients across the aortic valve of 70 mm Hg or more (Fig. 5–13).[15]

A characteristic of the murmur of aortic stenosis is that it increases its intensity after the compensatory pause of a premature beat. A larger volume of blood has to pass through the narrowed and fixed orifice of the aortic valve, increasing the velocity of flow and with it the intensity of the murmur. This process can be demonstrated clearly with an echophonocardiogram at the level of the aortic valve (Fig. 5–14). Another application of echophonocardiography in aortic stenosis is for the elucidation of systolic clicks. A *systolic ejection click* is characteristic of the bicuspid aortic valve and occurs at the time of maximal anterior excursion of the anterior aortic leaflet (Fig. 5–15).

5.2 AORTIC INSUFFICIENCY

Aortic insufficiency may result from aortic valve disease or from disease of the aortic root.

Common causes of valvular aortic insufficiency include (1) rheumatic aortic insufficiency (always associated with mitral valve disease), (2) infective endocarditis, (3) congenital deformities, and (4) aortic valve prolapse.

The most common cause of aortic insufficiency secondary to disease of the aorta are (1) syphilitic aortitis, (2) Marfan's syndrome, (3) dissecting aneurysms of the aorta, and (4) ankylosing spondylitis. These abnormalities are discussed in Chapter 6.

Echocardiographic Diagnosis

The echocardiographic diagnosis of aortic insufficiency is indirect and is based on several findings:

1. *Diastolic Flutter of the Mitral Valve.* High-frequency vibrations of the anterior (Figs. 5–16, 5–17) and occasionally the posterior mitral leaflets are characteristic of aortic insufficiency. These vibrations are produced by turbulence that is created by the regurgitant jet into the left ventricular outflow tract and mitral valve. The vibrations are usually of a similar frequency in any given patient but may vary significantly from patient to patient (Fig. 5–18). They occur mainly during the first two thirds of diastole and may be absent if diastole is very short (Fig. 5–19). Registering the echocardiogram at faster paper speed makes recognition of the diastolic flutter easier (Fig. 5–20). Maneuvers that increase the degree of aortic insufficiency, such as hand grip, increase the amplitude of the diastolic flutter. The inhalation of amyl nitrate may make the flutter disappear (Fig. 5–21). With two-dimensional echocardiography, only high-amplitude vibrations can be recognized.

2. *Diastolic Flutter of the Interventricular Septum.* Diastolic flutter of the interventricular septum (Fig. 5–22)[16–18] is relatively unusual but has the same connotation as mitral valve flutter (Fig. 5–23). This finding is particularly helpful in rheumatic mitral valve disease in which the fibrotic mitral leaflets often do not demonstrate diastolic flutter in the presence of associated aortic insufficiency (Fig. 5–24).

3. *Decreased Mitral Valve Opening.* The regurgitant jet may directly hit the anterior mitral leaflet and decrease its motion. With M-mode echocardiography this process is seen as a decreased early diastolic excursion of the mitral valve to the point where the E point may be absent (Fig. 5–25). With two-dimensional echocardiography this process appears as an abnormal short-axis configuration of the anterior mitral valve, which is pushed posteriorly. The mitral valve is pushed posteriorly only with severe aortic insufficiency. In the long-axis parasternal view, the anterior leaflet excursion is limited by a large mitral-to-septal separation (Fig. 5–26).

4. Diastolic Flutter of the Aortic Valve. This is a very specific, but not so sensitive, finding in aortic insufficiency (Fig. 5–27). It often occurs in the presence of infective endocarditis or with flail aortic valve.

5. Leaflet Thickening. Most patients with aortic insufficiency have some degree of increased aortic leaflet thickening (Fig. 5–28). This is particularly common in patients with rheumatic carditis.

6. Dilated Aortic Root. Variable degrees of aortic root dilatation are seen in most patients with aortic insufficiency (Fig. 5–28).

7. Left Ventricular Volume Overload. Patients with moderate or severe aortic insufficiency have increased end-diastolic and end-systolic diameters of the left ventricle and exaggerated septal and posterior wall motion (Fig. 5–29).[19]

8. Abnormal Septal Motion. An exaggerated early diastolic "dip" can be seen in recordings from some patients with moderate or severe aortic insufficiency (Fig. 5–30).

9. Lack of Leaflet Coaptation. In some patients with aortic insufficiency the M-mode echocardiogram shows lack of leaflet coaptation during diastole (Fig. 5–31). This is a nonspecific finding. In Marfan's syndrome, lack of leaflet coaptation may be apparent in the short-axis view (Fig. 5–32). This is probably the only direct echocardiographic finding of aortic insufficiency.

10. Premature Mitral Closure. In patients with acute aortic insufficiency, the rapidly regurgitant flow of blood from the aorta can raise left ventricular pressure to the point of producing mitral closure before the beginning of ventricular systole.[20, 21] The C point of the mitral valve occurs before the Q wave of the electrocardiogram (Fig. 5–33). Occasionally, examination of a patient with severe chronic aortic insufficiency may reveal similar findings.

Another cause of premature mitral closure is first-degree atrioventricular block (Fig. 5–34). This fact should be taken into account when premature mitral closure is observed in patients with aortic insufficiency.

11. Premature Aortic Valve Opening. Occasionally the diastolic pressure may be so great with severe aortic insufficiency that the aortic valve may open prematurely (Fig. 5–35).[22, 23]

12. Aortic Valve Prolapse. Some patients with mitral valve prolapse have associated aortic valve prolapse. Redundant aortic leaf-lets bulge into the left ventricular outflow tract during diastole. Most of these patients have aortic insufficiency.[24]

13. Flail Aortic Leaflets. High-frequency diastolic aortic valve flutter and echoes extending from the aortic valve into the left ventricular outflow tract in diastole are M-mode echocardiographic features useful in identification of flail aortic leaflets.[25]

Severity of Aortic Insufficiency

Echocardiography can provide helpful information regarding the severity of aortic insufficiency. The four most useful parameters are the degree of left ventricular volume overload, the left ventricular end-systolic diameter, the percentage of fractional shortening, and early mitral valve closure.

1. Degree of Left Ventricular Volume Overload. Echocardiography has been particularly useful in the follow-up of patients with chronic aortic insufficiency. The degree of volume overload of the left ventricle correlates with the degree of aortic insufficiency.

2. End-systolic Diameter of the Left Ventricle. A recommendation has been made to consider aortic valve replacement for patients with aortic insufficiency and end-systolic diameters greater than 55 mm.[26, 27] Patients with end-systolic dimensions of 50 to 54 mm should be observed by echocardiography every four or six months. Patients with end-systolic diameters smaller than 50 mm appear to be at lesser risk, and their progress could be safely followed by yearly echocardiograms. However, each patient with severe aortic regurgitation must be assessed individually, since there is no precise formula or measurement on which to base an unequivocal decision for the precise timing of surgery.

Furthermore, another group of investigators[28] has found that a preoperative end-systolic diameter equal to or greater than 55 mm does not preclude successful aortic valve replacement, as judged by long-term survival and symptomatic relief.

3. Percentage of Fractional Shortening. Depressed left ventricular function, as shown by fractional shortening of less than 25 per cent, has been found to be associated with an increased incidence of perioperative morbidity and late postoperative congestive heart failure and death (Figs. 5–36, 5–37).[27]

4. Early Closure of the Mitral Valve. In the presence of acute aortic insufficiency, this is a sign of severe hemodynamic compromise (Figs. 5–33, 5–35). Most patients who have this abnormally require early aortic valve replacement.[20, 21]

Conditions Complicating the Diagnosis

In the absence of aortic insufficiency, diastolic flutter can be seen on or around the mitral valve in these conditions; (1) when there are ruptured chordae tendineae; (2) in normal individuals (Fig. 5–38); (3) in the presence of atrial fibrillation; (4) at the level of the severed chordae tendineae after mitral valve replacement; and (5) when there is left ventricular thrombus (Fig. 5–39).

The characteristic diastolic flutter may not be seen in patients with aortic insufficiency in (1) mitral stenosis, (2) acute aortic insufficiency, or (3) severe aortic insufficiency with short diastole. With poor echocardiographic resolution, the diastolic flutter may be confused with the presence of thickened mitral leaflets.

Rarely, a patient with aortic insufficiency may have systolic anterior motion of the mitral valve (Fig. 5–40) that is similar to that seen in hypertrophic obstructive cardiomyopathy. Because the left ventricular outflow tract is not reduced in size and there is no septal hypertrophy, there is usually no difficulty in excluding a diagnosis of hypertrophic obstructive cardiomyopathy.

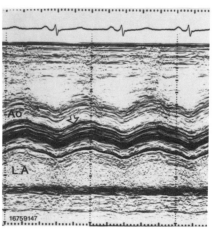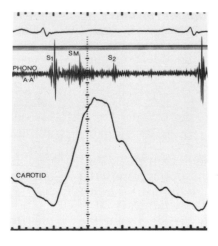

FIGURE 5–1
AORTIC STENOSIS
Marked thickening of the aortic leaflets (arrow) is demonstrated in a patient with severe aortic stenosis. No leaflet separation is evident. A phonocardiogram registers the typical diamond-shaped systolic ejection murmur. The carotid upstroke is delayed, with a U point at 240 msec. Ao = aorta; LA = left atrium.

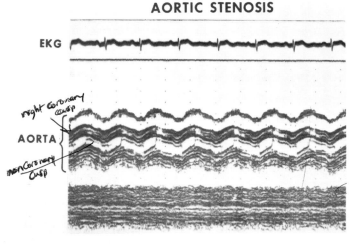

FIGURE 5–2
AORTIC STENOSIS
This echocardiogram demonstrates marked thickening of the right coronary cusp in a patient with aortic stenosis. The noncoronary cusp moves normally. The aortic root and left atrium are normal.

FIGURE 5–3
AORTIC STENOSIS
Long-axis parasternal view in a 92-year-old patient with senile fibro-calcific aortic stenosis. The horizontal arrows point to the thickened right and noncoronary cusps. The left ventricle (LV) is small, and the septum and the posterior wall are thickened. There is dilatation of the left atrium (LA). The small vertical arrows point to fibrotic chordae tendineae, which are a common finding in elderly patients. RV = right ventricle; Ao = aorta; MV = mitral valve.

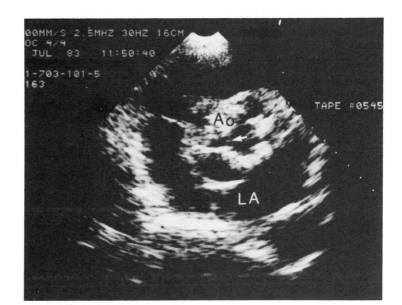

FIGURE 5–4
AORTIC STENOSIS
Left parasternal short-axis view at the level of the aorta in a 68-year-old man with mild aortic stenosis. Note the thickened leaflets and narrow aortic valve origin (arrow). Ao = aorta; LA = left atrium.

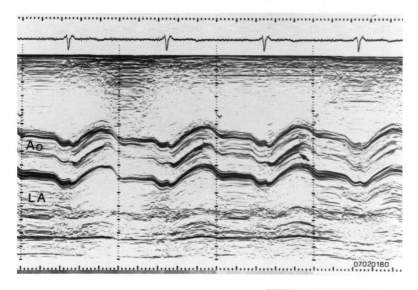

FIGURE 5–5
AORTIC STENOSIS, RESTRICTED LEAFLET MOTION
Echocardiogram at the level of the aorta in a patient with aortic stenosis and insufficiency. There is restricted leaflet motion with a maximal excursion of 1 cm. Ao = aorta; LA = left atrium.

FIGURE 5–6
AORTIC STENOSIS, RESTRICTED LEAFLET MOTION
Long-axis left parasternal view in a 46-year-old patient with severe aortic stenosis. There is mild dilatation of the left ventricle (LV) and left atrium (LA). The aortic leaflets are thickened and have markedly decreased systolic separation. Ao = aorta.

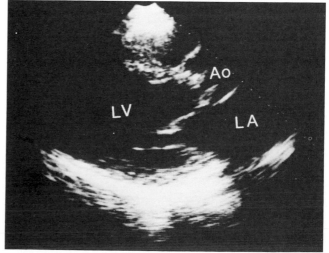

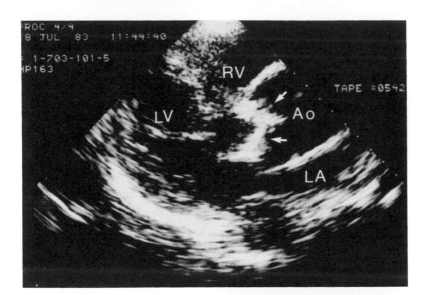

FIGURE 5–7
AORTIC STENOSIS
An echocardiogram from a patient with aortic stenosis demonstrates marked thickening of the aortic leaflets. There is also significant dilatation of the aortic root. RV = right ventricle; LV = left ventricle; Ao = aorta; LA = left atrium.

FIGURE 5–8
AORTIC STENOSIS, MAXIMAL CUSP SEPARATION
This long-axis left parasternal view during systole in the same patient as in Figure 5–7 shows aortic stenosis and restricted leaflet separation (about 8 mm). The aorta (Ao) is dilated. The left atrium (LA) and left ventricle (LV) are normal. RV = right ventricle.

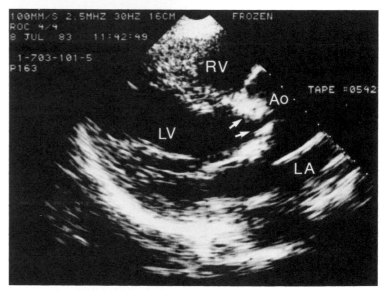

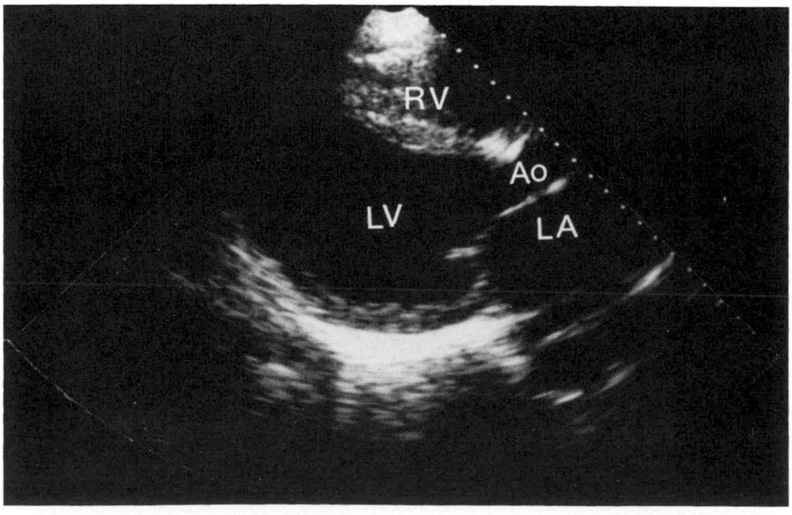

FIGURE 5–9
AORTIC STENOSIS, LEAFLET MOTION
Long-axis parasternal view in a patient with aortic stenosis and insufficiency. A thickened right coronary cusp is shown that during systole opens completely. This finding suggests the presence of only mild to moderate stenosis. In this patient, the aortic valve gradient was 50 mm Hg. RV = right ventricle; LV = left ventricle; Ao = aorta; LA = left atrium.

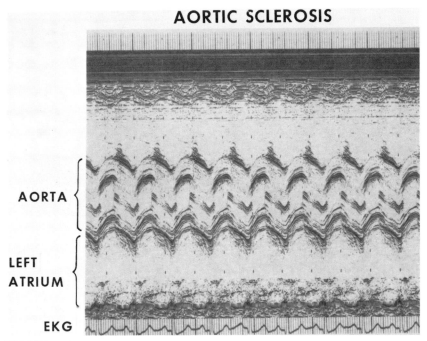

FIGURE 5–10
AORTIC SCLEROSIS
This echocardiogram of a patient with a systolic ejection murmur at the base
demonstrates thickening of the aortic leaflet, but with normal excursion. This
condition is characteristic of aortic sclerosis.

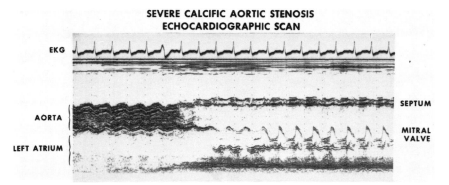

FIGURE 5–11
AORTIC ROOT CALCIFICATION
This M-mode echocardiographic scan from a patient with severe aortic stenosis
shows a densely calcified aortic root, which does not permit visualization of the
leaflets.

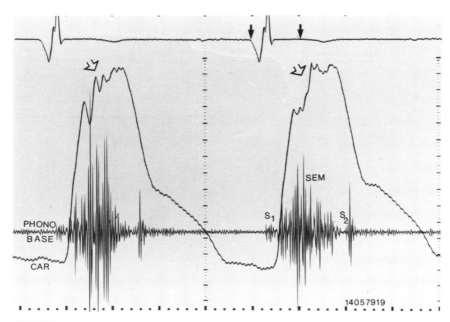

FIGURE 5–12

AORTIC STENOSIS

A phonocardiogram recorded at the left upper sternal border registers a systolic ejection murmur (SEM), which peaks at 200 msec after the Q wave on the electrocardiogram. The carotid pulse (CAR) shows the characteristic delayed upstroke and carotid shudder (*open arrows*). This patient had a bicuspid aortic valve with mild aortic insufficiency and a 50 mm Hg gradient across the aortic valve.

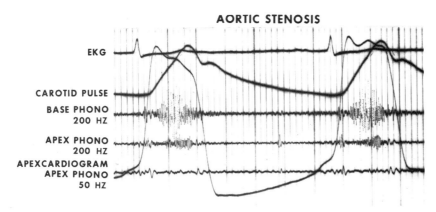

FIGURE 5–13

SEVERE AORTIC STENOSIS

Phonocardiogram and pulse recordings in a patient with severe aortic stenosis with a 100 mm Hg gradient. The U point of the carotid upstroke occurs at 280 msec. The peak of the murmur occurs at 260 msec after the Q wave on the electrocardiogram (EKG).

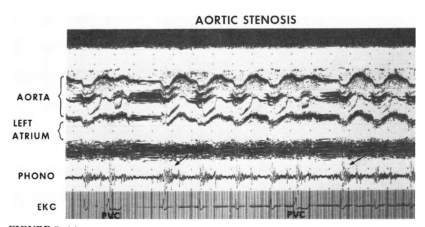

FIGURE 5–14
AORTIC STENOSIS
This echophonocardiogram from a patient with aortic stenosis illustrates how the intensity of the murmur increases after the compensatory pause of a premature ventricular contraction (PVC) *(arrows)*.

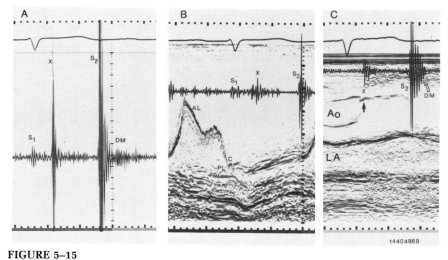

FIGURE 5–15
AORTIC STENOSIS, EJECTION CLICK
A systolic ejection click (X) is registered 120 msec after S_1 (panel A). Panel B shows the anterior (AL) and posterior (PL) mitral leaflets closing simultaneously with the first heart sound (S_1). The click occurs in early systole. Panel C shows the aortic valve opening *(black arrow)* coinciding with the click. A diastolic murmur (DM) follows the second heart sound. This echophonocardiogram was recorded from a 32-year-old man who had a bicuspid aortic valve, mild aortic stenosis, and moderate aortic insufficiency. Ao = aorta; LA = left atrium.

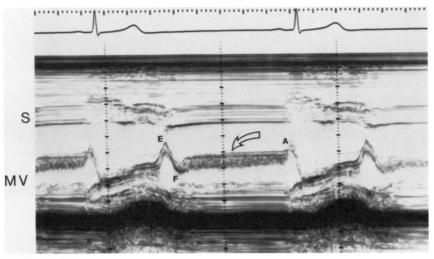

FIGURE 5–16
AORTIC INSUFFICIENCY
This M-mode echocardiogram of a patient with aortic insufficiency demonstrates the characteristic diastolic flutter of the anterior mitral valve (MV) leaflet *(arrow)*. S = septum.

FIGURE 5–17
AORTIC INSUFFICIENCY
Mixture of coarse and fine diastolic vibrations of the anterior mitral valve leaflet (A) in a patient with aortic insufficiency. P = posterior mitral valve leaflet.

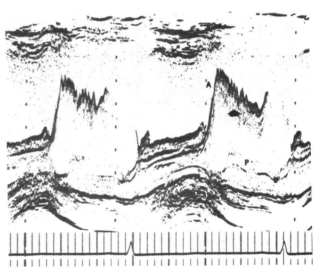

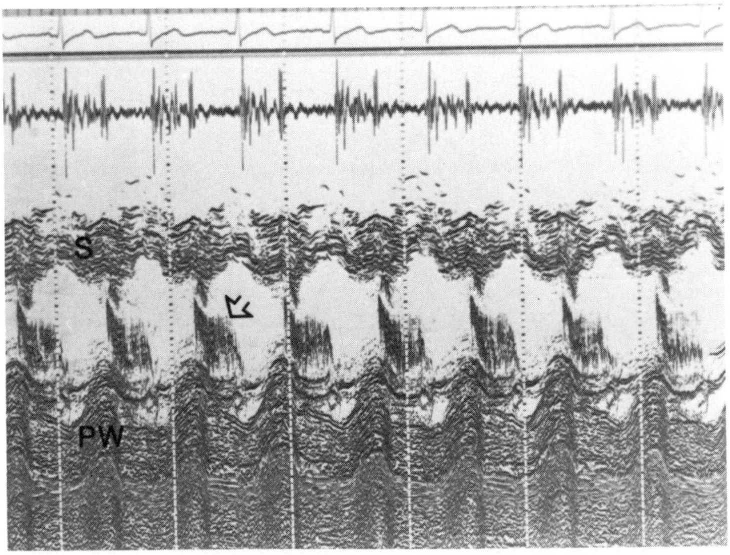

FIGURE 5–18
AORTIC INSUFFICIENCY
High-amplitude and high-frequency vibrations of the anterior mitral valve *(arrow)* were present in this patient with aortic insufficiency. Note the different types of mitral valve vibrations. S = septum; PW = posterior wall.

116

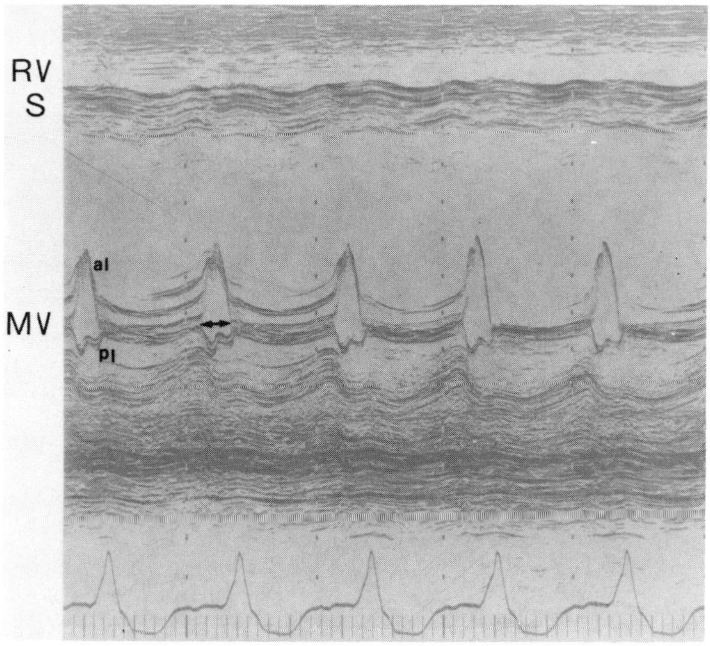

FIGURE 5–19
Aortic Insufficiency, Short Diastole
Echocardiogram at the level of the mitral valve (MV) recorded in a patient with severe aortic insufficiency. Diastole is markedly shortened (arrows), and the characteristic diastolic flutter of the mitral valve is not apparent. RV = right ventricle; S = septum; al = anterior leaflet; pl = posterior leaflet.

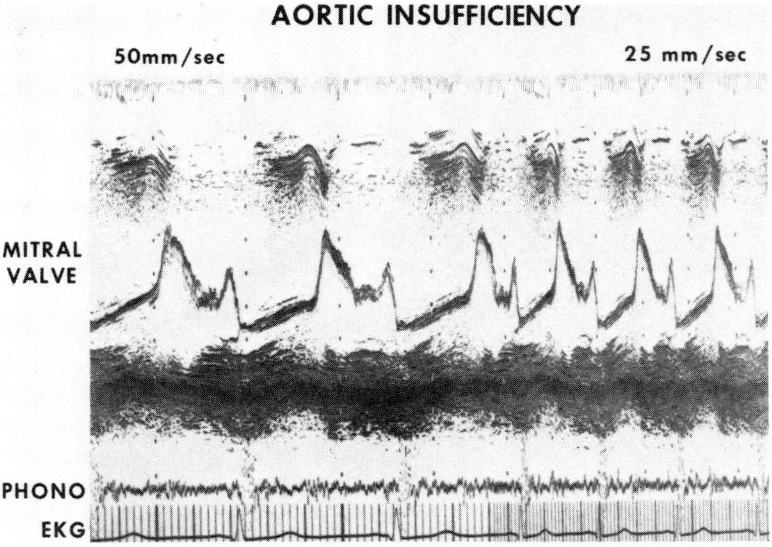

FIGURE 5–20
Aortic Insufficiency
The diastolic vibrations of the mitral valve in a patient with aortic insufficiency are easy to identify at a paper speed of 50 mm per second. At a speed of 25 mm per second the flutter may be confused with mild leaflet thickening.

FIGURE 5–21
Aortic Insufficiency
Echocardiograms from a patient with aortic insufficiency demonstrate increased amplitude of the diastolic flutter coinciding with hand grip and its disappearance after amyl nitrate administration.

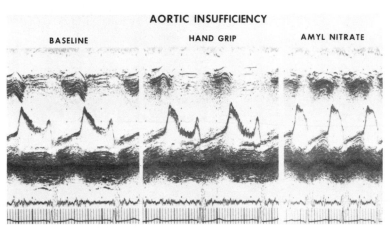

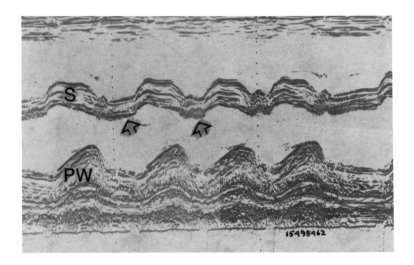

FIGURE 5–22
AORTIC INSUFFICIENCY
The arrrow points to diastolic vibrations in the interventricular septum (S) of a patient with aortic insufficiency. There is also evidence of right ventricular volume overload, as demonstrated by the enlarged right ventricle and paradoxic septal motion. PW = posterior wall.

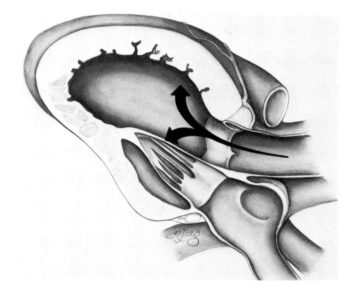

FIGURE 5–23
AORTIC INSUFFICIENCY
This diagram demonstrates the direction of the regurgitant jet that produces the septal and anterior mitral leaflet vibrations in aortic insufficiency.

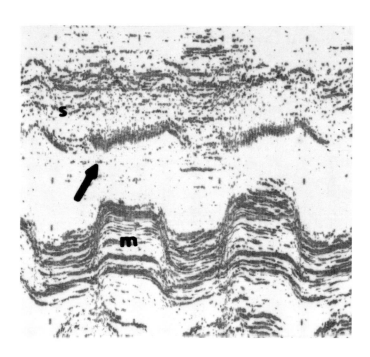

FIGURE 5–24
AORTIC INSUFFICIENCY, MITRAL STENOSIS
Diastolic vibrations of the interventricular septum (S) are evident *(arrows)* in this recording from a patient with mitral stenosis and aortic insufficiency. The thickened mitral leaflets do not show the characteristic diastolic vibrations of aortic insufficiency. M = mitral valve.

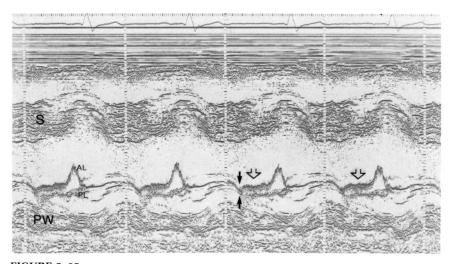

FIGURE 5–25
AORTIC INSUFFICIENCY
An echocardiogram from a 67-year-old man with bicuspid aortic valve and severe (4/4+) aortic insufficiency. The two black arrows point to the beginning of diastole, in which there is very little opening motion of the leaflets. The open arrow points to diastolic vibrations of both anterior (AL) and posterior (PL) leaflets. Maximal leaflet excursion occurs at the time of atrial systole. S = septum; PW = posterior wall.

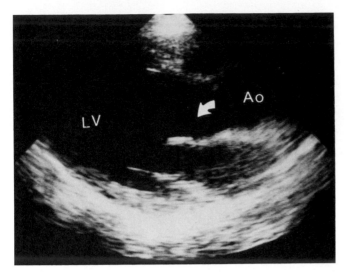

FIGURE 5–26
AORTIC INSUFFICIENCY
Long-axis parasternal view in a 38-year-old patient with severe aortic insufficiency. The left ventricle (LV) is enlarged. The opening of the mitral valve is restricted. The distance from the mitral valve to the septum is increased. The white arrow depicts the possible path of the aortic regurgitant flow as it pushes the mitral valve posteriorly. Ao = aorta.

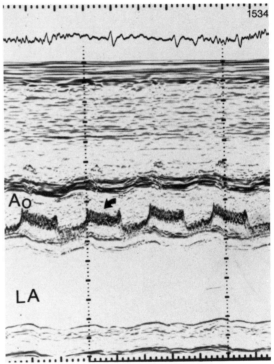

FIGURE 5–27
AORTIC INSUFFICIENCY, DIASTOLIC FLUTTER OF THE AORTIC VALVE
Echocardiogram of the aortic valve in a 50-year-old man with bacterial endocarditis and severe aortic insufficiency. The arrow points to diastolic flutter of the aortic valve, which is a very specific but insensitive finding in aortic insufficiency. Ao = aorta; LA = left atrium.

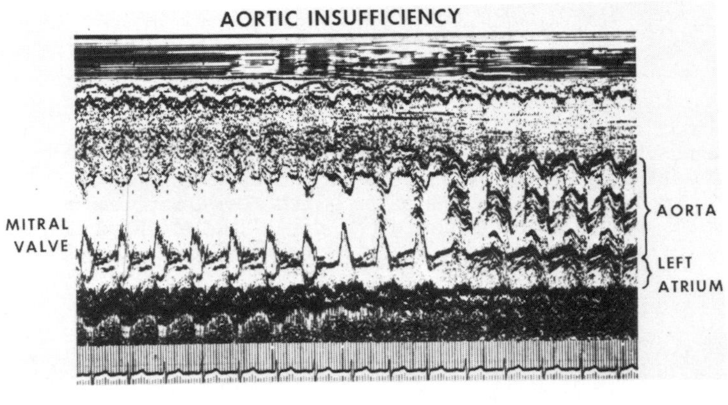

FIGURE 5–28
AORTIC INSUFFICIENCY
Significant aortic leaflet thickening was present in this patient with severe aortic insufficiency. The aortic root is also markedly dilated. There are increased end-systolic and end-diastolic left ventricular diameters and diastolic flutter of the mitral valve.

FIGURE 5–29
AORTIC INSUFFICIENCY, LEFT VENTRICULAR OVERLOAD
The left ventricular (LV) end-diastolic and end-systolic diameters are significantly increased (7 cm and 5 cm, respectively) in this patient with severe aortic insufficiency secondary to bacterial endocarditis. Also note the exaggerated septal excursion, which is a finding characteristic of left ventricular volume overload. RV = right ventricle; S = septum; PW = posterior wall.

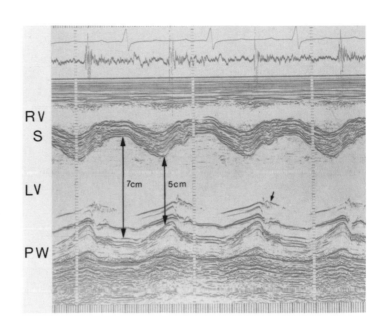

FIGURE 5–30
AORTIC INSUFFICIENCY, ABNORMAL SEPTAL MOTION
The large black arrow points to an exaggerated early diastolic "dip" in the interventricular septum (S) in a patient who had severe aortic insufficiency. LV = ventricle; PW = posterior wall.

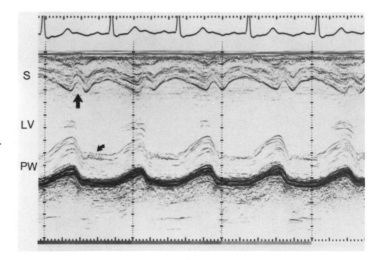

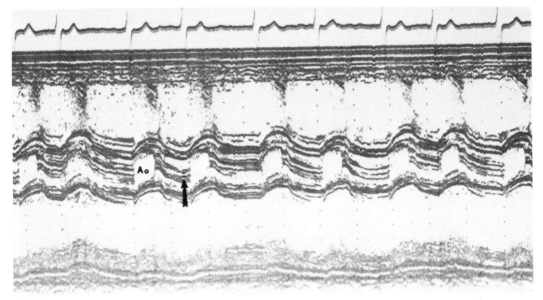

FIGURE 5–31
AORTIC INSUFFICIENCY, LACK OF LEAFLET COAPTATION
A recording from a patient with aortic insufficiency shows lack of aortic leaflet coaptation during diastole (arrow). This is a nonspecific finding. Ao = aorta.

FIGURE 5–32
AORTIC INSUFFICIENCY, MARFAN'S SYNDROME
Short-axis parasternal views during diastole and systole in a patient with Marfan's syndrome. The small arrows point to lack of leaflet coaptation during diastole. Ao = aorta; LA = left atrium.

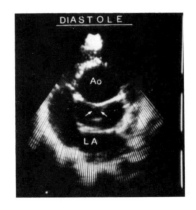
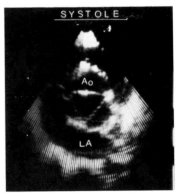

ACUTE AORTIC INSUFFICIENCY

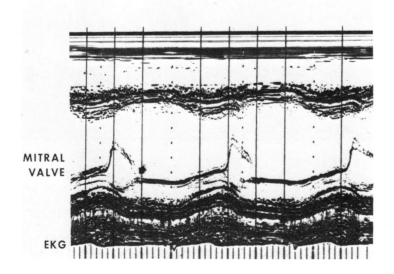

FIGURE 5–33
ACUTE AORTIC INSUFFICIENCY
Premature closure of the mitral valve is shown in a patient with acute aortic insufficiency. The black arrow points to the closure of the mitral valve, which occurs about 160 msec before the ventricular complex (QRS) in the electrocardiogram.

FIGURE 5–34
PREMATURE CLOSURE OF THE MI-
TRAL VALVE, FIRST-DEGREE ATRIO-
VENTRICULAR BLOCK
Premature closure of the mitral
valve is apparent in a patient
with first-degree atrioventricular
block and no aortic insufficiency. The lower arrow points
to the mitral closure, which occurs after the P wave on the
electrocardiogram and much
earlier than the ventricular complex (QRS) *(large arrow)*. S =
septum; AL = anterior leaflet;
PL = posterior leaflet.

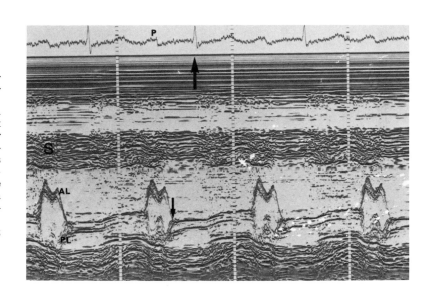

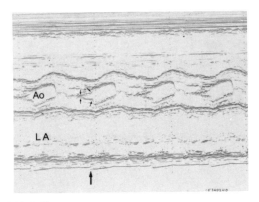
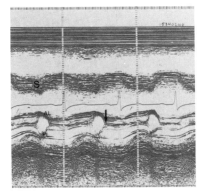

FIGURE 5–35
SEVERE AORTIC INSUFFICIENCY, PREMATURE AORTIC VALVE OPENING
Aortic and mitral valve echocardiograms from a 41-year-old patient with severe aortic
insufficiency secondary to subacute bacterial endocarditis. Left ventricular pressures were
98/50 mm Hg. Note the premature opening of the aortic valve *(small arrows)*, which occurs
before the beginning of the ventricular complex (QRS) *(large arrow)*. The echocardiogram
of the mitral valve shows premature closure of its leaflets. Ao = aorta; LA = left atrium;
S = septum.

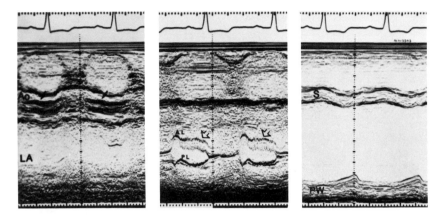

FIGURE 5–36

AORTIC INSUFFICIENCY, IMPAIRED LEFT VENTRICULAR FUNCTION

Echocardiogram from a 27-year-old man with aortic stenosis (50 mm Hg gradient) and moderate aortic insufficiency. The aortic valve is thickened and has decreased excursion. Diastolic flutter of the anterior mitral leaflet (AL) is evident (open arrows). There are increased end-systolic (6 cm) and end-diastolic (7.8 cm) left ventricular dimensions, with 22 per cent fractional shortening. Ao = aorta; LA = left atrium; PL = posterior leaflet; S = septum; PW = posterior wall.

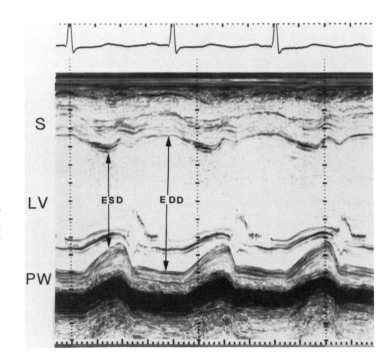

FIGURE 5–37

AORTIC INSUFFICIENCY, NORMAL LEFT VENTRICULAR FUNCTION

Echocardiogram from a patient with severe aortic insufficiency, dilated left ventricular end-diastolic (EDD) (7.6 cm) and end-systolic (ESD) (5 cm) diameters, but preserved left ventricular function with 34 per cent fractional shortening. S = septum; LV = left ventricle; PW = posterior wall.

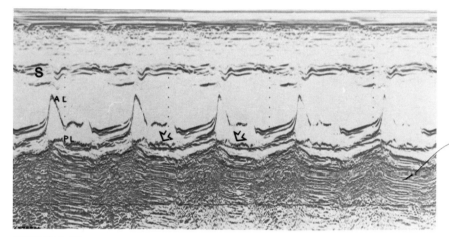

FIGURE 5–38
DIASTOLIC FLUTTER OF MITRAL VALVE WITHOUT AORTIC INSUFFICIENCY
M-mode echocardiogram from a 17-year-old boy with syncopal episodes secondary to hyperventilation. Results of cardiac examination were normal; specifically, there was no aortic insufficiency. The open arrows point to diastolic vibrations of the posterior mitral leaflet (PL). These vibrations occasionally are seen in normal individuals. S = septum; AL = anterior leaflet.

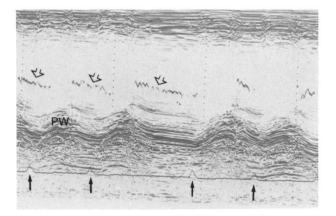

FIGURE 5–39
FLUTTERING OF A LEFT VENTRICULAR THROMBUS
An echocardiogram at the left ventricular level shows a structure with high-amplitude vibrations *(open arrows)* that resemble those seen in the mitral valves of patients with aortic insufficiency. However, closer inspection reveals that there is no relationship between the ventricular (QRS) complex of the electrocardiogram *(black arrows)* and the timing of motion of the vibrating structure. With two-dimensional echocardiography, it was possible to identify this structure as a mural thrombus. The patient did not have aortic insufficiency. PW = posterior wall.

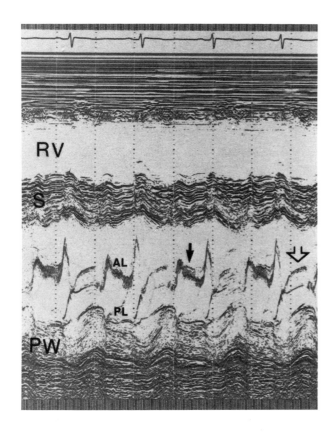

FIGURE 5–40
AORTIC INSUFFICIENCY WITH SYSTOLIC ANTERIOR
MOVEMENT OF THE MITRAL VALVE
This echocardiogram, recorded at the level of the
mitral valve in a patient with aortic insufficiency,
demonstrates mild systolic anterior motion of the
mitral valve *(open arrow)*. The black arrow points
to diastolic flutter of the mitral valve. RV = right
ventricle; S = septum; PW = posterior wall; AL
= anterior leaflet; PL = posterior leaflet.

6 THE AORTA AND DISEASES OF THE AORTA

6.1 ANATOMIC CONSIDERATIONS

The aorta can be divided anatomically into three segments:

1. Ascending Aorta or Aortic Root. The ascending aorta in a normal adult is about 3 cm wide at its origin at the level of the aortic valve and extends 5 to 6 cm superiorly to form the aortic arch. It lies behind the pulmonary trunk and is in front of the left atrium and right main stem bronchus.

2. Aortic Arch. This is a direct continuation of the aortic root without any clear anatomically differentiating landmarks. The aortic arch assumes an almost direct anteroposterior orientation in the superior mediastinum, in which its highest point is roughly 2 to 3 cm below the upper border of the sternum. The arch of the aorta gives rise to the innominate left common carotid and left subclavian arteries.

3. Descending Aorta. The descending aorta is the continuation of the aortic arch. The point at which the descending aorta and aortic arch join is called the *isthmus.* At its origin, the descending aorta lies to the left of the vertebral column. As it descends, it curves toward the right and lies directly in front of the vertebral column. The diaphragm divides the descending aorta into the thoracic and abdominal portions. In the abdomen, the descending aorta is anterior to the vertebral column and to the left of the inferior vena cava.

6.2 ECHOCARDIOGRAPHIC EXAMINATION OF THE AORTA

1. Ascending Aorta. With M-mode echocardiography the aortic walls appear as two strong echo-producing structures that move parallel to each other, anteriorly during systole and posteriorly during diastole.[1] At the base of the aorta, the aortic valve can be seen with its characteristic boxlike appearance (Fig. 6–1). It is at this level that the diameter of the aortic root is measured during diastole. With M-mode echocardiography it is possible to examine only the ascending aorta at the level of the leaflets and only 1 to 2 cm above that plane. M-mode echocardiography can be used to assess accurately the aortic root diameter.[2]

With two-dimensional echocardiography it is possible to examine the ascending aorta in a more complete way. The area of the aortic ring, the sinuses of Valsalva, and the tubular portion of the ascending aorta can be examined in detail in both the long (Fig. 6–2) and the short axes (Fig. 6–3). In diastole, soon after the aortic valve has closed, a slight bulge of the sinuses of Valsalva can be observed.

2. Aortic Arch. Although the aortic arch can be seen with M-mode echocardiography from the suprasternal window, two-dimensional echocardiography allows a much better characterization of this portion of the

127

aorta. With the transducer positioned on the suprasternal area, the sector plane can be aligned to the long axis of the aortic arch so that most of the arch can be visualized. The origins of the innominate, left common carotid, and left subclavian arteries can be seen. The descending part of the arch is more difficult to visualize, and only rarely can the area below the isthmus of the aorta be seen.

It is also possible to align the sector plane so that a short-axis view of the arch can be visualized, in which case the right pulmonary artery is seen in its long diameter.

3. Descending Aorta. With M-mode echocardiography (Fig. 6–4), the descending aorta may be recorded posteriorly to the left atrial or left ventricular walls.[3]

With two-dimensional echocardiography in the long-axis left parasternal view, the descending aorta appears as a circular structure behind the atrioventricular groove (Figs. 6–5, 6–6). By proper scan plane angulation, it may be possible to obtain the long-axis view of the descending aorta, which appears as a tubular structure behind the left ventricle (Fig. 6–7).[4] In the short-axis parasternal view, the descending aorta is seen as a circular structure, with its position shifting from left to right as the scan plane is moved inferiorly (Figs. 6–8 to 6–10). This orientation, described later, can be used to differentiate pleural from pericardial effusion.[5] From the subcostal window, it is possible to image the abdominal aorta, which is situated parallel and medial to the inferior vena cava. The abdominal aorta can be distinguished from the inferior vena cava by the characteristic systolic pulsations of the former. B-mode two-dimensional echocardiography is the preferred method to evaluate the abdominal aorta.[6]

6.3 ANEURYSMS OF THE AORTA

Classification. Aortic aneurysms can be classified according to five categories:
1. Arteriosclerotic
2. Syphilitic
3. Aortic dissection
   a. Type I: ascending aorta, aortic arch, and descending aorta
   b. Type II: ascending aorta
   c. Type III: descending aorta
4. Sinus of Valsalva aneurysm
5. Marfan's syndrome

6.4 ARTERIOSCLEROTIC AORTIC ANEURYSMS

The most common aortic aneurysms are atherosclerotic in origin. They are fusiform—that is, they involve the entire circumference of the aorta.

Echocardiographically, arteriosclerotic aortic aneurysms are seen as dilatations of the aortic root.[7] The left atrium is often compressed, producing a marked difference in the size relation between the aorta and the left atrium (Figs. 6–11, 6–12). The aortic diameter is larger than 4 cm. The aortic valve in its open position is still quite distant from the aortic walls and often has an early notch that is believed to be induced by eddy currents that partially close the valve in early systole. Systolic expansion of the aortic walls may be present. The diagnosis of aortic root dilatation can also be made by using a right parasternal approach.[8]

Aneurysms of the aortic arch and descending aorta are more difficult to define echocardiographically. A modified apical view has been used to visualize descending aortic aneurysms.[9]

6.5 SYPHILITIC AORTIC ANEURYSMS

There are no specific echocardiographic findings associated with the syphilitic aneurysm. Syphilitic aneurysms usually involve the ascending aorta, in which they are indistinguishable from arteriosclerotic aneurysms.

6.6 AORTIC DISSECTION

Aortic dissections are characterized by a tear of the intima and inner media that serves as an entrance point to a false channel that runs parallel to the longitudinal axis of the aorta. An exit or distal tear is present in only about 10 per cent of patients and usually appears in the abdominal aorta. The proximal or entrance tear is in the ascending aorta in approximately 70 per cent of the cases, in the arch in 10 per cent, and in the descending aorta in 20 per cent. A cross section of the aorta at the level of the dissection shows an outer layer composed of the adventitia and the outer media, a false lumen, an inner layer consisting of the inner media and intima, and the true lumen in the center.[10]

Longitudinally the dissection can be limited to the ascending aorta (DeBakey Type I), can extend from the ascending aortic aorta all the way to the abdominal aorta (DeBakey Type II), or can start in the descending aorta (DeBakey Type III). In cross section the dissection usually involves half of the aortic circumference or less. In the DeBakey Type I and II dissections, the portion of the aortic circumference involved is the right lateral wall and the greater curvature.

Despite the many reports of the value of echocardiography in the diagnosis of dissecting aneurysms,[11–16] this technique has not been very useful to the author in the recognition or management of patients with aortic dissection. Many studies have reported false-negative and false-positive results. Theoretically, it should be possible to recognize the intimal flap in any of the three regions of the aorta and hence to make the correct diagnosis and classification.

Echocardiographically, dissecting aneurysms are characterized by:

1. Dilatation of the aorta (greater than 42 mm) (Fig. 6–13).

2. Increased anterior or posterior aortic wall thickness, or both (15 mm or more).

3. The outer wall being thicker than the inner wall (Fig. 6–14).

4. An intimal flap (Figs. 6–15 to 6–19) that is seen as a thin structure medial to the strong echoes of the media and adventitia, which form the outer aortic wall. The aortic leaflets are seen in a position medial to the intima. In the M-mode echocardiogram, this flap occasionally is observed to oscillate throughout the cardiac cycle.[17]

5. Aortic insufficiency is frequently seen in DeBakey Type I or Type II dissection.

6. Mid-systolic closure of the aortic valve (Fig. 6–19).

False-positive findings can be seen if there is sclerosis of the aortic root or even if the echocardiographic beam transects the aorta at an angle.[18, 19] Dilatation of the sinus of Valsalva can also produce M-mode echocardiographic images that resemble those of aortic dissection.

The use of suprasternal echocardiography for the diagnosis of dissection has been described.[20]

6.7 ANEURYSM OF THE SINUS OF VALSALVA

The frequency with which the sinuses of Valsalva are affected by aneurysm varies.[21]

The right coronary sinus is affected in 69 per cent of cases and usually protrudes into the right ventricle or the right atrium. The noncoronary sinus is affected in 26 per cent of cases and usually protrudes into the right atrium. The left coronary sinus is affected in 5 per cent of cases. Associated anomalies include bicuspid aortic valve, ventricular septal defect, and coarctation of the aorta.

The echocardiographic findings depend on which sinus of Valsalva is affected[22, 23] and whether it is intact or has ruptured.[24, 25] Excessive echoes may be found in the vicinity of the right ventricular outflow tract (Fig. 6–20). Evidence of right ventricular or left ventricular volume overload is present when sinuses rupture. Premature opening of the pulmonic valve has been described in association with sinus of Valsalva aneurysm causing rupture into the right atrium.[26] With two-dimensional echocardiography, the walls of the sinus of Valsalva become thin and dilated. This finding is best observed in the short-axis view. In some patients the dilated sinuses may protrude into the right ventricular outflow tract (Figs. 6–21, 6–22), in which they may simulate primary right-sided valvular heart disease.[27] Dissection of the interventricular septum by a congenital sinus of Valsalva aneurysm is a rare lesion that can be diagnosed by echocardiography.[28]

6.8 MARFAN'S SYNDROME

Cardiovascular Abnormalities

The cardiovascular abnormalities seen in patients with Marfan's syndrome include fusiform aneurysm of the ascending aorta, aortic regurgitation, aortic dissection, mitral valve prolapse, and calcification of the mitral annulus.[29, 30]

1. Fusiform Aneurysm of the Ascending Aorta. Marked dilatation of the ascending aorta at the level of the sinus of Valsalva and at the origin of the tubular portion is a common finding in patients with Marfan's syndrome.

2. Aortic Regurgitation. This condition usually is associated with severe dilatation of the aortic root that makes leaflet coaptation inadequate. Myxomatous degeneration of the aortic leaflets is another possible cause of aortic insufficiency.

3. Aortic Dissection. This condition tends to affect an aorta that previously was normal in size.

4. Mitral Valve Prolapse. The great majority of patients with Marfan's syndrome have myxomatous degeneration of the mitral valve with or without mitral insufficiency. A dilated mitral ring is also frequently seen and usually indicates the presence of mitral insufficiency.

5. Calcification of the Mitral Annulus. This development has been reported as a common finding in patients with Marfan's syndrome.

Echocardiographic Findings

In patients with Marfan's syndrome, echocardiography may demonstrate aortic root dilatation, aortic insufficiency, lack of leaflet coaptation, or mitral valve prolapse.

1. Aortic Root Dilatation. Moderate to severe aortic root dilatation is a common finding in patients with Marfan's syndrome.[31-33] This finding can be characterized by both M-mode (Figs. 6–23, 6–24) and two-dimensional echocardiography (Figs. 6–25, 6–26). The latter method permits better evaluation of the degree of involvement of the aorta in its longitudinal axis (Fig. 6–27) and better evaluation of the sinus of Valsalva, which often has aneurysmal dilatation (Fig. 6–28). The aortic walls often appear thin. The aortic leaflets remain far away from the aortic walls during systole.

2. Aortic Insufficiency. In the presence of aortic insufficiency, the usual M-mode echocardiographic findings of diastolic flutter of the mitral valve are seen. There may also be evidence of left ventricular volume overload (Fig. 6–23).

3. Lack of Leaflet Coaptation. Marfan's syndrome is one of the few abnormalities in which the direct echocardiographic diagnosis of aortic insufficiency can be made by observing lack of leaflet coaptation. This condition is demonstrated by two-dimensional echocardiography in the short-axis view at the level of the aortic ring. In diastole the leaflets can be seen to come close together, but because of the markedly dilated aortic ring there is an open space between the leaflets (Fig. 6–28).

4. Mitral Valve Prolapse. Pansystolic prolapse of the mitral valve is a common finding in patients with Marfan's syndrome.[34] The association of severe dilatation of the aortic root with pansystolic mitral valve prolapse is highly suggestive of Marfan's syndrome (Fig. 6–29). With two-dimensional echocardiography the apical four- and five-chamber views permit demonstration of mitral valve prolapse and dilatation of the aortic root (Fig. 6–30).

6.9 ANKYLOSING SPONDYLITIS

Discrete areas of increased bright echo recordings below the left or noncoronary cusps that are suggestive of a subaortic "bump" have been described in patients with ankylosing spondylitis. Aortic root dilatation does not occur without aortic regurgitation.[35]

FIGURE 6–1
ASCENDING AORTA, M-MODE
Echocardiogram of the ascending aorta at the level of the aortic valve. Note the systolic anterior motion of the anterior (A Ao W) and posterior (P Ao W) aortic walls. The aortic valve with its characteristic boxlike appearance is seen within the walls. The left atrium is behind the aorta. RCC – right coronary cusp; NCC – noncoronary cusp.

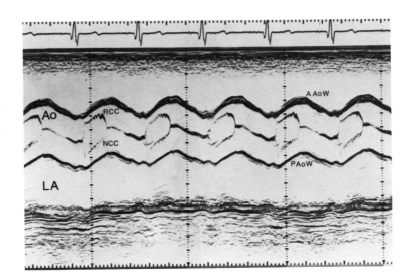

FIGURE 6–2
ASCENDING AORTA, LONG-AXIS PARASTERNAL VIEW
Echocardiogram of the ascending aorta showing (1) the aortic ring, (2) the sinus of Valsalva (right coronary and noncoronary), and (3) the tubular portion. RV = right ventricle; LV = left ventricle; Ao = aorta; LA = left atrium.

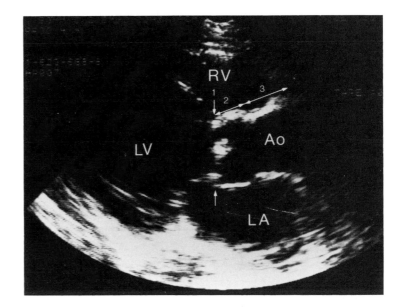

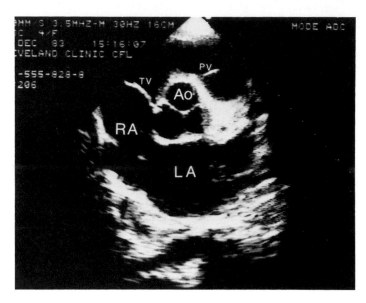

FIGURE 6–3
ASCENDING AORTA, SHORT-AXIS PARASTER-NAL VIEW
This diastolic frame shows the aortic valve in a closed position and a slight bulge of the sinuses of Valsalva. RA = right atrium; Ao = aorta; LA = left atrium; TV = tricuspid valve; PV = pulmonic valve.

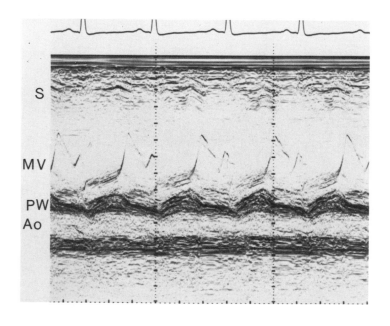

FIGURE 6–4
DESCENDING AORTA
This echocardiogram recorded at the level of the mitral valve (MV) shows an echo-free space behind the posterior wall (PW) of the left ventricle that simulates a pericardial effusion but actually corresponds to the descending aorta (Ao). This situation can be observed better on the two-dimensional echocardiogram, as shown in Figure 6–5.

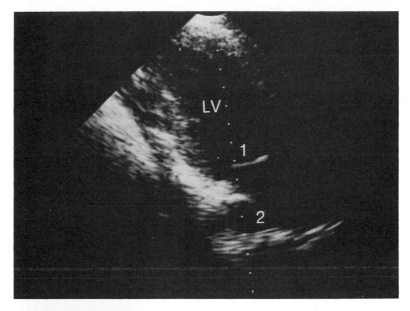

FIGURE 6–5
DESCENDING AORTA
This long-axis left parasternal view shows the descending aorta (2), which appears as a circular echo-free structure behind the atrioventricular groove. The mitral valve (1) is visible within the left ventricular cavity.

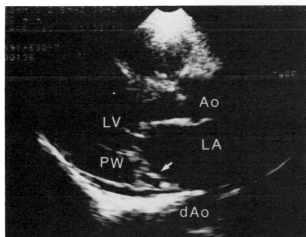

FIGURE 6–6
DESCENDING AORTA
This long-axis left parasternal view demonstrates the descending aorta (dAo) behind the left atrium (LA). The arrow points to the coronary sinus, which can be differentiated from the descending aorta in that it is smaller and moves in concert with the posterior wall (PW) of the left ventricle (LV). Ao = aorta.

FIGURE 6–7
DESCENDING AORTA
This long-axis left parasternal view shows the descending aorta (dAo) in its long-axis behind the left ventricle (LV). Note the tubular shape of the descending aorta at this level. Ao = aorta; LA = left atrium.

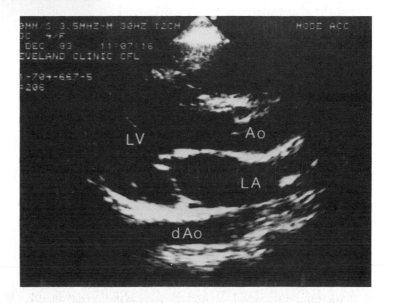

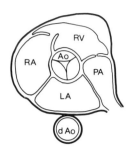

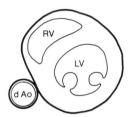

FIGURE 6–8
DESCENDING AORTA
These short-axis views at the levels of the aorta (Ao), mitral valve (MV), and papillary muscle demonstrate the shift to the right of the descending aorta (dAo) as the position of the cross-sectional plane becomes more inferior. RV = right ventricle; RA = right atrium; PA = pulmonary artery; LA = left atrium; LV = left ventricle.

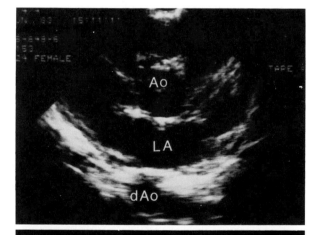

FIGURE 6–9
DESCENDING AORTA
Short-axis left parasternal view at the level of the aorta (Ao). The descending aorta (dAo) is posterior to the left atrium (LA) at about 6 o'clock of the atrial circumference.

FIGURE 6–10
DESCENDING AORTA
Short-axis left parasternal view at the papillary muscle level. The descending aorta (dAo) has shifted to the left, being situated at about 7 o'clock of the ventricular circumference. LV = left ventricle.

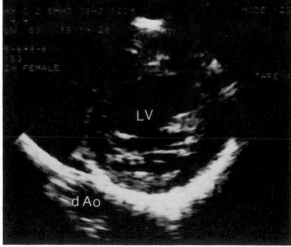

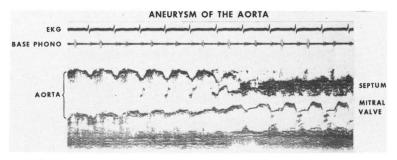

FIGURE 6–11
ARTERIOSCLEROTIC AORTIC ANEURYSM
An echocardiographic scan from the aorta to the mitral valve demonstrates marked dilatation of the aortic root and compression of the left atrium. The aortic valve does not come near to the aortic walls during systole.

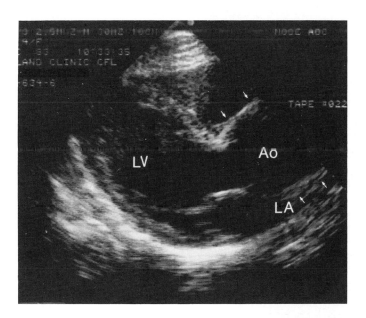

FIGURE 6–12
ARTERIOSCLEROTIC AORTIC ANEURYSM
This long-axis parasternal view demonstrates aneurysmal dilatation of the aorta (Ao) *(arrows)*. The dilatation is more pronounced above the aortic valve in the tubular region of the aorta. LV = left ventricle; LA = left atrium.

FIGURE 6–13
AORTIC DISSECTION
Long-axis left parasternal view in a 55-year-old man with DeBakey Type I aortic dissection and severe aortic insufficiency. There is marked aortic root dilatation (7 cm), as evidenced by the distance from the anterior (a) to the posterior (p) walls of the aorta (Ao). The arrow points to the intimal flap. RV = right ventricle; LV = left ventricle; LA = left atrium.

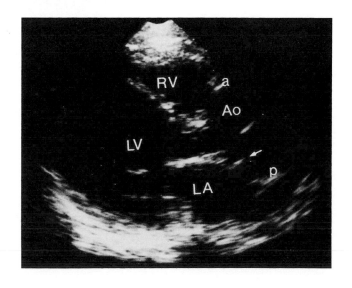

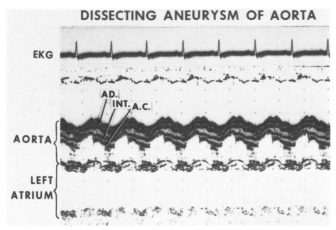

DISSECTING ANEURYSM OF AORTA

FIGURE 6–14
AORTIC DISSECTION
Echocardiogram at the aortic level in a patient with a dissecting aneurysm of the aorta. The outer wall, which corresponds to the adventitia, is much thicker than the intima. AD. = adventia; INT. = intima; A.C. = aortic cusps.

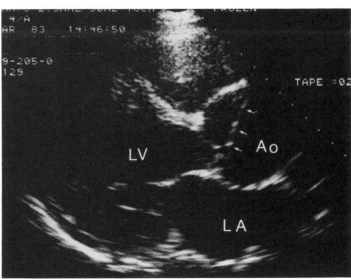

FIGURE 6–15
AORTIC DISSECTION, INTIMAL FLAP
Long-axis left parasternal view in a patient with DeBakey Type II dissecting aneurysm. The intimal flat is indicated by the arrows. The aorta (Ao) is dilated. LV = left ventricle; LA = left atrium.

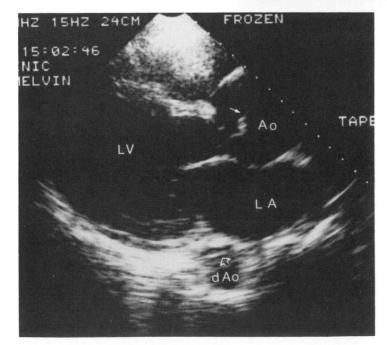

FIGURE 6–16
AORTIC DISSECTION, INTIMAL FLAP
Long-axis left parasternal view in the same patient as in Figure 6–15. The intimal flap can be seen in the ascending aorta (Ao) (*small arrow*), as well as in the descending aorta (dAo) (*open arrow*). There is also significant left ventricular dilatation secondary to severe aortic insufficiency. LV = left ventricle; LA = left atrium.

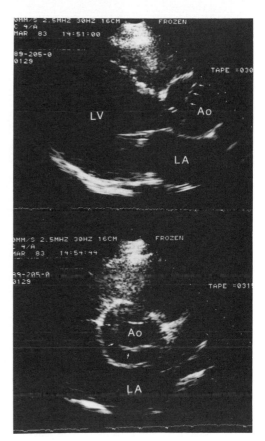

FIGURE 6–17
AORTIC DISSECTION, INTIMAL FLAP
Long- and short-axis left parasternal views in the same patient
as in Figure 6–15. The small arrows point to the intimal flap.
In the short-axis view the intimal flap appears along the right
border of the aortic circumference. LV = left ventricle; Ao =
aorta; LA = left atrium.

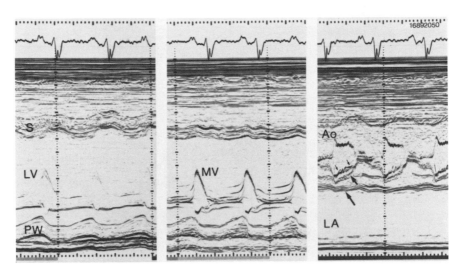

FIGURE 6–18
AORTIC DISSECTION
M-mode echocardiograms recorded from the same patient as in Figure 6–15. Significant
left ventricular dilatation and dysfunction are demonstrated in panel A. Panel B shows
a shortened diastole, as evidenced by the early closure of the mitral valve. Panel C is at
the aortic valve level and shows the intimal flap (medium-sized arrow). S = septum;
LV = left ventricle; PW = posterior wall; MV = mitral valve; Ao = aorta; LA = left
atrium.

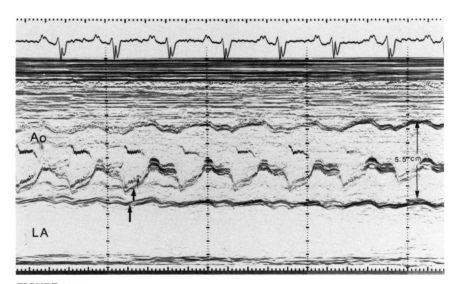

FIGURE 6–19
AORTIC DISSECTION
M-mode echocardiogram of the aorta in the same patient as in Figure 6–15. Note the dilatation of the aortic root. The large arrow points to the posterior aortic wall; the medium-sized arrow points to the intimal flap; and the small arrow points to the noncoronary cusp of the aortic valve. There is early to mid-systolic closure of the aortic valve. Ao = aorta; LA = left atrium.

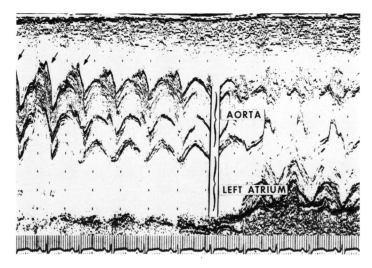

FIGURE 6–20
SINUS OF VALSALVA ANEURYSM
Echocardiographic scan from the aortic root to the left ventricle. A "cloud" of echoes is seen in the anterior wall of the aorta and protrudes into the right ventricular outflow tract (arrows).

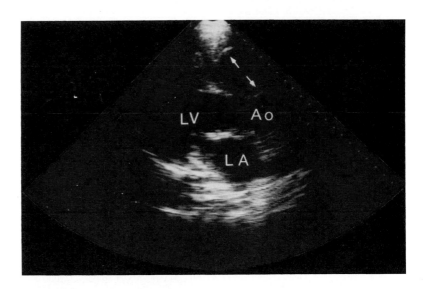

FIGURE 6–21
SINUS OF VALSALVA ANEURYSM
Long-axis left parasternal view in a patient with a large sinus of Valsalva aneurysm originating on the right coronary sinus and protruding into the right ventricular outflow tract. The arrows point to the anterior and posterior borders of the circular aneurysm. LV = left ventricle; Ao = aorta; LA — left atrium.

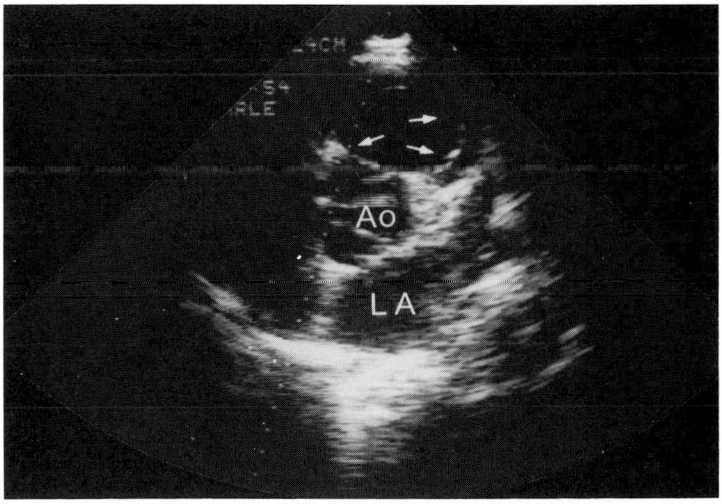

FIGURE 6–22
SINUS OF VALSALVA ANEURYSM
Short-axis left parasternal view in the same patient as in Figure 6–21. The circular shape of the aneurysm (arrows) can be seen anterior to the aorta (Ao) and protruding into the right ventricular outflow tract. LA = left atrium.

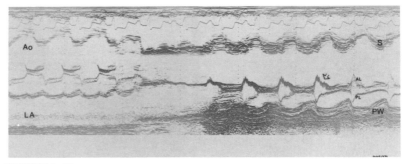

FIGURE 6–23
MARFAN'S SYNDROME
Echocardiographic scan from the aorta to the left ventricle in a 23-year-old man with Marfan's syndrome and severe aortic insufficiency. Marked dilatation of the aortic root is apparent. The open arrow points to diastolic flutter of the mitral valve secondary to aortic insufficiency. The left ventricle is dilated. Ao = aorta; LA = left atrium; S = septum; AL = anterior leaflet; PL = posterior leaflet; PW = posterior wall.

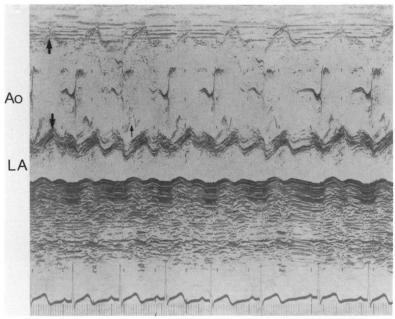

FIGURE 6–24
MARFAN'S SYNDROME
Echocardiogram at the level of the aorta in a 13-year-old boy with Marfan's syndrome. The aorta (Ao) is markedly dilated (*arrows*), and the left atrium (LA) is compressed. There is mid-systolic closure of the aortic valve (*small arrow*), which is a common finding in aneurysmal dilatation of the aorta.

FIGURE 6–25
MARFAN'S SYNDROME
Long-axis parasternal view in a patient with Marfan's syndrome. There is mild aortic root dilatation (5 cm). The noncoronary sinus of the Valsalva is seen to protrude into the left atrium (LA). Ao = aorta; LV = left ventricle.

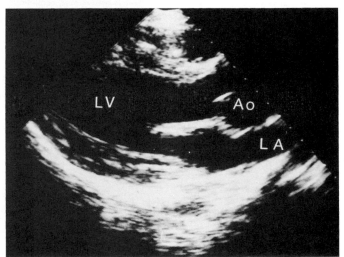

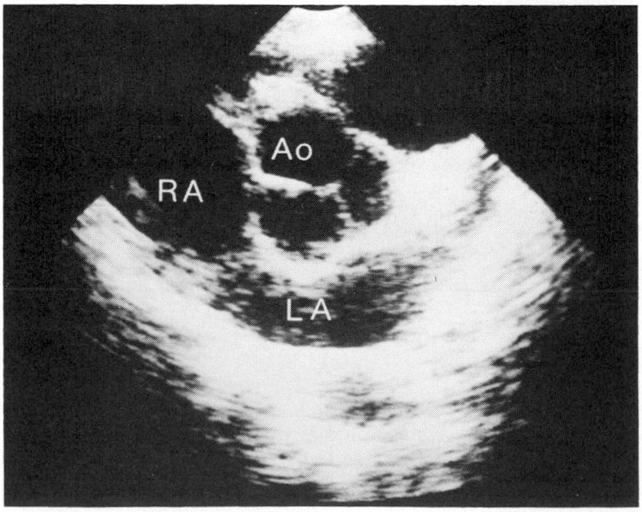

FIGURE 6–26
MARFAN'S SYNDROME
Short-axis parasternal view in the same patient as in Figure 6–25. Dilatation of the aortic root can be observed with prominent right and noncoronary sinuses of Valsalva. RA = right atrium; Ao = aorta; LA = left atrium.

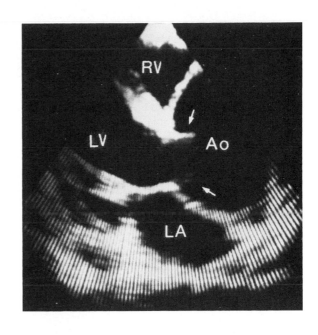

FIGURE 6–27
MARFAN'S SYNDROME
This long-axis left parasternal view shows aneurysmal dilatation of the aortic root. The arrows point to the aortic valve leaflets, which during systole remain at a significant distance from the aortic walls. RV = right ventricle; LV = left ventricle; Ao = aorta; LA = left atrium

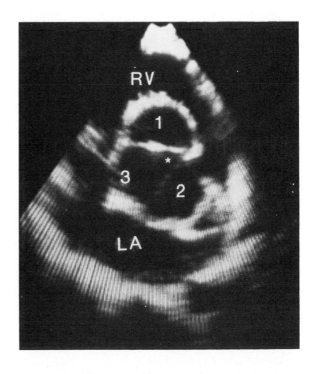

FIGURE 6–28
MARFAN'S SYNDROME
This short-axis parasternal view demonstrates marked dilatation of the right (1), left (2), and noncoronary (3) sinuses of Valsalva. Although this is a diastolic frame, there is lack of leaflet coaptation (*asterisk*). RV = right ventricle; LA = left atrium.

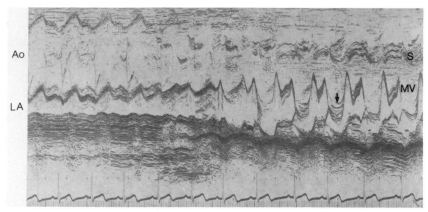

FIGURE 6–29
MARFAN'S SYNDROME
This echocardiographic scan from the aorta to the mitral valve (MV) shows the characteristic findings of Marfan's syndrome: aneurysmal dilatation of the aorta (Ao) and pansystolic prolapse of the mitral valve. LA = left atrium; S = septum.

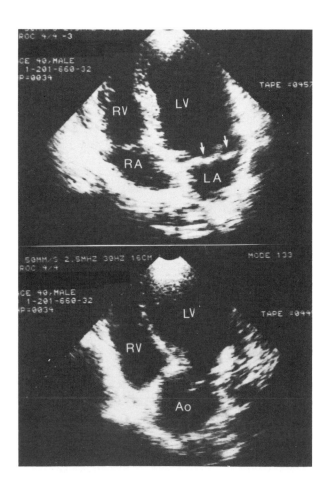

FIGURE 6–30
MARFAN'S SYNDROME
Apical views in a 40-year-old man with Marfan's syndrome demonstrate mitral valve prolapse (arrows) and aneurysmal dilatation of the arota (Ao). RV = right ventricle; LV = left ventricle; RA = right atrium; LA = left atrium.

7 TRICUSPID VALVE DISEASE

7.1 TRICUSPID STENOSIS

Tricuspid stenosis can be caused by (1) rheumatic heart disease, (2) malignant carcinoid, (3) endocardial fibroelastosis,[1] and (4) congenital diseases.

Rheumatic tricuspid stenosis is always associated with mitral stenosis, and often aortic stenosis is present as well. As in all other rheumatic valvular diseases, there is diffuse thickening of the leaflets, with more change in the free edges. Calcium deposits are rare. The normal tricuspid valve area is about 6 to 7 sq cm. Clinically important tricuspid stenosis occurs with a valve area of 1.5 sq cm or less. A stenotic tricuspid valve is nearly always considered incompetent.

Echocardiographically, four abnormalities have been observed in patients with tricuspid stenosis: decreased diastolic slope, thickened leaflets, diastolic doming, and decreased orifice size.[2–4]

1. Decreased Diastolic Slope. This finding is compatible with but not diagnostic of tricuspid stenosis (Figs. 7–1, 7–2). Also, a normal or nearly normal E to F slope does not rule out tricuspid stenosis.

2. Thickened Leaflets. The degree of leaflet thickening in tricuspid stenosis is not as marked as that of mitral stenosis. Dense fibrosis and calcifications are rare.

3. Diastolic Doming. Restricted excursion of the leaflet tips with preserved motion of the body of the leaflets leads to diastolic doming. This condition can be observed with two-dimensional echocardiography from the short-axis parasternal view at the level of the aorta or from the long-axis parasternal view of the inflow tract of the right ventricle.

4. Decreased Orifice Size. It is likely that in a stenotic tricuspid valve the orifice size is small. However, the echocardiographic recording of this abnormality has not yet proved practical.

7.2 TRICUSPID INSUFFICIENCY

Tricuspid insufficiency can be functional or organic. Functional tricuspid insufficiency occurs with pulmonary hypertension and right ventricular dilatation and infarction.

Organic tricuspid insufficiency can be seen in (1) rheumatic heart disease, (2) bacterial endocarditis, (3) carcinoid syndrome, (4) trauma, (5) Ebstein's anomaly, (6) common atrioventricular canal, (7) tricuspid valve prolapse, and (7) ruptured chordae tendineae.

Echocardiography is not a very useful method to directly detect the presence of tricuspid insufficiency. However, it may show the presence of abnormalities that can cause organic tricuspid insufficiency.[5, 6] Also, there are several indirect echocardiographic findings that can be useful in inferring the presence of tricuspid regurgitation. These include right ventricular volume overload, right atrial volume overload, dilated and pulsatile inferior vena cava, regurgitant contrast material, and thickened leaflets.

1. *Right Ventricular Volume Overload.* Tricuspid insufficiency causes dilatation of the right ventricle and paradoxic septal motion (Fig. 7–3).

2. *Right Atrial Volume Overload.* This condition is evident as a dilated right atrium with systolic expansion and bowing of the interatrial septum toward the left atrium.

3. *Dilated and Pulsatile Inferior Vena Cava.* With significant tricuspid insufficiency there is dilatation and systolic expansion of the inferior vena cava and the hepatic veins (Fig. 7–4). This condition can be visualized best with two-dimensional echocardiography from the subcostal window.

4. *Regurgitant Contrast Material.* With contrast echocardiography, after the injection of contrast material into an upper extremity vein, the appearance of regurgitant contrast material in the inferior vena cava and hepatic veins during systole is characteristic of tricuspid regurgitation.[7, 8] Two-dimensional echocardiography permits visualization of the microbubbles with great detail (Figs. 7–5, 7–6), but since the timing of the appearance of the contrast material is crucial, a simultaneously recorded M-mode echocardiogram provides useful information (Fig. 7–7).

Cardiac tamponade and severe right ventricular failure may produce regurgitant contrast material in the inferior vena cava, but this usually occurs during diastole.

5. *Thickened Leaflets.* Patients with rheumatic tricuspid insufficiency may have echocardiograms indistinguishable from those of patients with tricuspid stenosis (Fig. 7–8).

Carcinoid heart disease frequently involves the tricuspid valve, which on two-dimensional echocardiography appears thickened and retracted (Figs. 7–9, 7–10). If there is associated tricuspid insufficiency, this can be demonstrated by contrast echocardiography (Fig. 7–11). Phonocardiography and pulse tracings can be of additional assistance to evaluate tricuspid involvement in carcinoid heart disease (Fig. 7–12).

7.3 TRICUSPID VALVE PROLAPSE

Tricuspid valve prolapse appears to affect primarily the septal and anterior leaflets. It is often associated with mitral valve prolapse (Figs. 7–13 to 7–15)[9, 10] but may occur independently in rare cases.

With M-mode echocardiography,[11] there is late or holosystolic hammocking of the anterior leaflet. As in mitral valve prolapse, the leaflets may appear somewhat redundant. The main problem with the M-mode echocardiographic diagnosis of tricuspid valve prolapse is that to record the tricuspid valve, excessive angulation of the transducer may be necessary, and this in itself may create the echocardiographic appearance of prolapse even in a normal valve.

The association between septal defect and prolapse of the tricuspid valve has been reported.[12]

With two-dimensional echocardiography,[13, 14] it is possible to observe not only the leaflet motion but the plane of the tricuspid valve. Tricuspid valve prolapse is defined as superior bowing of one or two tricuspid leaflets into the right atrium above the tricuspid ring (Fig. 7–16). The best views in which to study this phenomenon are the apical four-chamber and the long-axis parasternal views of the right ventricular inflow tract.

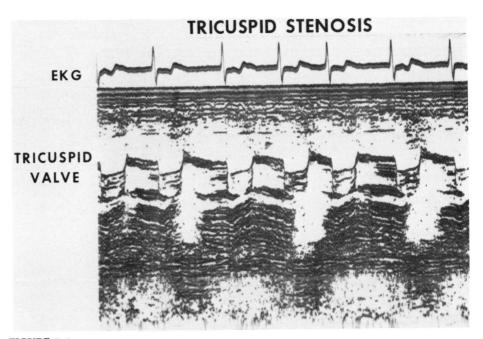

FIGURE 7–1
TRICUSPID STENOSIS
Echocardiogram of the tricuspid valve in a patient with rheumatic heart disease with mitral and tricuspid stenosis. The E to F slope is reduced. The motion of the posterior leaflet is paradoxic, and there is increased leaflet thickness.

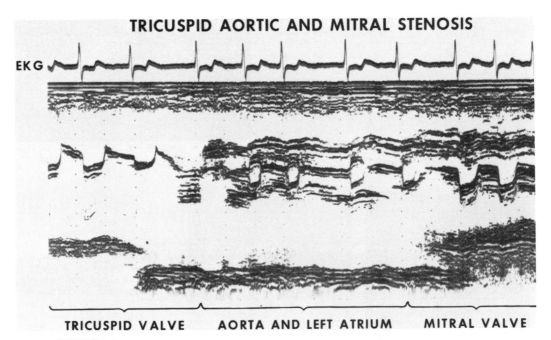

FIGURE 7–2
TRICUSPID STENOSIS
An echocardiographic scan from the same patient as in Figure 7–1 shows tricuspid and mitral stenosis. The leaflet thickening is much more pronounced in the mitral valve.

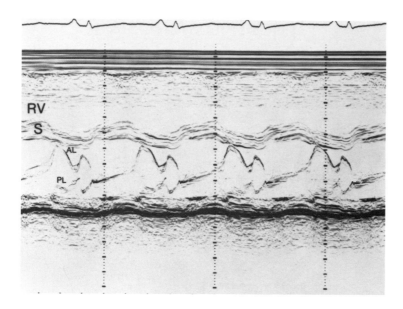

FIGURE 7–3
TRICUSPID INSUFFICIENCY, RIGHT VEN-
TRICULAR VOLUME OVERLOAD
An echocardiogram at the right and
left ventricular levels demonstrates
dilatation of the right ventricle (RV)
and abnormal septal motion in a
patient with tricuspid insufficiency
secondary to carcinoid heart disease. S = septum; AL = anterior
leaflet; PL = posterior leaflet.

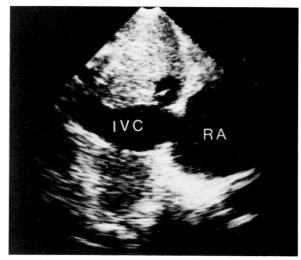

FIGURE 7–4
TRICUSPID INSUFFICIENCY, DILATED INFERIOR VENA CAVA
Subcostal view of the inferior vena cava in a 79-
year-old woman with rheumatic tricuspid insufficiency. The inferior vena cava (IVC) is quite dilated
(2 cm diameter). RA = right atrium.

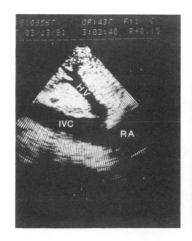
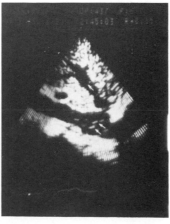

FIGURE 7–5
TRICUSPID INSUFFICIENCY, CONTRAST
STUDY
Subcostal echocardiographic scans of
the long axis of the inferior vena cava
before and after a peripheral injection
of normal saline solution. The small
arrows point to microbubbles filling the
dilated inferior vena cava (IVC) and
hepatic vein (HV). RA = right atrium.

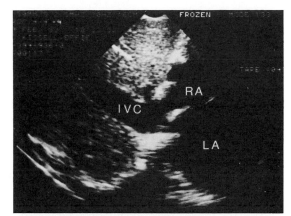

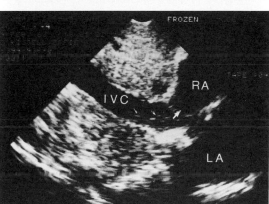

FIGURE 7–6
TRICUSPID INSUFFICIENCY, CONTRAST STUDY
Subcostal echocardiographic scan of the long axis of
the inferior vena cava in a 60-year-old patient with
severe tricuspid insufficiency secondary to rheumatic
heart disease. The arrow points to microbubbles passing from the right atrium (RA) to the inferior vena
cava (IVC). LA = left atrium.

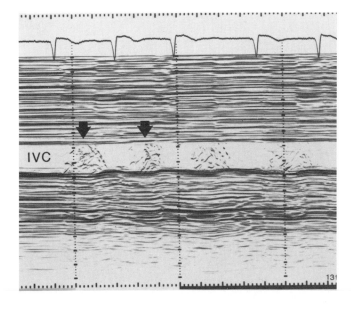

FIGURE 7–7
TRICUSPID INSUFFICIENCY, CONTRAST STUDY
Echocardiogram at the level of the inferior
vena cava (IVC) in a patient with tricuspid
insufficiency after the injection of contrast
material in a peripheral vein. The echocardi-
ogaphic recording of contrast material appears
in the inferior vena cava with each systole
(arrows).

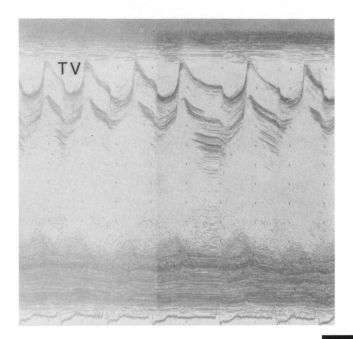

FIGURE 7–8
RHEUMATIC TRICUSPID INSUFFICIENCY
Recording from a 53-year-old woman with tricuspid insufficiency of rheuamtic origin. The tricuspid valve (TV) is very similar to that of patients with tricuspid stenosis.

FIGURE 7–9
CARCINOID HEART DISEASE
Apical four-chamber view in a 52-year-old woman with severe right ventricular failure secondary to carcinoid tricuspid valve disease. At cardiac catheterization there was severe tricuspid valve insufficiency without stenosis and a 10 mm Hg gradient across the pulmonic valve. Note the thickened and somewhat domed tricuspid valve (TV) (arrows). RV = right ventricle; LV = left ventricle; RA = right atrium; LA = left atrium.

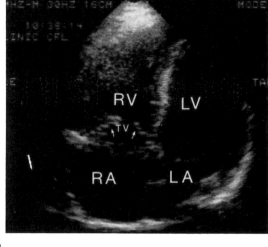

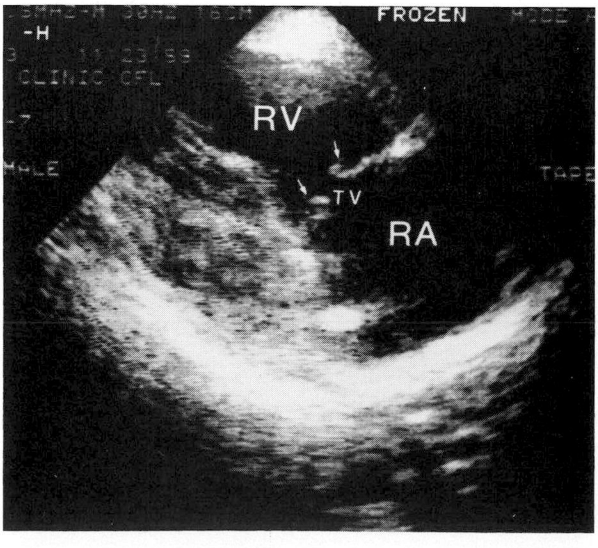

FIGURE 7–10
CARCINOID HEART DISEASE
Left parasternal long-axis view of the right ventricular inflow tract in the same patient as in Figure 7–9. Note the thickened and retracted tricuspid valve (TV) leaflets (arrows).

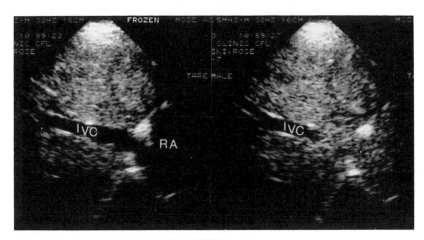

FIGURE 7–11
CARCINOID HEART DISEASE
Subcostal view of the long axis of the inferior vena cava (IVC) before and after injection of contrast material in the same patient as in Figure 7–9. Note how the right atrium (RA) and proximal IVC are filled with microbubbles.

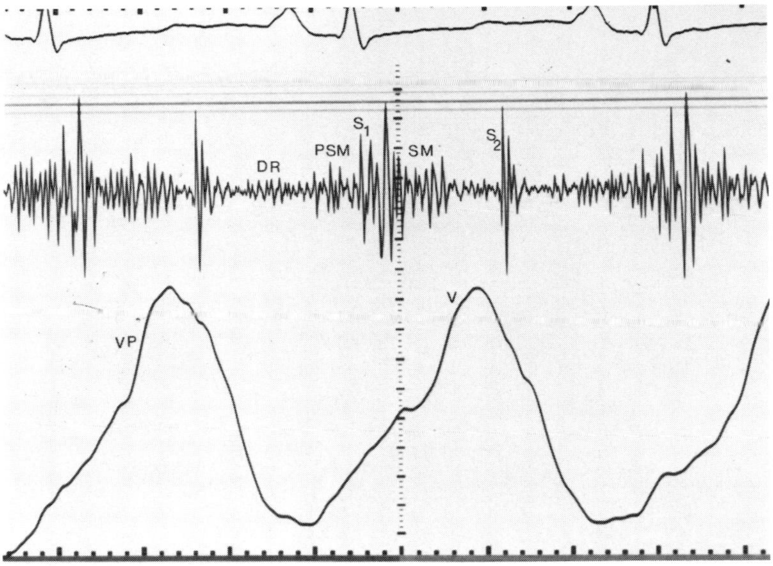

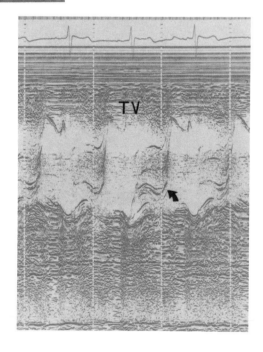

FIGURE 7–12
CARCINOID HEART DISEASE
Phonocardiogram at the left lower sternal border in the same patient as in Figure 7–9. A presystolic murmur (PSM) follows a diastolic rumble (DR). There is also a systolic murmur (SM). The venous pulse (VP) shows large *v* waves. Although the phonocardiogram suggested combined tricuspid stenosis and insufficiency, no gradient across the tricuspid valve was measured at the time of catheterization.

FIGURE 7–13
TRICUSPID AND MITRAL VALVE PROLAPSE
Echocardiogram recorded at the level of the tricuspid valve (TV) in a 78-year-old woman. The arrows point to the late systolic tricuspid prolapse.

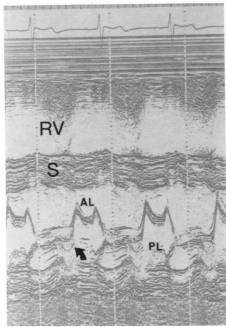

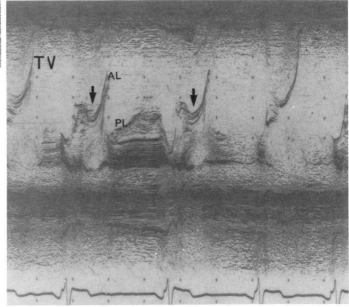

FIGURE 7–14
TRICUSPID AND MITRAL VALVE PROLAPSE
Echocardiogram of the mitral valve in the same patient as in Figure 7–13. The arrow points to mitral valve prolapse. RV = right ventricle; S = septum; AL = anterior leaflet; PL = posterior leaflet.

FIGURE 7–15
TRICUSPID VALVE PROLAPSE
Late systolic hammocking of the tricuspid valve (TV) is shown (arrows) in a patient with dextrocardia and mitral and tricuspid valve prolapse. Al = anterior leaflet; PL = posterior leaflet.

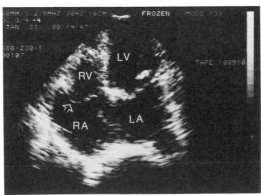

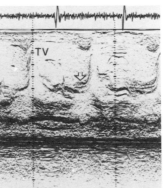

FIGURE 7–16
TRICUSPID PROLAPSE
This apical four-chamber view in a patient with tricuspid prolapse demonstrates superior arcing of the tricuspid valve. The M-mode echocardiogram also shows tricuspid prolapse (open arrow). RV = right ventricle; LV = left ventricle; RA = right atrium; LA = left atrium.

8 PULMONIC VALVE AND PULMONARY ARTERY

8.1 PULMONARY HYPERTENSION

Three types of abnormalities in the M-mode echocardiogram of the pulmonic valve suggest pulmonary hypertension: absent or diminished *a* wave, decreased E to F slope, and mid-systolic closure.[1-5]

1. Absent or Diminished a Wave. The *a* wave of the pulmonic valve is produced by the atrial kick and hence is temporarily related to the P wave on the electrocardiogram (Fig. 8–1). The absence of the *a* wave is a frequent finding in the presence of pulmonary hypertension and presumably is caused by elevated diastolic pulmonary artery pressure (Fig. 8–2). With pulmonary hypertension and severe right ventricular failure, the *a* wave may reappear, but it will be broader and deeper (Fig. 8–3). This change is related to an increased end-diastolic right ventricular pressure, which may equalize the diastolic pulmonary arterial pressure during atrial systole.

Severe pulmonary hypertension with a significant *a* dip on the pulmonic valve echocardiogram has been described.[6]

2. Decreased E to F Slope. This finding often is seen in patients with pulmonary hypertension but is rather nonspecific (Fig. 8–4).

3. Mid-Systolic Closure. This is a valuable sign of pulmonary hypertension. It is often but not necessarily associated with mid-systolic flutter (Figs. 8–2, 8–4).

Mid-systolic notching of the pulmonic valve has also been described in the absence of pulmonary hypertension.[7] Other abnormalities that can be seen with echocardiography in the presence of pulmonary hypertension include increased right ventricular and septal wall thickness. Abnormalities of septal motion are also common. With M-mode echocardiography, the interventricular septum is seen to move paradoxically with a rapid and sharp diastolic posterior motion (Fig. 8–5). With two-dimensional echocardiography, abnormalities of the septal contour are noted. In the short-axis view, the circumference of the left ventricle is distorted by flattening of the interventricular septum (Figs. 8–6, 8–7). There is some correlation between the degree of pulmonary hypertension and the degree of contour deformity. In the long-axis view, the left ventricle appears compressed by the enlarged right ventricle (Figs. 8–8, 8–9).

Abnormalities of the tricuspid valve are frequently seen with pulmonary hypertension. The E to F slope is reduced, and if there is increased right ventricular end-diastolic pressure, there may be a prominent B notch.[8] Right-sided systolic time intervals have been used to estimate right ventricular systolic pressure.[9, 10]

In some patients there is lack of correlation between echocardiographic pulmonic valve morphology and pulmonary arterial pressure.[11]

8.2 PRIMARY PULMONARY HYPERTENSION

The diagnosis of primary pulmonary hypertension is one of exclusion. Echocardiography is an important tool in the diagnosis. The echocardiographic signs of pulmonary hypertension discussed previously are present (Figs. 8–10, 8–11). Other forms of valvular or myocardial disease can be excluded by echocardiography. Contrast echocardiography permits the exclusion of an intracardiac shunt as the cause of pulmonary hypertension (Figs. 8–12, 8–13). A relatively high incidence of echocardiographic mitral valve prolapse has been found in patients with primary pulmonary hypertension (Fig. 8–14).

8.3 PULMONIC STENOSIS

Congenital valvular and infundibular pulmonic stenosis are by far the most common forms of this disorder.[12] These forms are discussed in Chapter 16.

Rheumatic pulmonic stenosis is extremely rare and is always associated with rheumatic mitral valve disease.

Obstruction of the right ventricular outflow tract can also be seen in malignant carcinoid. Rarely, an aneurysm of the sinus of Valsalva produces obstruction in the right ventricular outflow tract.

8.4 PULMONIC INSUFFICIENCY

The most common cause of pulmonic insufficiency is dilatation of the valve ring secondary to pulmonary hypertension or dilatation of the pulmonary artery. Other causes include infective endocarditis, rheumatic involvement, and congenital abnormalities.

Diastolic flutter of the tricuspid valve is the characteristic echocardiographic finding of pulmonic insufficiency (Fig. 8–15). This condition, similar to the flutter seen in the mitral valve in aortic insufficiency, is of high frequency. It is observed best in the anterior leaflet but can be seen in the posterior leaflet as well (Fig. 8–16). The pattern of right ventricular volume overload is usually present (Fig. 8–17).

When pulmonic insufficiency is caused by pulmonary hypertension, the echocardiographic findings of the latter abnormality are also present.

8.5 PULMONARY ARTERY DILATATION

Pulmonary artery dilatation can be seen in (1) pulmonary hypertension, (2) conditions associated with increased pulmonary blood flow, (3) poststenotic dilatation in pulmonic stenosis, and (4) idiopathic conditions.

Echocardiographically, the best projection to demonstrate this abnormality is the left parasternal short-axis view at the level of the great vessels (Figs. 8–18 to 8–20).

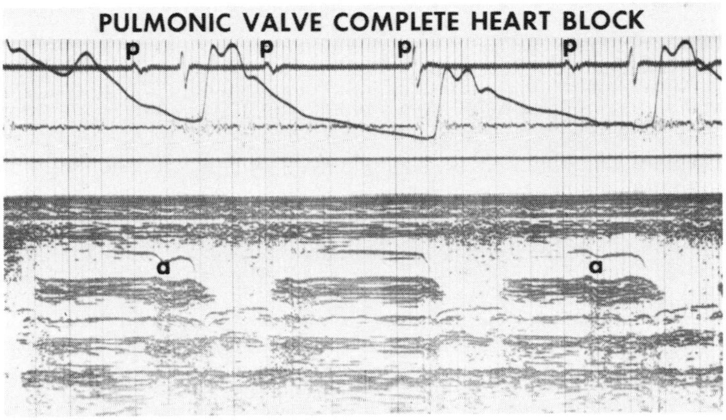

PULMONIC VALVE COMPLETE HEART BLOCK

FIGURE 8–1
PULMONIC VALVE, COMPLETE HEART BLOCK
An echocardiogram of the pulmonic valve in a patient with complete heart block demonstrates the variable position of the *a* wave in the pulmonic valve tracing in relation to the *P* wave of the electrocardiogram.

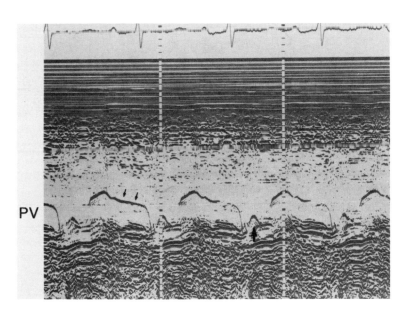

PV

FIGURE 8–2
PULMONARY HYPERTENSION
Pulmonic valve echocardiogram from a 28-year-old woman with primary pulmonary hypertension (pulmonary artery pressure of 95/10 mm Hg). The small arrows point to the area where the *a* wave should have been. As can be seen, the E to F slope does not have the normal indentation produced by the atrial kick. The large black arrow points to mid-systolic closure of the pulmonic valve (PV)—another finding common in pulmonary hypertension.

PULMONARY HYPERTENSION RIGHT VENTRICULAR FAILURE

FIGURE 8–3
PULMONARY HYPERTENSION, RIGHT VENTRICULAR FAILURE
With pulmonary hypertension and right ventricular failure, the *a* wave may reappear, but it is broader and deeper than the normal *a* wave (*arrow*).

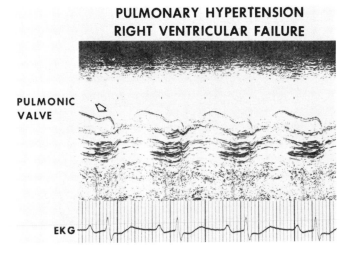

PULMONIC VALVE

EKG

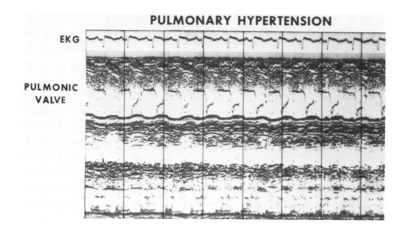

PULMONARY HYPERTENSION

EKG

PULMONIC
VALVE

FIGURE 8–4
PULMONARY HYPERTENSION
An obviously flat E to F slope of the pulmonic valve is apparent in this patient with pulmonary hypertension. The *a* wave is absent, and mid-systolic closure of the pulmonic valve is also present.

FIGURE 8–5
PULMONARY HYPERTENSION, ABNORMAL SEPTAL MOTION
This echocardiogram demonstrates marked dilatation of the right ventricle (RV) and abnormal septal motion. The black arrow points to paradoxic septal motion occurring in early systole. The open arrow points to an abnormal sharp diastolic posterior motion of the septum (S). These abnormalities are characteristic of pressure overload of the right ventricle. LV = left ventricle; PW = posterior wall.

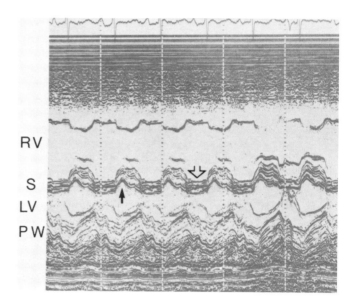

RV

S

LV

PW

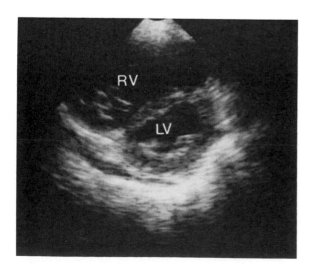

RV

LV

FIGURE 8–6
PULMONARY HYPERTENSION, FLATTENED SEPTUM
Short-axis systolic view at the level of the mitral valve in a 24-year-old patient with pulmonary hypertension (pulmonary artery pressure of 75/36 mm Hg). The circumference of the left ventricle (LV) is distorted by flattening of the interventricular septum. There is also marked dilatation of the right ventricle (RV).

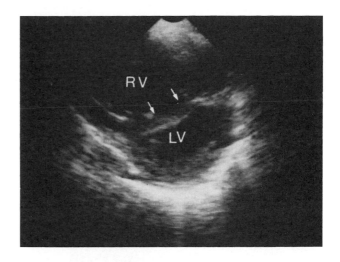

FIGURE 8–7
PULMONARY HYPERTENSION
Diastolic view in the same patient as in Figure 8–6. Note the marked distortion of the left ventricular shape produced by flattening of the interventricular septum *(arrows)*. LV = left ventricle; RV = right ventricle.

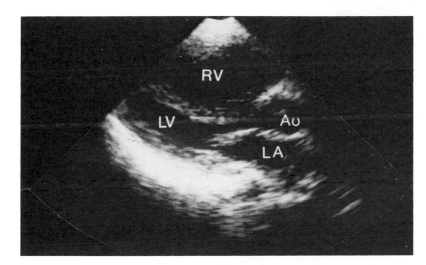

FIGURE 8–8
PULMONARY HYPERTENSION, FLAT-TENED SEPTUM
Long-axis parasternal view of the left ventricle (LV) in the same patient as in Figure 8–6. The left ventricle appears compressed by a large right ventricle (RV) that pushes the interventricular septum posteriorly. Ao = aorta; LA = left atrium.

FIGURE 8–9
PULMONARY HYPERTENSION, COM-PRESSED LEFT VENTRICLE
Long-axis parasternal view in a 27-year-old man with primary pulmonary hypertension (pulmonary artery pressure of 150/80 mm Hg). There is severe dilatation of the right ventricle (RV), which pushes the interventricular septum toward the left ventricular cavity, making this chamber rather small. A pericardial effusion (pe) is seen behind the left ventricle (LV). AO = aorta.

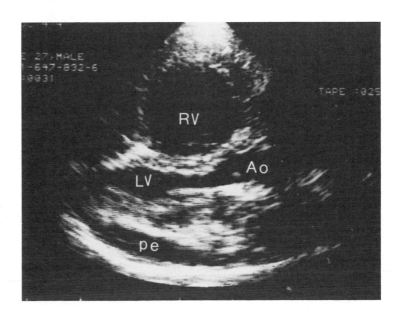

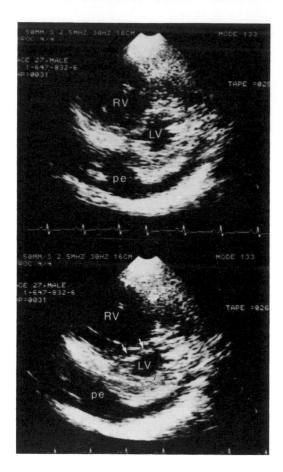

FIGURE 8–10
PRIMARY PULMONARY HYPERTENSION
Short-axis parasternal views at the level of the left ventricle (LV) in the same patient as in Figure 8–9. The abnormal contour of the left ventricle with flattening of the septum during diastole (*arrows*) is apparent. RV = right ventricle; pe = pericardial effusion.

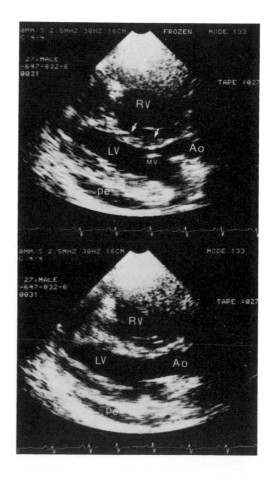

FIGURE 8–11
PRIMARY PULMONARY HYPERTENSION
Long-axis parasternal view at the left ventricular level in the same patient as in Figure 8–9. The encroachment on the left ventricle (LV) by the septum as it is pushed by the right ventricle (RV) is more apparent during diastole (*arrows*). Ao = aorta; MV = mitral valve; pe = pericardial effusion.

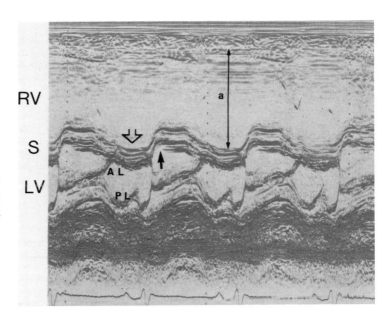

FIGURE 8–12
PRIMARY PULMONARY HYPERTENSION
Echocardiogram at the level of the mitral valve in a 49-year-old man with recurrent pulmonary embolism (pulmonary artery pressure of 95/40 mm Hg). The right ventricle (RV) is markedly dilated (*arrow a = 4.5 cm*). There is abnormal septal motion (*arrows*) and compression of the left ventricle (LV) with decreased mitral valve motion. S = septum; AL = anterior leaflet; PL = posterior leaflet.

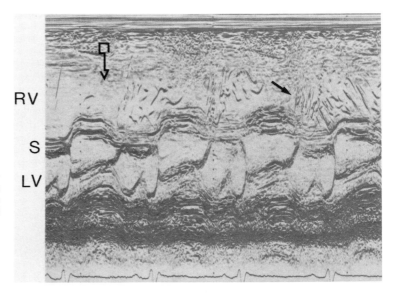

FIGURE 8–13
PRIMARY PULMONARY HYPERTENSION
Echocardiogram recorded in the same patient and at the same level as in Figure 8–12 after injections of normal saline solution into a peripheral vein (*open arrow*). As the bolus arrives in the right ventricle (RV) (*black arrow*), the echocardiographic contrast material can be seen to stay in the right side of the heart—a finding that excludes the presence of a right-to-left shunt. S = septum; LV = left ventricle.

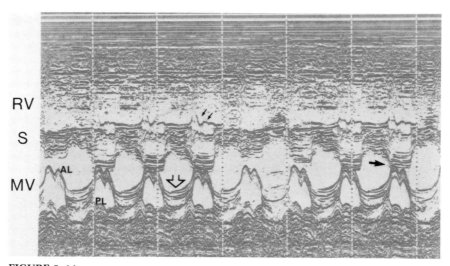

FIGURE 8–14
PRIMARY PULMONARY HYPERTENSION, MITRAL VALVE PROLAPSE
This echocardiogram recorded at the level of the mitral valve (MV) in a patient with primary pulmonary hypertension demonstrates pansystolic prolapse of the mitral valve (open arrow). The small arrows point to the tricuspid valve, and the black horizontal arrow points to mitral septal coaptation, which is a frequent finding of both primary pulmonary hypertension and mitral valve prolapse. RV = right ventricle; S = septum; AL = anterior leaflet; PL = posterior leaflet.

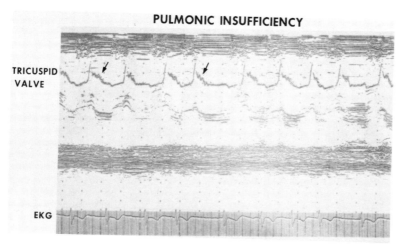

FIGURE 8–15
PULMONIC INSUFFICIENCY
Echocardiogram of the tricuspid valve in a patient with pulmonic insufficiency. Diastolic flutter of the anterior leaflet can be seen (arrows).

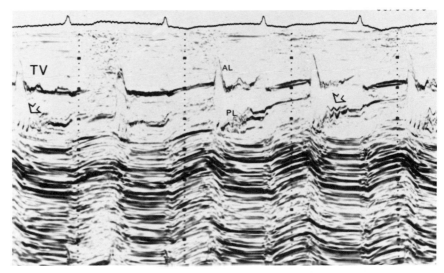

FIGURE 8–16
PULMONIC INSUFFICIENCY
Echocardiogram of the tricuspid valve (TV) in a 62-year-old man with mitral valve disease, pulmonic hypertension, and pulmonic insufficiency. Diastolic flutter of the anterior (AL) and posterior (PL) tricuspid leaflets is apparent. The flutter in the posterior leaflet (open arrows) is coarser and more visible.

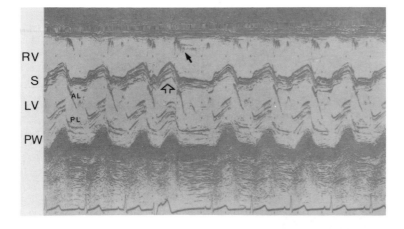

FIGURE 8–17
PULMONIC INSUFFICIENCY
This echocardiogram from a patient with pulmonic insufficiency demonstrates flutter of the tricuspid valve (black arrow) and right ventricular volume overload, as shown by the abnormal septal motion (open arrow) and the enlarged right ventricle (RV). S = septum; LV = left ventricle; PW = posterior wall; AL = anterior mitral leaflet; PL = posterior mitral leaflet.

FIGURE 8–18
PULMONARY ARTERY ANEURYSM
Short-axis parasternal view at the level of the great vessels in a 62-year-old woman with an aneurysm of the pulmonary artery. Pulmonary artery pressure was 55 mm Hg at catheterization. A large echo-free space recorded to the left of the aorta (Ao) corresponds to the aneurysm of the pulmonary artery (PA).

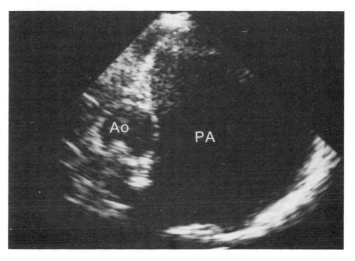

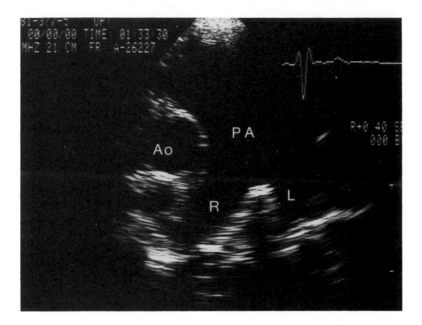

FIGURE 8–19
PULMONARY ARTERY DILATATION
Short-axis left parasternal view at the level of the pulmonary artery (PA) bifurcation in a patient with marked dilatation of the pulmonary artery secondary to pulmonary hypertension. The patient had a ventricular septal defect with pulmonary vascular obstructive disease. Ao = aorta; R = right ventricle; L = left ventricle.

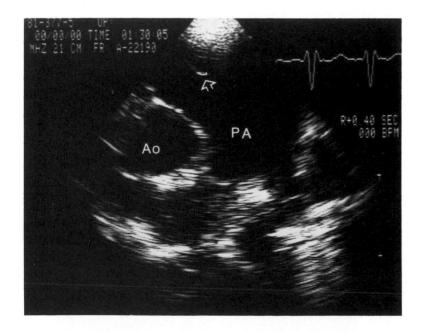

FIGURE 8–20
PULMONARY ARTERY DILATATION
An echocardiogram recorded from the same patient as in Figure 8–19 but at a lower level again demonstrates marked dilatation of the pulmonary artery (PA). The arrow points to the pulmonic valve. Ao = aorta.

9 INFECTIVE ENDOCARDITIS

9.1 GENERAL CONSIDERATIONS

Vegetations are the characteristic lesions in infective endocarditis. They are engrafted most frequently in the aortic and mitral leaflets, less often in the pulmonic and tricuspid valves (especially in drug addicts), and rarely in the endocardium of the ventricles, atria, or great vessels.[1] These vegetations usually are located in valves altered by heart disease, but they also may be found on apparently normal surfaces. The vegetations are usually found on the ventricular surface of the aortic valve in aortic insufficiency, with satellite lesions in the anterior mitral leaflet. They are found on the atrial surface of the mitral leaflets in mitral insufficiency.

Vegetations on the mitral valve may extend to the chordae tendineae and papillary muscles. Ruptured chordae tendineae is a frequent complication of this process.

Progression and extension of the infection may also lead to *ring abscess, mycotic aneurysm, myocardial abscess,* and *fenestration* and *perforation of the leaflets.* Detachment of part of the leaflet from its annulus may occur. Another group of intracardiac complications includes the formation of fistulae and aneurysm of the sinus of Valsalva. Septal defect pericarditis and cardiac tamponade may also occur.

9.2 ECHOCARDIOGRAPHIC FINDINGS

Echocardiography plays an important role not only in the diagnosis and management of patients with infective endocarditis,[2–7] but also in the detection or confirmation of the presence of conditions for which antibiotic prophylaxis for infective endocarditis is reccommended. It can also be of value in the diagnosis of culture-negative endocarditis.[8]

Both M-mode and two-dimensional echocardiography have been useful in the detection of vegetations.[9–13] Vegetations as small as 3 mm in diameter can be recognized by M-mode echocardiography. Echocardiography does not permit the differentiation between active and healed vegetations, but in a given patient with endocarditis the vegetations become smaller and more echodense with the healing process.[14, 15] Organized or calcified vegetations may be easier to detect than fresh ones.

Pre-existing valvular heart disease may obscure the presence of a vegetation, particularly in mitral valve prolapse and rheumatic mitral valve disease. Furthermore, endocarditis may destroy the valve before a distinct vegetation is formed. The sensitivity of M-mode echocardiography to detect vegetations has been found to be between 40 and 50 per cent. Thus, the failure to dem-

161

onstrate vegetations by M-mode echocardiography cannot be used to rule out a diagnosis of infective endocarditis. The specificity of M-mode echocardiography for the diagnosis of infective endocarditis is very good except in the presence of myxomatous valvular degeneration.

Mitral Valve Vegetations

Mitral valve vegetations have one or more of five echocardiographic characteristics:

1. "Shaggy" Echoes Attached to the Mitral Valve. Mitral valve vegetations appear as "shaggy" echoes attached to, but not restricting the motion of, the anterior or posterior leaflets, or both (Figs. 9–1, 9–2). These abnormal echoes are observed more clearly during diastole but can also be seen during systole. Since most of the vegetations are attached to the atrial surfaces of the leaflets, the vegetations are seen best in the inflow tract of the left ventricle. With two-dimensional echocardiography, the vegetations are seen as a mass of echoes attached to the atrial surface of the valve (Fig. 9–3). With the short-axis view, it is possible to further define the position of the vegetation in the valve (Fig. 9–4).

2. Vegetations Prolapsing into the Left Atrium. Large vegetations may be seen to prolapse into the left atrium during systole and into the left ventricle during diastole. This type of vegetation may be difficult to differentiate from a left atrial mass (Figs. 9–5, 9–6).[16]

3. Vegetations Extending from the Aortic Valve. Vegetations that are seeded in the mitral valve from aortic valve endocarditis are present in the base of the anterior leaflet's ventricular surface (Figs. 9–7, 9–8). These vegetations are visible in the left ventricular outflow tract during systole.

4. Ruptured Chordae Tendineae. Ruptured chordae are a frequent complication of mitral valve endocarditis (Figs. 9–9 to 9–11). When this condition is present, "shaggy" echoes with fine flutter are seen during systole, and often the vegetation or part of the leaflet is observable in the left atrium. Fine flutter may also be seen at this time. In some patients, these abnormalities are clear enough to make a definite diagnosis of endocarditis. This is particularly true if both the "shaggy" echoes recorded by M-mode echocardiography and the diastolic masses attached to the leaflets are seen on two-dimensional echocardiography. In some cases only a probable or possible diagnosis should be made if the abnormalities are not distinct.

5. Natural History of Vegetations. Serial echocardiographic studies of a patient with mitral valve vegetations may demonstrate complete or partial disappearance of the abnormal echoes—as in embolic dislodgment of vegetation. Serial echocardiograms can also show progressive fibrosis and diminution in size occurring with healing of a vegetation (Figs. 9–12, 9–13).

Aortic Valve Vegetations

Aortic valve vegetations have a number of characteristics:

1. Irregular or "Shaggy" Thickening of the Aortic Leaflets. Without systolic restriction of valve motion, this finding is highly suggestive of infective endocarditis.[17–22] During diastole multiple linear or coalescent echoes are seen (Fig. 9–14). In some patients an irregular mass of echoes fills most of the aortic root during diastole. This condition is usual in the presence of large vegetations.

2. Diastolic Flutter of the Aortic Valve. Partial destruction of one or more cusps is a complication of infective endocarditis (Fig. 9–15). This condition is seen with M-mode echocardiography as coarse or fine diastolic vibrations. The leaflet is usually eccentric, often toward the posterior aortic wall.

3. A Mass of Echoes in the Left Ventricular Outflow Tract. With a large vegetation that prolapses into the left ventricular outflow tract, a mass of echoes is seen during diastole (Fig. 9–16). The mass appears behind the interventricular septum and in front of the anterior mitral valve, which has the characteristic diastolic flutter. In the presence of severe and acute aortic insufficiency, the mitral valve is observed to close prematurely.

4. Direct Visualization of Vegetation. With two-dimensional echocardiography, the vegetations appear as distinct masses or clumps of echoes attached to the aortic leaflets on their ventricular surfaces (Figs. 9–17, 9–18). In cross section it is possible to determine which and how many of the leaflets are affected by the endocarditis.

5. Flail Aortic Leaflets. Valvular necrosis is common in endocarditis of the aortic valve. This condition may produce leaflet perforation, fenestration, and a completely torn flail leaflet. With a fenestrated valve or a flail leaflet, the valves—or part of them—are seen to swing freely into the left ventricular outflow tract during diastole (Fig. 9–19).[23, 24] It may be possible to observe the vegetations attached to the leaflets.

6. Secondary Effects of Aortic Insufficiency. These secondary effects include (a) diastolic flutter of the mitral valve, (b) left ventricular volume overload, and (c) premature closure of the mitral valve (acute aortic insufficiency).

Tricuspid Valve Vegetations

The tricuspid valve, usually an uncommon site of infection, is the most frequently involved valve in intravenous drug users. *Staphylococcus aureus* is the predominant infecting organism. Two-dimensional echocardiography is superior to M-mode echocardiography in detecting tricuspid vegetation,[25–27] in part because of the relative difficulty of recording the tricuspid valve by M-mode echocardiography. Tricuspid vegetations are usually larger than left-sided vegetations. The tricuspid vegetations appear as a diffuse mass of echoes that is attached to one of the leaflets on either the atrial or the ventricular surface. Characteristically these vegetations are extremely mobile (Fig. 9–20).

With M-mode echocardiography[28, 29] the tricuspid leaflets are thickened and have the characteristic mass of "shaggy" echoes attached (Fig. 9–21). A large vegetation can be difficult to differentiate from a right atrial tumor. As the infective process progresses, rupture of chordae may occur, with portions of the leaflets becoming flail and prolapsing into the right atrium. Tricuspid insufficiency with the pattern of right ventricular volume overload is almost always present.

Pulmonic Valve Vegetations

The pulmonic valve is the least frequently infected valve in endocarditis. Pulmonic valve vegetations appear as "shaggy" mobile masses[30–34] attached to one of the pulmonic leaflets (Figs. 9–22, 9–23). Rapid vibrations of the leaflets can produce a fuzzy appearance.

Two-dimensional echocardiography pro-vides better visualization of the pulmonic valve and yields more positive study results than M-mode echocardiography (Fig. 9–24).

Occasionally, the atriopulmonary sulcus is hyperactive and may give the false impression of a mass behind the posterior pulmonary leaflet.

9.3 NONVALVULAR ENDOCARDITIS

Forms of endocarditis involving other sites include (1) pacemaker endocarditis (in the atrium and ventricle) (Fig. 9–25),[35] (2) atrial endocarditis (Fig. 9–26), (3) coarctation of the aorta, and (4) patent ductus arteriosus.

Prosthetic valve endocarditis is discussed in Chapter 10.

9.4 VALVE RING ABSCESS

Valve ring abscess is an uncommon but serious complication of endocarditis. Abscesses may be present in as many as one third of patients who die from endocarditis and are usually in the aortic ring area. Necropsies of 74 patients with endocarditis studied by Arnett and Roberts revealed that 22 had aortic ring abscess and only 2 had mitral ring abscess. Of 22 patients with prosthetic valve endocarditis, 15 had aortic and 7 had mitral ring abscess.[36, 37]

Ring abscess of the aortic valve appears in M-mode echocardiography as double echoes in the aortic wall. However, these findings are nonspecific and can be seen in aortic dissection and atherosclerotic aortas.

With two-dimensional echocardiography,[38–40] the diagnosis of valve ring myocardial abscess is made by identifying an abnormal echolucent cavity in the perivalvular tissue in several tomographic sections. This technique also allows for the determination of the actual distribution and extension of the abscess cavity. When the abscess extends into the interventricular septum, thickening in this area is evident. The area of the abscess is highly reflective and may appear speckled internally.

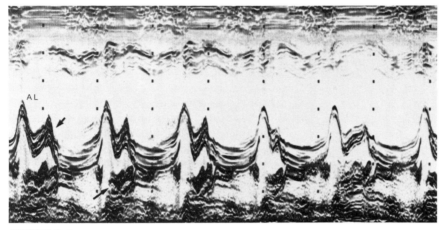

FIGURE 9–1
MITRAL VALVE VEGETATIONS
This echocardiogram of the mitral valve shows "shaggy" echoes attached to the posterior mitral leaflet (long arrow). These echoes are characteristic of vegetations in patients with infective endocarditis. The anterior leaflet is also thickened (small arrow), and there is pansystolic prolapse of the mitral valve.

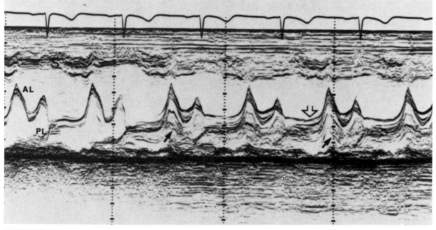

FIGURE 9–2
MITRAL VALVE VEGETATIONS
Variable leaflet thickness is shown in this echocardiogram of the mitral valve in a patient with infective endocarditis. Only the areas affected by the vegetation (black arrows) appear thickened in echocardiographic recordings. The open arrow points to coexisting mitral valve prolapse.

FIGURE 9–3
MITRAL VALVE VEGETATIONS
Long-axis parasternal view in a patient with infective endocarditis. A mass of echoes *(large arrow)* is visible in the inflow tract of the left ventricle (LV) attached to the mitral valve. The small arrow points to a thickened anterior leaflet. Ao = aorta; LA = left atrium.

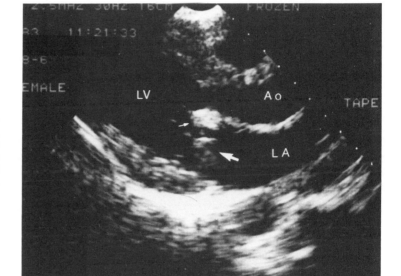
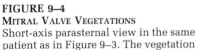

FIGURE 9–4
MITRAL VALVE VEGETATIONS
Short-axis parasternal view in the same patient as in Figure 9–3. The vegetation is attached to the mitral valve, close to the medial commissure *(arrow)*. S = septum; AL = anterior leaflet.

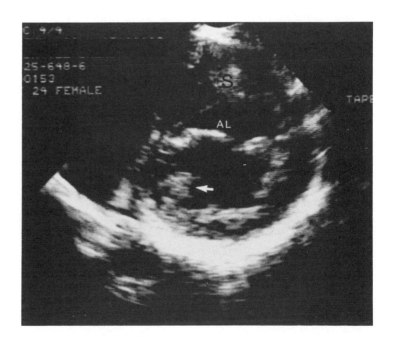

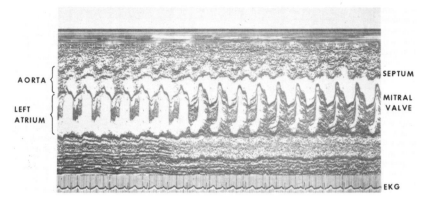

FIGURE 9–5
LARGE MITRAL VEGETATION PROLAPSING IN THE LEFT ATRIUM
Echocardiographic scan from the aorta to the left ventricle in a patient with a large mitral valve vegetation. A mass of echoes is seen in the left atrium during systole and attached to the mitral valve during diastole. This mass may be confused with a left atrial myxoma.

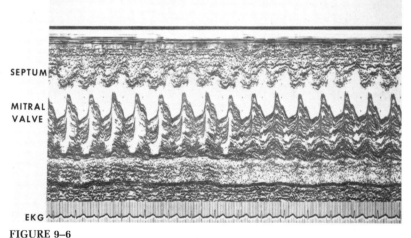

FIGURE 9–6
LARGE MITRAL VALVE VEGETATION
Echocardiographic scan from the base to the tip of the mitral valve in the same patient as in Figure 9–5. A mass of "shaggy" echoes attached to the anterior leaflet of the mitral valve is seen filling the mitral valve orifice close to its tip.

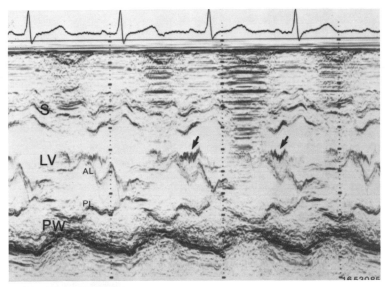

FIGURE 9–7
MITRAL VALVE VEGETATION EXTEND-
ING FROM THE AORTIC VALVE
M-mode echocardiogram of the mitral valve in a 19-year-old woman
with aortic insufficiency secondary
to bacterial endocarditis and a vegetation seeded in the anterior leaflet
(AL) of the mitral valve (arrows). S
= septum; LV = left ventricle; PW
= posterior wall; PL = posterior
leaflet.

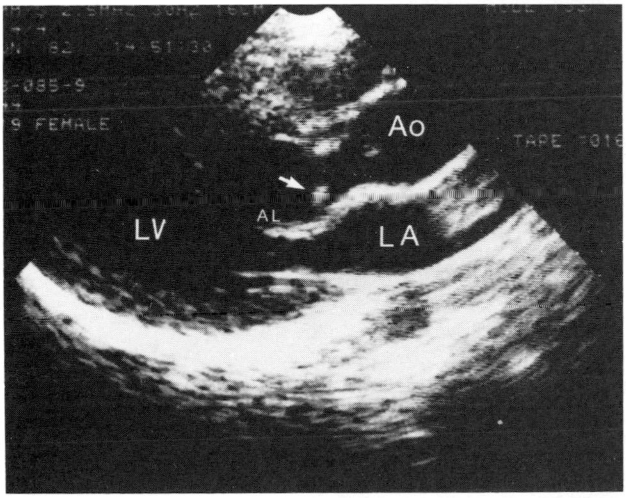

FIGURE 9–8
MITRAL VALVE VEGETATION EXTENDING FROM
THE AORTIC VALVE
Long-axis left parasternal view in the same
patient as in Figure 9–7. The arrow points to
the vegetation attached to the anterior mitral
valve in the outflow tract of the left ventricle
(LV). Ao = aorta; AL = anterior leaflet; LA
= left atrium.

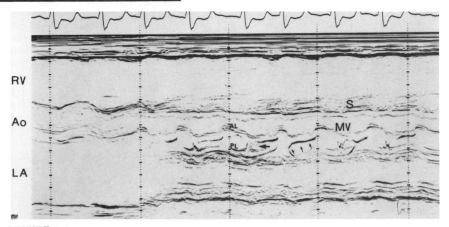

FIGURE 9–9
RUPTURED CHORDAE TENDINEAE
Echocardiographic scan from a 62-year-old man with infective endocarditis, severe
mitral regurgitation, and ruptured chordae tendineae. The arrows point to the "shaggy"
echoes with systolic vibrations produced by the vegetation in the ruptured chordae. RV
— right ventricle; Ao = aorta; LA = left atrium; AL = anterior leaflet; PL = posterior
leaflet; S = septum; MV = mitral valve.

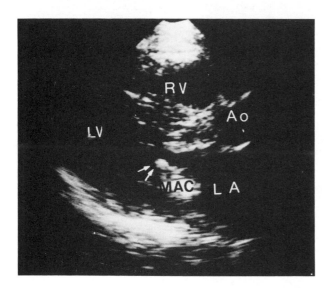

FIGURE 9–10
RUPTURED CHORDAE TENDINEAE
Long-axis left parasternal view in the same
patient as in Figure 9–9. This diastolic frame
shows a thickened posterior leaflet of the
mitral valve *(arrows)*. The patient also has
calcification of the mitral annulus (MAC). LV
= left ventricle; RV = right ventricle; Ao =
aorta; LA = left atrium.

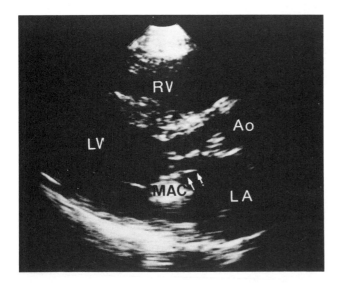

FIGURE 9–11
RUPTURED CHORDAE TENDINEAE
Systolic frame recorded in same patient as in
Figure 9–9. Note the rupture chordae prolapsing into the left atrium (LA) *(arrows)*. LV =
left ventricle; RV = right ventricle; Ao =
aorta; MAC = mitral annulus calcification.

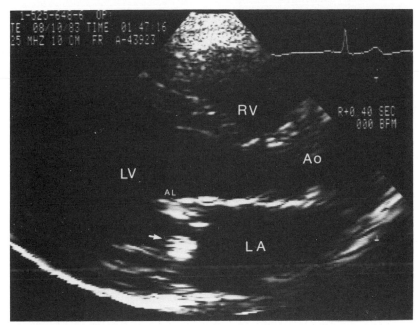

FIGURE 9–12
HEALED VEGETATION
Long-axis left parasternal view recorded one month later in the same patient as in Figure 9–3. The vegetation (*arrows*) is smaller, rounder, and more echodense. LV = left ventricle; RV = right ventricle; Ao = aorta; AL = anterior leaflet; LA = left atrium.

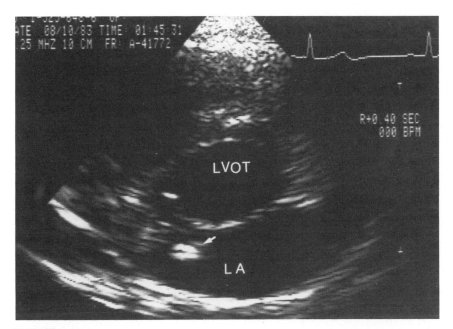

FIGURE 9–13
HEALED VEGETATION
Short-axis left parasternal view in same patient as in Figure 9–3. The vegetation (*arrow*) can be seen to prolapse into the left atrium (LA). LVOT = left ventricular outflow tract.

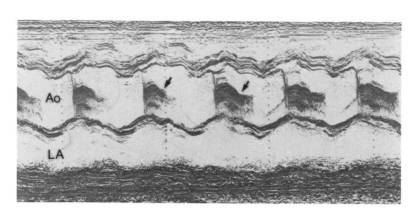

FIGURE 9–14
AORTIC VALVE VEGETATION
This tracing at the aortic valve level demonstrates multiple echoes during diastole *(arrows)*. The leaflet motion is not restricted. The patient had infective endocarditis with severe aortic insufficiency. Ao = aorta; LA = left atrium.

FIGURE 9–15
AORTIC VALVE VEGETATION
Echocardiogram of the aortic valve in a patient with infective endocarditis and a large vegetation in the aortic valve. The arrows point to the diastolic flutter that is commonly seen in endocarditis. RV = right ventricle; Ao = aorta; LA = left atrium; RCC = right coronary cusp; NCC = noncoronary cusp.

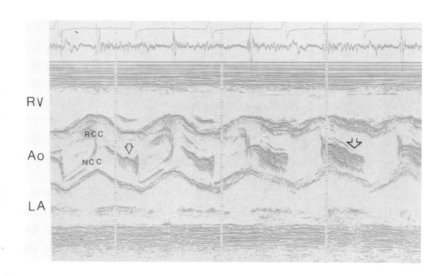

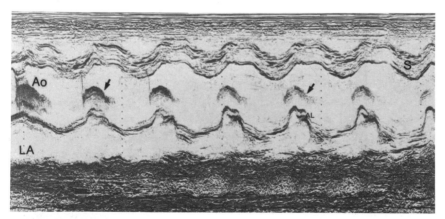

FIGURE 9–16
AORTIC VEGETATION PROLAPSING INTO THE LEFT VENTRICLE
Echocardiographic scan from the aorta to the left ventricle in a patient with a large aortic valve vegetation prolapsing into the left ventricle. A mass of "shaggy" echoes is seen in the outflow tract of the left ventricle *(arrows)*. Ao = aorta; LA = left atrium; AL = anterior leaflet.

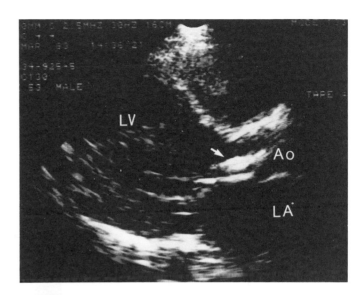

FIGURE 9–17
AORTIC VEGETATION
Long-axis left parasternal view in a 53-year-old man with endocarditis involving the aortic valve. A large vegetation is indicated by the arrow. At the time of surgery, this vegetation was found to be attached to the noncoronary cusp. LV = left ventricle; Ao = aorta; LA = left atrium.

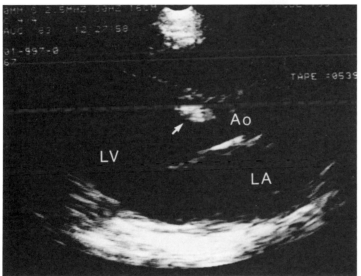

FIGURE 9–18
AORTIC VEGETATION
Long-axis left parasternal view in a patient with severe aortic insufficiency secondary to bacterial endocarditis. A vegetation is seen attached to the right coronary cusp (arrow). LV = left ventricle; Ao = aorta; LA = left atrium.

FIGURE 9–19
AORTIC VEGETATION, FLAIL LEAFLET
Echocardiographic scan from the aortic to the mitral valve level in a patient with endocarditis and severe aortic insufficiency secondary to flail leaflet. The black arrow points to diastolic vibrations of the aortic valve. The large arrow points to part of the flail leaflet prolapsing into the left ventricular outflow tract. Premature mitral valve (MV) closure was also present (vertical arrows). Ao = aorta; LA = left atrium.

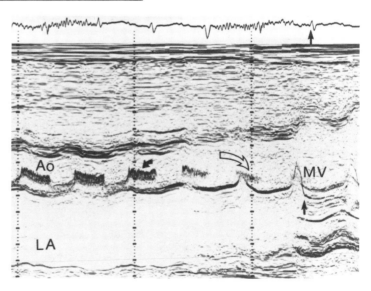

10.3 CAGED-BALL VALVES

All of the caged-ball valves look essentially the same with M-mode and two-dimensional echocardiography. To evaluate the motion of the ball the transducer should be parallel to the direction of the poppet displacement (Fig. 10–8). To evaluate the mitral prosthesis the transducer is placed in the left ventricular apex and is directed toward the left atrium. The prosthetic echoes closest to the transducer are those of the tip of the cage from one of the struts. The motion of this structure is similar to that of the mitral ring. Next to the mitral suture ring the anterior surface of the ball is seen to move in a pattern similar to that of mitral stenosis. During diastole the ball moves anteriorly, touching the strut and remaining close to it for the rest of diastole (Fig. 10–9). At the time of atrial systole, a slight separation may be seen between the poppet and the struts (Fig. 10–10). In the presence of atrial fibrillation, a long diastolic period may produce a more pronounced separation between poppet and strut (Fig. 10–11). The suture ring is situated posteriorly to the anterior border of the ball and moves in a direction parallel to the strut. The posterior border of the ball is seen as a line that moves in a manner similar to the anterior border. This echo recording is usually distant from the anterior border because the velocity of ultrasound passing through the poppet is different from that of ultrasound passing through heart tissue.

The aortic prosthesis can be evaluated best by placing the transducer on the right supraclavicular fossa and directing it toward the left ventricular outflow tract. The motion of the struts is less prominent than that of the mitral prosthesis. The anterior border of the ball has a motion similar to that of the anterior aortic leaflet in that it moves anteriorly toward the struts in systole and posteriorly during diastole (Fig. 10–12).

Two-dimensional echocardiography permits clearer observation of the spatial position of the prosthesis by allowing visualization of the suture ring and the cage. However, the highly reflective materials from which these components are made tend to oversaturate the images and thus make the definition of their different parts difficult. Multiple reverberations from the valve structure further distort the images. The poppet as a whole is difficult to identify, but parts of its anterior and posterior borders can be seen as two parallel lines from which M-mode readings can be obtained to study its motion (Fig. 10–13).

The difficulties of examining caged-ball valves by echocardiography limit the value of this technique to detect abnormalities in this type of prosthesis.

Often indirect signs such as left ventricular volume overload or diastolic flutter of the mitral valve must be used to detect periprosthetic aortic leak.

Prosthetic *valve dehiscence* is suggested by the observation of excessive rocking of the suture ring or by difference in motion of the anterior and posterior ball borders.

Thrombus in or around the prosthesis is difficult to identify because of the strong reflectivity of the echoes surrounding the prosthesis. Alterations may be noted in the ball motion with incomplete or absent opening of the ball (Fig. 10–14).[3]

Simultaneous recording of the tricuspid valve may aid in detecting abnormalities of the poppet motion of a prosthetic mitral valve (Figs. 10–15 to 10–17).

With *ball variance,* lack of ball-strut coaptation has been noted.[4]

Echophonocardiography permits the simultaneous recording of the poppet motion and the sound it produces during its closing and opening motion.[5, 6] In the mitral position, the closing click is much louder than the opening click, which can be single (Fig. 10–18) or multiple (Fig. 10–19).

In the presence of both mitral and tricuspid caged-ball prostheses, echophonocardiography may be useful to detect which opening click belongs to which prosthesis and in this way to define possible alterations in a specific prosthesis (Fig. 10–20). With prosthetic obstruction or severe mitral regurgitation, the opening click, which normally occurs from 70 to 110 msec after A_2, occurs within 50 msec, whereas a delay to longer than 170 msec suggests interference with poppet excursion. A simultaneous carotid pulse recording may show evidence of intermittent decrease in stroke volume (Fig. 10–21). With an aortic ball prosthesis, an opening ejection sound is recorded approximately 70 msec after S_1; this opening click is twice as loud as the closing click that occurs at the time of S_2.

A thrombus may encapsulate the cage but not directly affect the ball motion. In this situation the echocardiogram may appear normal.

10.4 CAGED-DISC VALVES

The echocardiographic appearance of caged-disc valves is very similar to that of caged-ball valves. The excursion of the disc is small, and only one line of echoes is seen to move behind the struts.[7]

Descriptions of echocardiographic abnormalities of this type of prosthesis are scant, but in general the abnormalities are similar to those seen with caged-ball valves.[8, 9]

10.5 TILTING-DISC VALVES

Björk-Shiley

In this type of prosthesis, the disc is tethered off center in a stellite cage and pivots 60 degrees during ejection. The normal disc excursion of the greater curvature varies with the size of the prosthesis. For the smaller size (17) the excursion is 9 mm; for the medium size (23) the excursion is 13 mm; and for the large size (31) the excursion is 17 mm. Since the opening of the disc is eccentric, the patterns of echoes reflected depend on the angle between the ultrasound beam and the disc. This relation makes the echocardiographic pattern quite variable.

Ideal alignment occurs when the plane of the opened disc is perpendicular to the echo scan. This may be accomplished by observing on the posteroanterior and lateral chest x-rays the position of the prosthesis in the chest and then attempting to place the transducer in a position that provides perpendicular imaging.[10] When the disc opens, the larger segment moves toward the transducer and inscribes a square pattern similar to that seen in the mitral valve of patients with mitral stenosis (Figs. 10–22, 10–23). The dense distal echoes seen during valve closure represent the distal position of the annulus behind the echoes arising from the fulcrum portion of the disc and its metallic strut hinges.

Because of the different echocardiographic patterns that may be present in an individual patient, special care must be taken to ascertain whether a decreased excursion is caused by varying alignment of the transducer or by valve dysfunction. It has been recommended that for each patient an initial echocardiogram recorded soon after surgery should be used as the control. This echocardiogram can serve as the basis for comparison if valve dysfunction is suspected.

With a thrombosed Björk-Shiley prosthesis, the amplitude of valve excursion is markedly reduced, as are the opening and closing rates of the disc.[11–16] Very dense echo-recordings posterior to the prosthesis can be noted.

The role of two-dimensional echocardiography in the evaluation of patients with Björk-Shiley prosthetic dysfunction has not been defined.

Lillehei-Kaster

The Lillehei-Kaster prosthesis in the mitral postion can be recorded clearly with M-mode echocardiography. The recording resembles a mitral stenosis pattern with a disc excursion of 7 to 12 mm and mean opening and closing velocities of 37.7 and 59.8 cm per second, respectively.[17, 18] Echophonocardiography shows an association between the opening of the mitral valve and a soft sound that follows the aortic component of the second sound by 0.05 to 0.09 second and that does not occur at the peak of the disc excursion, but at the onset. In about 50 per cent of patients, this opening sound cannot be recorded. The closing sound is made up of two components; the first corresponds to the onset of closure and the second to the end of closure.

10.6 BILEAFLET VALVES

St. Jude Medical

This low-profile bileaflet prosthesis is constructed of pyrolytic carbon. Two half discs are inserted at the valve suture ring.

An M-mode echocardiogram (Fig. 10–24) from the left parasternal border shows both leaflets and the anterior and posterior aspects of the valve ring, which are registered as four parallel lines.[19, 20] The appearance of the valve ring is somewhat similar to that of the normal aorta. The leaflets have an atrial systolic wave when the patient is in sinus rhythm. Leaflet flutter may be noted during long cycles. Gravitational effects promote early posterior leaflet closure when the plane of valve opening is perpendicular to the direction of gravity.

The St. Jude valve can also be studied by two-dimensional echocardiography.[21] It is possible to qualitatively assess ring motion as well as leaflet motion. Left ventricular outflow tract dimensions have confirmed the low-profile design of the prosthesis and indicate a low probability of contact with adjacent structures or of left ventricular outflow tract obstruction. An opening sound can be recorded 60 ± 12 msec after the onset of the ventricular (QRS) complex.

10.7 HOMOGRAFTS (ALLOGRAFTS)

Dura Mater. The dura mater prosthesis is mounted in the outer surface of the stents, which are easily recorded, especially in the aortic position, in which they may resemble a normal aortic valve.

10.8 HETEROGRAFTS

The most commonly used heterografts are the *Hancock* and the *Carpentier-Edwards valves.* The Hancock xenograft has three flexible polypropylene stents supported on a stellite ring. A glutaraldehyde-preserved porcine aortic valve is mounted inside the stents.

In the Carpentier-Edwards bioprosthesis, a porcine aortic valve is fitted on an elgiloy frame.

Porcine Valves

With M-mode echocardiography, the leaflets appear as a normal aortic valve, although there is decreased excursion. In the semilunar position, the boxlike appearance is seen during systole (Fig. 10–25). In the atrioventricular position, the boxlike appearance is seen during diastole (Figs. 10–26, 10–27). The leaflets are observed to move inside two parallel lines that represent the motion of two stents.[22–25]

With two-dimensional echocardiography, it is possible to recognize the stents, suture ring, and leaflets inside the prosthesis (Fig. 10–28). The leaflets have the characteristics of a normal aortic valve in that they are thin and are seen mainly during the closed position, in which they appear as a thin line parallel to the stents (Figs. 10–29, 10–30). In the short-axis view it is occasionally possible to visualize the three leaflets and the three stents, which appear as three strong echo-producing points (Fig. 10–31).

One of the disadvantages of the xenografts is that after six to seven years they tend to have tissue degeneration and calcification. This condition can be recognized by echocardiographic recordings showing increased echo returns from the leaflets, which lose their normal "thin" appearance and instead generate very pronounced echoes. Cusp mobility may be altered.[26] Systolic and diastolic flutter[27–30] of the cusps has been noted with mitral and tricuspid insufficiency (Figs. 10–32, 10–33).

With thrombus surrounding the stents, multiple, dense, and nonhomogeneous echoes can be seen attached to one of the stents or to the suture ring (Fig. 10–34).[31] The spatial orientation of two-dimensional echocardiography increases the possibility of detecting masses around the prosthesis. Thrombi in the left atrium can also be recognized with two-dimensional echocardiography.[32]

If there is a significant degree of *valve dehiscence,* this may be possible to observe with two-dimensional echocardiography. During systole and diastole, the angle of the prosthesis changes, and separation can be observed between the echoes from the ring of the prosthesis and the wall from which it has dehisced (Figs. 10–35, 10–36). There is increased rocking or erratic motion of the valve.

Bovine Valves

Ionescu-Shiley Prosthesis. This is a stented pericardial xenograft that is mounted in a solid and continuous metal ring with three struts. The leaflet motion can be visualized by echocardiography with greater ease than for the the other types of xenografts, probably because the stents are smaller and the leaflets are therefore not as secluded.[33]

10.9 AUTOGRAFT VALVES

Fascia lata. Stented fascia lata grafts in the mitral position have been evaluated with M-mode echocardiography.[34] The rate of diastolic closure of the cusps (E to F slope) has a significant correlation with the effective graft area and is usually suggestive of mild mitral stenosis.

10.10 PROSTHETIC VALVE ENDOCARDITIS

The relative risk of endocarditis following prosthetic valve implantation ranges from 1 to 4 per cent.[35] About two thirds of such cases occur about two months after surgery (late onset), whereas one third occur within two months of surgery (early onset).

The organisms involved in early onset endocarditis are usually more virulent (*Staphylococcus, Pseudomonas, Klebsiella*). In late onset endocarditis, the organisms that predominate are similar to those of natural valve endocarditis (*Streptococcus, Staphylococcus*). Valvular regurgitation around an aortic or mitral valve prosthesis may not produce a heart murmur, so that the diagnosis is difficult to determine clinically. Symptoms of congestive heart failure may be the only clue.

Echocardiography may aid in the diagnosis of prosthetic valve endocarditis by the demonstration of valve dehiscence or vegetations, or both.

Valve dehiscence can be detected in both mechanical and tissue prostheses. Vegetations are much easier to demonstrate in tissue prostheses. The strong echo reflections from a mechanical valve obtruder make the echocardiographic visualization of vegetation difficult. A large vegetation may compromise the motion of the poppet or disc, and this condition may be detected by echocardiography. A vegetation in a tissue prosthesis is seen as a mass of "shaggy" echoes attached to the leaflets (Figs. 10–37 to 10–42).

Prosthetic valve dehiscence can be diagnosed by two-dimensional echocardiography by demonstration of excessive rocking of the prosthetic suture ring. During part of the cardiac cycle lack of contact may be evident between the suture ring and the surrounding cardiac tissue.

Ring abscess can also be demonstrated by echocardiography.

In the absence of a heart murmur, secondary manifestations of ventricular volume overload may be visible in the echocardiogram and may serve as a clue for the diagnosis of perivalvular leak. Severed chordae that remain attached to the papillary muscles after mitral valve replacement may be recorded as highly mobile linear echoes with coarse or fine vibrations and can be confused with the presence of vegetations at that level (Figs. 10–43, 10–44).

10.11 CONDUITS

Conduits with or without a prosthetic valve have been used to replace part of a great artery or to bypass a stenotic area. The more widely used is the *Lillehie-Kaster conduit*. This conduit is often used to replace part of the ascending aorta in the presence of a large aneurysm.

Echocardiographically, the conduits appear as rigid and strong echo-producing structures (Fig. 10–45). They lack the normal systolic expansion seen in the normal aorta. When present, the prosthetic valve has the same characteristics as the regular Lillehei-Kaster valve.

10.12 CARPENTIER RING

The Carpentier ring is used in the tricuspid and mitral position and serves as a support for an annuloplasty.

With echocardiography, the Carpentier ring is seen as a dense band of echoes at the levels of the mitral or tricuspid rings.[36] In the mitral position, its echocardiographic appearance is very similar to that of mitral annulus calcification (Figs. 10–46, 10–47).

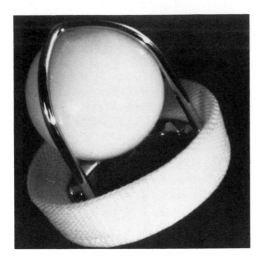

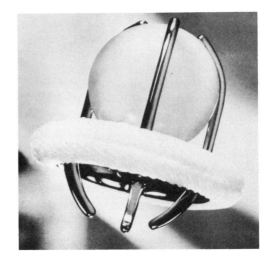

FIGURE 10–1
STARR-EDWARDS CAGED-BALL AORTIC VALVE
Note the wide sewing ring. The Silastic ball is in the open position against the struts of the stellite cage. The cage end is closed.

FIGURE 10–2
SMELOFF-CUTTER VALVE
This prosthetic valve has a double cage of titanium and a Teflon cloth sewing ring. Both cage ends are open.

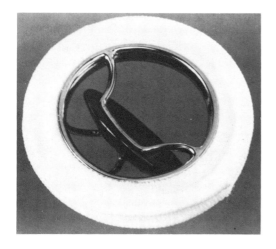

FIGURE 10–3
BJÖRK-SHILEY VALVE
This prosthetic valve has a tilting pyrolytic carbon disc, a stellite cage, and a Teflon cloth sewing ring. The valve opens to about 60 degrees.

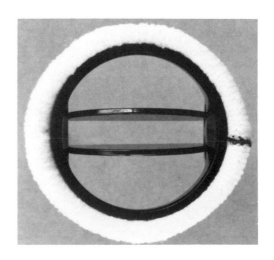

FIGURE 10–4
ST. JUDE MEDICAL CARDIAC VALVE
This low-profile prosthesis is constructed of pyrolytic carbon and has a bileaflet design that produces central flow.

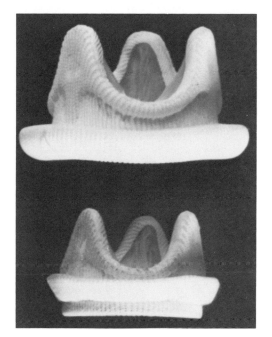

FIGURE 10–5
HANCOCK BIOPROSTHESIS
These glutaraldehyde-preserved porcine aortic xenografts are constructed with a stellite ring in the annulus and flexible polypropylene stents.

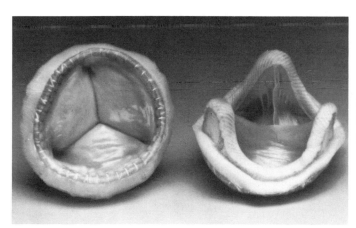

FIGURE 10–6
CARPENTIER-EDWARDS BIOPROSTHESIS
This bioprosthesis is fitted on a flexible elgiloy frame and covered with Teflon cloth.

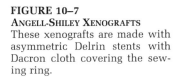

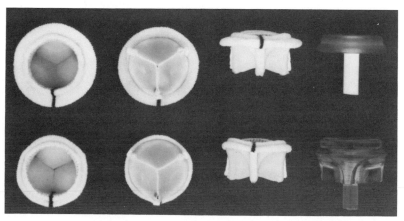

FIGURE 10–7
ANGELL-SHILEY XENOGRAFTS
These xenografts are made with asymmetric Delrin stents with Dacron cloth covering the sewing ring.

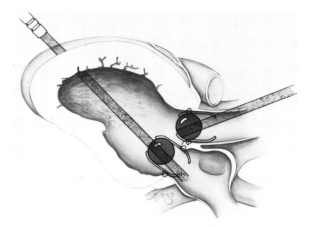

FIGURE 10–8
AORTIC AND MITRAL CAGED-BALL PROSTHESIS
This diagram demonstrates that to evaluate the motion of the mitral poppet with M-mode echocardiography the transducer must be placed at the apex, and to evaluate the motion of the aortic valve it must be placed in the suprasternal area.

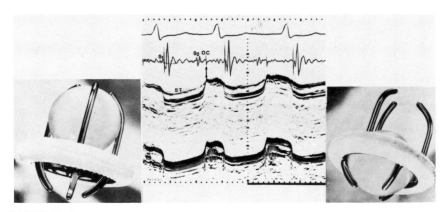

FIGURE 10–9
CAGED-BALL PROSTHESIS, MITRAL POSITION
Smeloff-Cutter mitral valve prosthesis during diastole and systole. The motion of the poppet against the struts and the suture ring is well demonstrated.

MITRAL SMELOFF CUTTER VALVE

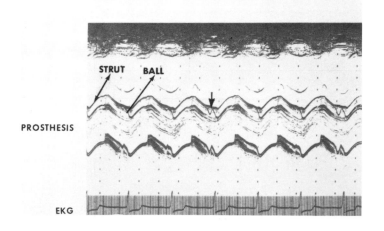

FIGURE 10–10
CAGED-BALL PROSTHESIS, ATRIAL SYSTOLE
There may be a brief separation during atrial systole between the poppet and the strut, as indicated by the black arrow.

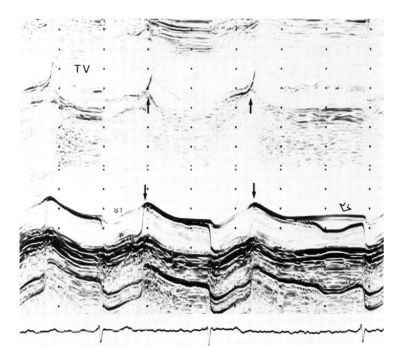

FIGURE 10–11

CAGED-BALL PROSTHESIS, ATRIAL FIBRILLATION

Patients with atrial fibrillation with a normally functioning caged-ball prosthesis may have a prolonged separation between the poppet and the struts during long diastolic periods, as indicated by the open arrow. TV = tricuspid valve; ST = strut, P = poppet.

STARR-EDWARDS AORTIC VALVE PROSTHESIS

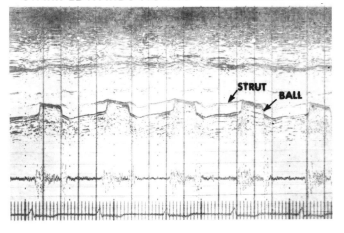

FIGURE 10–12

CAGED-BALL PROSTHESIS, AORTIC POSITION

Echocardiogram recorded from the supraclavicular fossa in a patient with a Starr-Edwards aortic valve prosthesis. The anterior border of the poppet is seen to move anteriorly and to touch the strut immediately after the ventricular complex (QRS) in the electrocardiogram. The anterior border of the poppet remains in contact with the strut for the rest of systole and moves back toward the suture ring at the beginning of diastole.

FIGURE 10–13

CAGED-BALL PROSTHESIS, MITRAL POSITION

Apical four-chamber view in a patient with a mitral caged-ball prosthesis. The inferior and superior borders of the poppet are visualized as two parallel lines (*arrows*). RV = right ventricle; RA = right atrium; ST = strut; LA = left atrium.

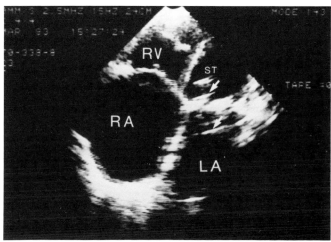

SMELOFF CUTTER VALVES

MITRAL

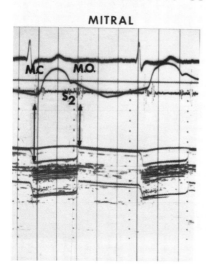

TRICUSPID

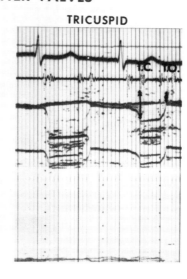

FIGURE 10–20
MITRAL AND TRICUSPID CAGED-BALL VALVES
Echophonocardiography of the mitral and tricuspid prosthetic valves helps to identify which opening and closing clicks belong to which valve. The point of contact between each poppet and its corresponding strut or suture ring can be clearly delineated by simultaneous recording of the phonocardiogram and the prosthetic valve echocardiogram. M.C. = mitral valve closure; M.O. = mitral valve opening.

MALFUNCTION OF BALL VALVE

FIGURE 10–21
THROMBOSED MITRAL PROSTHESIS
Simultaneous recording of an echocardiogram and the carotid pulse shows evidence of intermittent decrease in stroke volume (white arrow) coinciding with failure of the poppet to open.

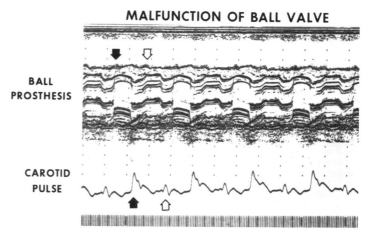

BALL PROSTHESIS

CAROTID PULSE

AORTIC BJÖRK-SHILEY PROSTHESIS

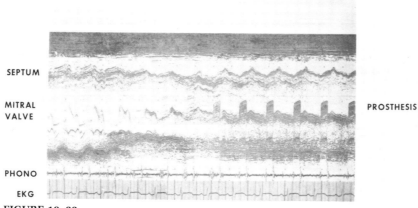

SEPTUM

MITRAL VALVE

PROSTHESIS

PHONO

EKG

FIGURE 10–22
AORTIC BJÖRK-SHILEY PROSTHESIS
Echocardiographic scan from the mitral valve to the aorta. The aortic prosthesis is recorded behind the anterior wall of the aorta and appears as a mass of echoes moving toward the transducer during systole.

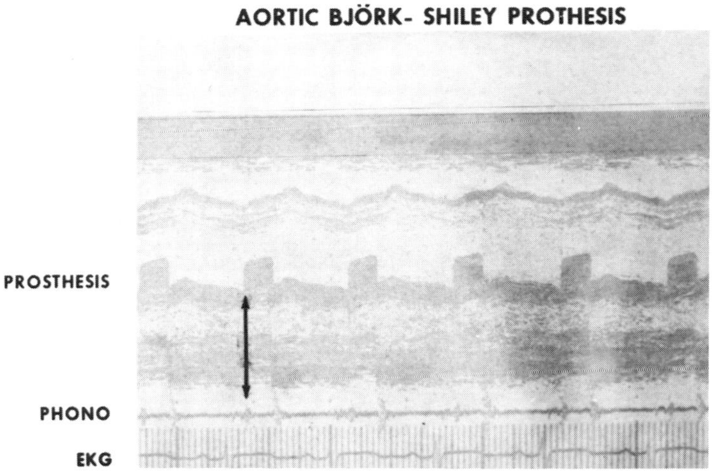

AORTIC BJÖRK- SHILEY PROTHESIS

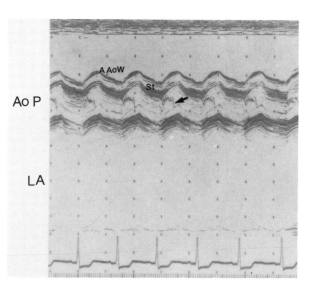

FIGURE 10–23
AORTIC BJÖRK-SHILEY PROSTHESIS
An echocardiogram from the same patient as in Figure 10–22 demonstrates the presence of an opening click *(arrow)* as the disc reaches its maximal anterior point.

PROSTHESIS

PHONO

EKG

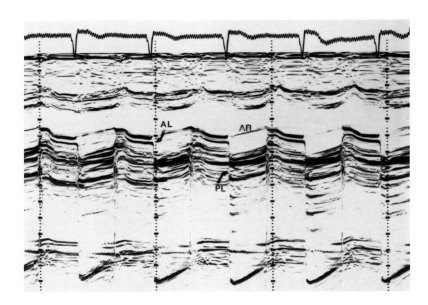

AL

AR

PL

FIGURE 10 24
ST. JUDE PROSTHETIC VALVE
Echocardiogram of the normal St. Jude prosthesis in the mitral position. AR = anterior ring; AL = anterior leaflet; PL = posterior leaflet.

FIGURE 10–25
PORCINE VALVE, AORTIC POSITION
Echocardiogram of a normally functioning Hancock prosthesis. The arrow points to the boxlike structure that is similar to a native aortic valve but with decreased excursion. This structure is situated posterior to a strut (St) and to the anterior aortic wall (AAoW). The left atrium (LA) is markedly dilated because of associated mitral valve disease. Ao P = aortic prosthesis.

A AoW

St

Ao P

LA

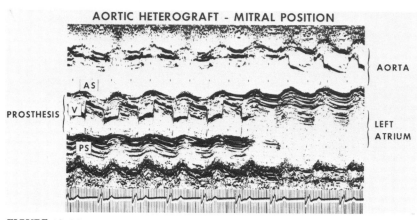

FIGURE 10–26
Porcine Valve, Mitral Position
Echocardiographic scan from the left ventricle to the aorta in a patient with a normally functioning Hancock mitral prosthesis. Note the similar appearances of the mitral and aortic valves. AS = anterior stent; PS = posterior stent; V = valvular leaflets.

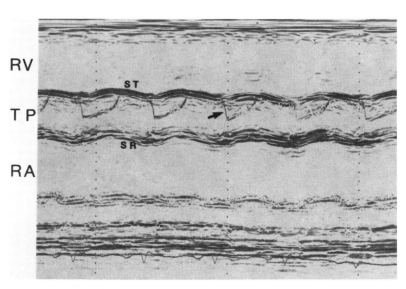

FIGURE 10–27
Porcine Valve, Tricuspid Position
Echocardiogram of a normal Hancock tricuspid valve. An anterior strut (ST), the suture ring (SR), and a leaflet (arrow) are clearly recorded. RV = right ventricle; TP = tricuspid prosthesis; RA = right atrium.

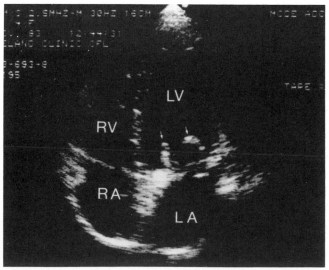

FIGURE 10–28
Porcine Valve, Mitral Position
Apical four-chamber view in a 56-year-old man with a normal Carpentier-Edwards (29 mm) mitral prosthesis. Anterior and posterior struts are clearly seen (arrows). The leaflet tissue and suture ring are not clearly observable in this figure. RV = right ventricle; LV = left ventricle; RA = right atrium; LA = left atrium.

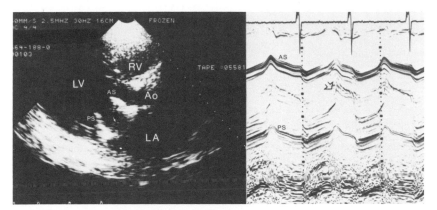

FIGURE 10–29
PORCINE VALVE, MITRAL POSITION
Long-axis left parasternal view and M-mode echocardiogram in a 60-year-old patient with a normally functioning Hancock (31 mm) prosthesis. Note the anterior (AS) and posterior (PS) struts as well as the leaflet tissue (arrows). RV = right ventricle; LV = left ventricle; Ao = aorta; LA = left atrium.

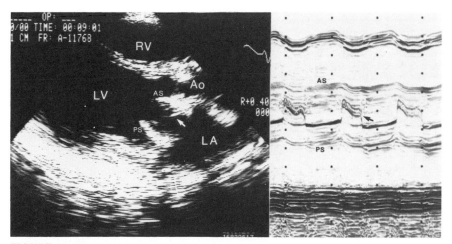

FIGURE 10–30
PORCINE VALVE, MITRAL POSITION
Long-axis left parasternal view and M-mode echocardiogram in a 60-year-old patient with a normally functioning #33 Carpentier-Edwards prosthesis. Note the similarity in appearance with the Hancock prosthesis shown in Figure 10–29. The arrows point to the leaflets. RV = right ventricle; LV = left ventricle; Ao = aorta; LA = left atrium; AS = anterior strut; PS = posterior strut.

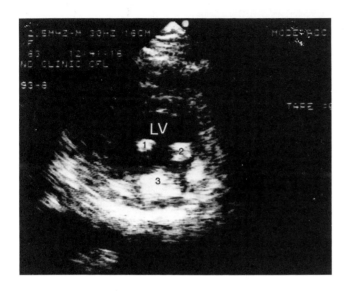

FIGURE 10–31
PORCINE VALVE, MITRAL POSITION
Short-axis left parasternal view at the level of
the tip of the prosthesis. The stents appear as
circular structures within the left ventricular
cavity and are numbered 1, 2, and 3. LV =
left ventricle.

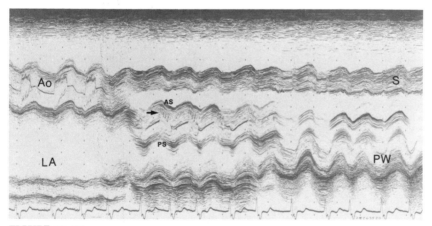

FIGURE 10–32
PORCINE VALVE DYSFUNCTION
Echocardiographic scan from the aorta (Ao) to the left ventricle in a patient with a
Hancock mitral valve prosthesis and severe mitral regurgitation. Note the systolic
flutter (arrow) of the mitral prosthesis, which is suggestive of leaflet degeneration.
LA = left atrium; S = septum; PW = posterior wall; AS = anterior strut, PS =
posterior strut.

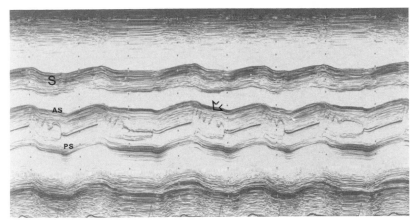

FIGURE 10–33
PORCINE VALVE DYSFUNCTION
An echocardiogram from the same patient as in Figure 10–32 but recorded at a faster speed demonstrates more clearly the systolic flutter of the prosthetic leaflet (*arrow*). This type of vibration in the mitral position always denotes prosthetic dysfunction. S = septum; AS = anterior strut; PS = posterior strut.

FIGURE 10–34
THROMBOSED PORCINE VALVE
Apical four-chamber view in a 22-year-old woman with a malfunctioning porcine valve. There is a thrombus at the level of the suture ring reflected by a large "cloud" of echoes. The arrows point to the struts. RV = right ventricle; LV = left ventricle; S = septum; RA = right atrium; LA = left atrium.

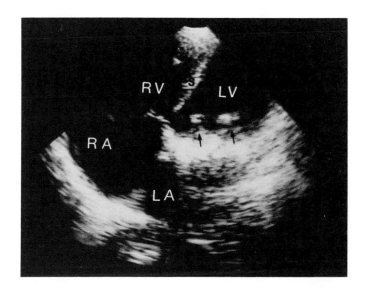

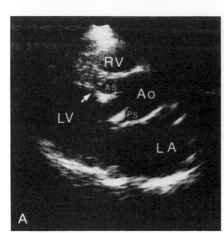
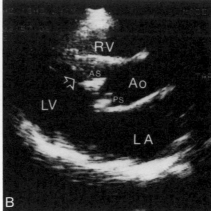

FIGURE 10–35
PORCINE VALVE DEHISCENCE
Left parasternal long-axis view in a patient with dehiscence of a porcine aortic prosthesis. During systole (A) the anterior stent (AS) is close to the septum (small arrow). During diastole (B) there is a significant separation between the two structures (open arrow). RV = right ventricle; LV = left ventricle; Ao = aorta; LA = left atrium; PS = posterior stent.

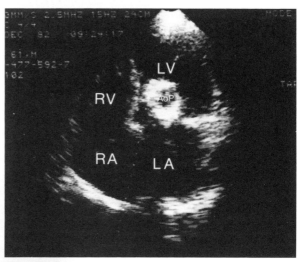

FIGURE 10–36
PORCINE VALVE DEHISCENCE
Apical four-chamber view in the same patient as in Figure 10–35. The aortic prosthesis (AoP) is seen to prolapse into the left ventricular outflow tract. LV = left ventricle; RV = right ventricle; RA = right atrium; LA = left atrium.

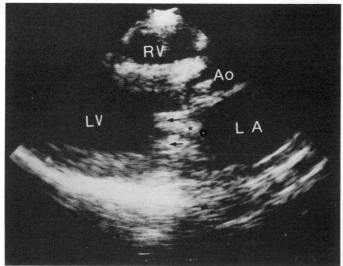
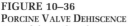

FIGURE 10–37
PORCINE VALVE VEGETATION
Long-axis left parasternal view in a 31-year-old patient with Hancock mitral and aortic valves and bacterial endocarditis. A large vegetation (*) is seen in the mitral prosthesis behind the anterior stent. RV = right ventricle; LV = left ventricle; Ao = aorta; LA = left atrium.

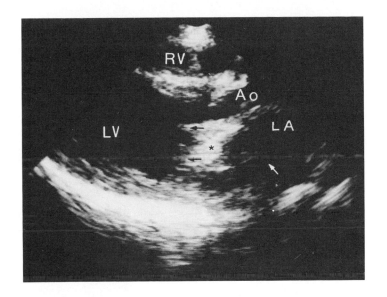

FIGURE 10–38
PORCINE VALVE VEGETATION
A long-axis left parasternal view in the same patient as in Figure 10–37. The fine linear echo pattern in the left atrium (LA) *(white arrow)* is probably related to parts of the affected leaflet or to a vegetation prolapsing into the left atrium. The asterisk indicates the vegetation. The black arrows point to the anterior and posterior stents. RV = right ventricle; LV = left ventricle; Ao = aorta.

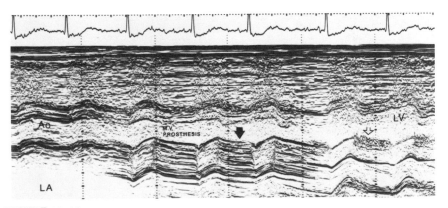

FIGURE 10–39
PORCINE VALVE VEGETATION
Echocardiographic scan from the aorta to the left ventricle in a patient with fungal endocarditis and a large vegetation in a Hancock mitral valve. A mass of echoes is seen at the level of the prosthesis *(black arrow)*. This mass protrudes into the left ventricle (LV), in which it has high-frequency vibrations *(white arrow)*. Ao = aorta; LA = left atrium; M.V. = mitral valve.

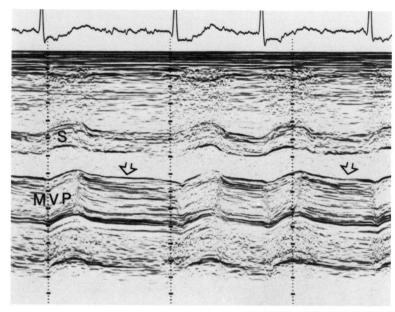

FIGURE 10–40
PORCINE VALVE VEGETATION
An echocardiogram recorded in the same patient as in Figure 10–39 at the level of the mitral valve prosthesis (MVP) shows linear echoes attached to the leaflets that indicate a large vegetation (arrows). S = septum.

FIGURE 10–41
PORCINE VALVE VEGETATION
This long-axis left parasternal view shows large vegetation (arrow) attached to the mitral prosthetic valve and prolapsing into the left ventricle (LV) in diastole. RV = right ventricle; Ao = aorta; LA = left atrium.

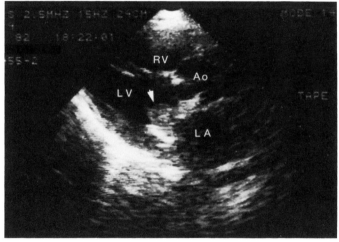

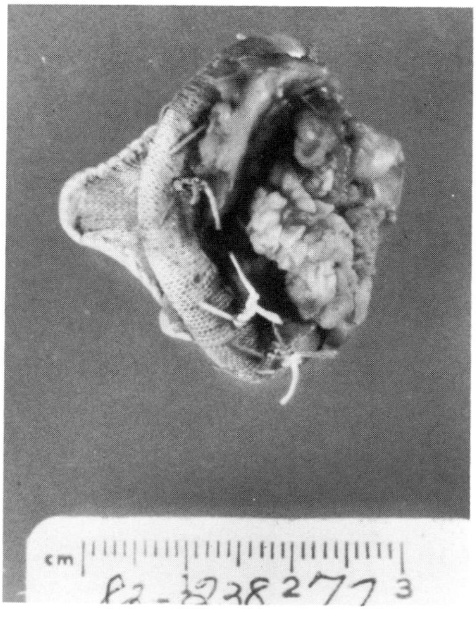

FIGURE 10–42
PORCINE VALVE VEGETATION
Anatomic specimen from the patient who had the vegetation viewed in Figures 10–39 to 10–41. A large verrucous vegetation can be seen attached to the porcine valve.

oc
si

di
fr
(I
vi
Fi

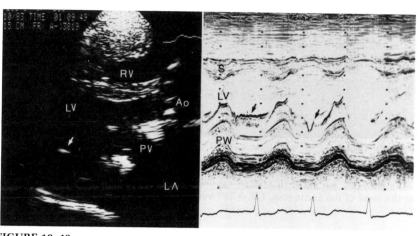

FIGURE 10–43
MITRAL VALVE REPLACEMENT, SEVERED CHORDAE
M-mode and left parasternal long-axis echocardiograms from a patient with mitral valve replacement show a fine structure close to the posterior wall (PW) *(arrows)*. This structure has a chaotic motion and represents the severed chordae that remain after mitral valve replacement and that are a normal finding. RV = right ventricle, LV = left ventricle; Ao = aorta; PV = prosthetic valve; LA = left atrium; S = septum.

lc
is
a
th
v
c

FIGURE 10–44
MITRAL VALVE REPLACEMENT, SEVERED CHORDAE
M-mode echocardiogram recorded after mitral valve replacement in a 54-year-old patient. The arrows point to a structure with high-frequency vibrations that represents severed chordae. The patient did not have aortic insufficiency. S = septum; LV = left ventricle; PW = posterior wall.

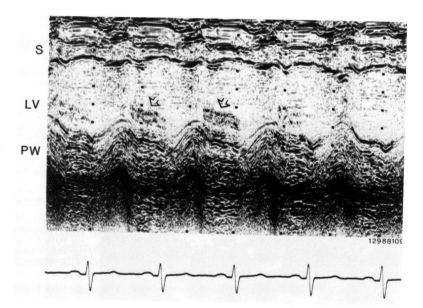

m
fr
ta
se
T

si
a
le
sh
re
to
b
m
st
v

The left ventricular walls can be analyzed from a number of orientations by two-dimensional echocardiography.

The Apex. The apex can be visualized best from any of the apical views (Fig. 11–14). It usually cannot be seen from the long-axis parasternal or short-axis parasternal views.

The Interventricular Septum. This area can be visualized best from the apical four-chamber view (Fig. 11–15). The base of the septum can also be seen clearly from the parasternal long and short axes.

Anterior Wall. The best view in which to visualize the anterior wall is the apical two-chamber view (Fig. 11–16). The second best is the short-axis parasternal view.

Lateral Wall. The lateral wall can be seen best from the apical four-chamber view (Fig. 11–17). It can also be observed from the parasternal short axis.

Inferior Wall. The inferior wall can be viewed best in the apical two-chamber view but can also be evaluated from the parasternal short- and long-axis views (Fig. 11–18).

11.2 LEFT VENTRICULAR HYPERTROPHY

After the age of two, heart weight remains stable at about 0.45 per cent of body weight. Normal left ventricular mass may range from 185 grams in average-sized individuals to 220 grams in persons with large body size or high levels of physical activity. Left ventricular hypertrophy is defined as an increase of left ventricular mass above this normal level.[29]

Left ventricular hypertrophy may be induced by many causes. A prevailing theory is that myocardial hypertrophy regulates the size, shape, and wall thickness of the cardiac chambers to keep wall tension within normal limits. This idea can be expressed mathematically by Laplace's law in which

$$T = P \times r/2\ WT$$

or

$$P = T \times 2\ WT/r$$

where P = pressure, T = tension, and WT = wall thickness.

A constant pressure overload (as in hypertension or aortic stenosis) would produce concentric left ventricular hypertrophy with an increase in relative wall thickness (wall thickness divided by chamber radius) sufficient to keep peak wall tension within normal limits.

With continuous volume overload (as in aortic insufficiency) eccentric left ventricular hypertrophy is induced with an increase in wall thickness proportional to the increase in diameter, which brings about a magnification of the left ventricle and a normal relative wall thickness. Myocardial failure may also be a stimulus to left ventricular hypertrophy by a simple mechanism of volume overload. In heart failure there is dilatation of the left ventricle; hence to decrease wall stress, wall thickness of the ventricle must increase. The left ventricular hypertrophy seen in endurance athletes *(physiologic left ventricular hypertrophy)* is also an eccentric hypertrophy related to increased stroke volume.

Left ventricular hypertrophy can be diagnosed echocardiographically by demonstrating increased wall thickness, increased left ventricular mass, small left ventricular size, large papillary muscles, prominent trabeculae carneae, and decreased left ventricular compliance.

Increased Wall Thickness. Echocardiography is probably the best method by which to determine left ventricular wall thickness. Left ventricular hypertrophy can be detected with relative ease by both M-mode and two-dimensional echocardiography.[30, 31]

With M-mode echocardiography, both the septum and the posterior wall are found to be thickened (Figs. 11–19, 11–20) so that they measure more than 12 mm during diastole. The ratio of septal to posterior wall thickness is usually 1:1, but occasionally some hypertensive patients have disproportionate septal hypertrophy.[32] An M-mode echocardiogram derived from a line of the sector scanner is probably the best means of measuring wall thickness. Two-dimensional echocardiography permits a broader evaluation of wall thickness (Fig. 11–21) and may permit visualization of thickened walls outside the M-mode pathway.

Increased Left Ventricular Mass. As discussed previously, measurements of left ventricular wall thickness can be used to estimate the size of the myocardial shell surrounding the left ventricular chamber. When both M-mode and two-dimensional echocardiograms are used, regression equations for calculation of left ventricular mass show that in the presence of left ventricular hypertrophy this mass is greater than the upper limits of normal.

Small Left Ventricular Size. Patients with concentric left ventricular hypertrophy usually have small left ventricular cavities, and both the end-systolic and end-diastolic diameters are reduced. Patients with eccentric left ventricular hypertrophy have large ventricular cavities (Fig. 11–22). Since there is usually a "magnification" of the left ventricle and a normal relative wall thickness in such patients, the increased wall thickness may not be as apparent as in patients with concentric left ventricular hypertrophy.

Large Papillary Muscles. Although there has been no study in which the echocardiographic size or mass of the papillary muscles was measured, their increased size is an obvious qualitative finding on two-dimensional echocardiography (Fig. 11–23). They are very prominent in all views and fill a significant part of the left ventricular cavity.

Prominent Trabeculae Carneae. A frequent finding in left ventricular hypertrophy is an increase in size of the trabeculae carneae in the endocardial surface of the left ventricle. This condition creates multiple parallel lines in the M-mode recording of the posterior wall endocardium and may make difficult the measurement of posterior wall thickness (Fig. 11–24).

On two-dimensional echocardiography, the trabeculae carneae produce a very prominent and highly reflective image of the endocardium (Fig. 11–25).

Decreased Left Ventricular Compliance. Patients with left ventricular hypertrophy often have a decreased E to F slope of the mitral valve and decreased diastolic posterior wall velocity. Both signs are suggestive of decreased left ventricular compliance.[33]

With the aid of a minicomputer, it is possible to measure the rate of change of the ventricular dimensions throughout the cardiac cycle. Abnormal changes in left ventricular filling, probably related to decreased compliance, have been described in patients with left ventricular hypertrophy.

11.3 LEFT VENTRICULAR SIZE AND FUNCTION IN SYSTEMIC HYPERTENSION

Several echocardiographic abnormalities have been described in hypertensive subjects (Fig. 11–26).[34–38] These include (1) left ventricular hypertrophy, (2) left atrial enlargement, (3) left ventricular dilatation, (4) decreased E to F slope of the mitral valve, (5) decreased left ventricular ejection fraction, (6) disproportionate septal thickening, and (7) decreased left atrial emptying index.[39]

11.4 LEFT VENTRICULAR SIZE AND FUNCTION IN ATHLETES

Several studies have shown alterations in left ventricular size, mass, and function in professional athletes.[40–42] The most common findings include enlargement of the left ventricular end-diastolic dimension and increased septal and posterior left ventricular wall thickness (Fig. 11–27).

Exercise training has been associated with an increase in stroke volume that is suggestive of an enhanced contractile state.[43]

11.5 CARDIOMYOPATHIES

Cardiomyopathies are diseases that primarily affect the heart muscle and are not the result of congenital, valvular, hypertensive, or ischemic diseases. A variety of schemes has been used to classify the cardiomyopathies. For this discussion the functional classification is used with the recognition that there is some overlap. Three functional categories have been described: (1) congestive cardiomyopathy, (2) hypertrophic cardiomyopathy, and (3) restrictive cardiomyopathy.

Congestive Cardiomyopathy

Congestive cardiomyopathy is characterized by impaired left ventricular systolic function with dilatation of all four chambers of the heart, particularly of the left ventricle. There may also be some degree of left ventricular hypertrophy, but the increase in wall thickness is inadequate for the degree of ventricular dilatation. Left and right ventricular thrombi are common. The contractility of the left ventricle is diffusely decreased, permitting differentiation from coronary artery disease, in which there is segmental dysfunction. The cardiac valves are normal by definition, but mild nonspecific leaflet thickening is not unusual.

In most patients with congestive cardiomyopathy, the echocardiogram shows cardiac enlargement, global left ventricular dysfunction, decreased stroke volume, and evidence of increased diastolic pressure.

Cardiac Enlargement. Most patients with congestive cardiomyopathy have at least moderate left ventricular dilatation (Fig. 11–28) with increased end-systolic and end-diastolic dimensions.[44] On two-dimensional echocardiography, a globular type of dilatation is often apparent (Figs. 11–29 to 11–32). The left atrium is also enlarged in the majority of patients. Right ventricular and right atrial enlargement are common.

Left ventricular hypertrophy, when present, is not a prominent feature and is always inadequate for the degree of left ventricular dilatation present.

A small pericardial effusion is often seen behind the posterior left ventricular wall.

Global Left Ventricular Dysfunction. Typically, in congestive cardiomyopathy diffuse and symmetrically reduced contractility of the left ventricular walls is observed. The percentage of fractional shortening is reduced below 30 per cent. All or most derived indices of left ventricular function are reduced. There is decreased ejection fraction, circumferential fiber shortening, and posterior wall velocity (Fig. 11–33).

Decreased Stroke Volume. The usual echocardiographic manifestations of decreased stroke volume are frequently seen. These include (a) decreased total amplitude of the mitral valve (Fig. 11–34), (b) decreased D to E slope, (c) decreased mitral valve stroke volume, (d) gradual closure of the aortic valve during systole, (e) decreased aortic wall amplitude (Fig. 11–35), and (f) increased (greater than 7 mm) mitral E point septal separation. In the two-dimensional echocardiogram, the mitral valve orifice appears narrowed on the short-axis left parasternal view (Fig. 11–36).

Increased Diastolic Pressure. Indirect evidence of increased left ventricular end-diastolic pressure is frequently observed with the presence of a B notch in the mitral valve (Fig. 11–37).

Differential Diagnosis

Although global left ventricular dysfunction is suggestive of primary congestive cardiomyopathy, the end-stage left ventricle of many conditions may have the same echo-cardiographic appearance. Echocardiographically, severe coronary artery disease with severe left ventricular dysfunction may be indistinguishable from primary myocardial disease. Hence, severe coronary artery disease cannot be excluded by echocardiography.

Severe aortic insufficiency with severe left ventricular dysfunction can also give an echocardiographic appearance of the left ventricle that is similar to that of congestive cardiomyopathy. With severe aortic insufficiency, diastole may be foreshortened, and the characteristic diastolic flutter of the mitral valve may not be apparent.

Abnormalities of septal motion, such as those seen with left bundle branch block or after open-heart surgery, make the measurement of the percentage of fractional shortening—an important echocardiographic parameter of left ventricular function—difficult or impossible to measure.

Patients with mild left ventricular dysfunction may have echocardiograms that are normal or nearly normal in appearance. The evaluation of left ventricular function by echocardiography is based on adequate visualization of the endocardial surface motion. If the surface is not well registered, then it is not possible to make this evaluation.

Hypertrophic Cardiomyopathy

The term hypertrophic cardiomyopathy denotes a group of diseases characterized by *idiopathic left ventricular hypertrophy* that is genetically transmitted as an autosomal dominant trait with a high degree of penetrance.[45, 46]

The pattern of hypertrophy is distinctive in that there is disproportionate involvement of the interventricular septum when compared with the posterior and anterolateral walls of the left ventricle. In some cases hypertrophy preferentially affects the cardiac apex (apical hypertrophy of the heart), and in some cases it affects the free wall of the left ventricle more than the septum. These cases are the exception rather than the rule. Symmetric thickening of the left ventricle can also occur.

Conditions of septal hypertrophy other than hypertrophic cardiomyopathy include: (a) fetal state or in (b) neonates and infants, (c) left ventricular hypertrophy, (d) right ventricular hypertrophy, and (e) coronary artery disease. The latter condition may cause abnormal septal thickness relative to the posterior wall.

Left ventricular outflow tract obstruction may be present. When present, the obstruction is dynamic in the sense that it appears after ejection has started. There is decreased left ventricular compliance related to increased wall stiffness in patients with hypertrophic cardiomyopathy.

Other abnormalities frequently found in patients with hypertrophic cardiomyopathy include a dilated left atrium, a thickened mitral valve, and a mural plaque in the left ventricular outflow tract. The presence of a mural plaque presumably is related to the trauma of the anterior mitral leaflet opposing the septum during early diastole and during systole.

At the microscopic level, a bizarre form of myocardial fiber hypertrophy and disarray[47] is commonly found in the interventricular septum of patients with hypertrophic cardiomyopathy. This form may be the cause of the "sparkling" effect observed with two-dimensional echocardiography in some patients with hypertrophic cardiomyopathy.

Several investigators[48-50] have reviewed the echocardiographic findings in hypertrophic cardiomyopathy (Figs. 11–38 to 11–43). These include asymmetric septal hypertrophy, apical hypertrophy, hypertrophy in unusual locations, systolic anterior mitral valve motion, aortic valve mid-systolic notching, small left ventricular outflow tract size, decreased left ventricular compliance, and left atrial enlargement.

Asymmetric Septal Hypertrophy (ASH).[51] This is by far the most common form of ventricular hypertrophy seen in patients with hypertrophic cardiomyopathy (Figs. 11–44, 11–45). With M-mode echocardiography, asymmetric septal hypertrophy is defined as a septum to posterior wall ratio of more than 1.2 to 1, measured at the level of the mitral valve. The interventricular septum must also measure at least 1.3 mm in thickness. The term asymmetric septal hypertrophy is reserved for those cases in which there is no apparent cause for the septal hypertrophy. If there is a cause, such as right ventricular hypertrophy or coronary artery disease, to explain a discrepancy in septal as opposed to posterior wall thickness, the term *disproportionate septal hypertrophy* is used.

The term asymmetric septal hypertrophy was initially introduced as an echocardi-

ographic marker of hypertrophic cardiomyopathy. Since the original description it has become obvious that although this is a sensitive parameter for the diagnosis of this entity it is not specific enough to be pathognomonic. Therefore, the more general and descriptive term septal hypertrophy may be preferred. Three forms of septal hypertrophy have been described by two-dimensional echocardiography: hypertrophy at the base of the septum, in its middle portion, and in its apical section. In some patients the septum protrudes into the right ventricular outflow tract. The septum is often hypokinetic and may have a peculiar reflective pattern at the level of maximal thickness (Fig. 11–46). A mural plaque in the outflow tract occasionally can be seen.

Apical Hypertrophy. In a small number of patients with hypertrophic cardiomyopathy, the hypertrophy is confined primarily to the region of the left ventricular apex (Figs. 11–47, 11–48).[52, 53] The basal half of the interventricular septum is of normal thickness. Portions of the left ventricular free wall are often thickened.

Hypertrophy in Unusual Locations. In some patients with hypertrophic cardiomyopathy, there may be areas of ventricular hypertrophy that are missed in a routine M-mode echocardiogram (Fig. 11–49).[54] Only two-dimensional echocardiography permits the detection of focal hypertrophy when this involves localized areas of anterolateral wall and posterior ventricular septum.

Systolic Anterior Motion of the Mitral Valve (SAM). Systolic anterior motion of the mitral valve is best evaluated by M-mode echocardiography when both the anterior and the posterior mitral leaflets are observed.[55] SAM is seen as an abrupt anterior motion of the mitral valve that starts a short time after the closure of the mitral valve (C point), lasts throughout systole, and ends just before mitral opening (D point) (Fig. 11–50). Multiple echoes are often but not necessarily seen within the arc made by the mitral valve during systole. This SAM is independent of the posterior wall motion. There are many degrees of SAM (Figs. 11–51 to 11–53). In the most severe form, there is mitral-septal contact during a significant part of systole (Fig. 11–54). Patients with this type of SAM usually have a gradient at rest.[56] The degree of systolic anterior motion augments after a premature ventricular contraction (Fig. 11–55).

Patients with latent obstruction have a mild degree of SAM when there is either no mitral-septal contact during systole or when such contact occurs for only a short part of systole. Some patients with latent obstruction have no SAM at rest, and SAM becomes apparent only after amyl nitrate administration (Fig. 11–56).

In patients with pericardial effusion, care must be taken in the interpretation of the systolic anterior motion, since the swinging of the heart may produce pseudosystolic anterior motion. Occasionally, hypertrophic cardiomyopathy and pericardial effusion may be observed (Fig. 11–57).

In normal individuals chordae tendineae may move into the left ventricular outflow tract and simulate systolic anterior motion of the mitral valve. In general, the chordae tendineae do not approximate the septum, and the outflow tract is normal in size (Figs. 11–58, 11–59).

Patients with *nonobstructive hypertrophic cardiomyopathy* have no SAM at rest or after provocation (Figs. 11–60 to 11–62). Some patients have severe hypertrophic cardiomyopathy without obstruction (Figs. 11–63 to 11–65).

Aortic Valve Mid-Systolic Notching. This phenomenon is seen on M-mode echocardiography as a mid-systolic semiclosure of the aortic valve.[57] This finding often is associated with coarse leaflet flutter. After semiclosure the valves move back to a fully open position (Figs. 11–66, 11–67). This appears to be a specific and sensitive echocardiographic finding in patients with the obstructive form of hypertrophic cardiomyopathy.

Small Left Ventricular Outflow Tract Size. The left ventricular outflow tract diameter that is seen with two-dimensional echocardiography or measured by M-mode echocardiography as the distance between the left side of the septum and the initial systolic echo of the mitral valve (C point) appears small.

Decreased Left Ventricular Compliance. Patients with hypertrophic cardiomyopathy have small and stiff left ventricles. The mitral E to F slope is usually reduced (Fig. 11–68). The left ventricular cavity is small, and the diastolic filling pattern of the left ventricle is altered.[58]

Left Atrial Enlargement. This is a common finding in patients with hypertrophic obstructive cardiomyopathy. It is probably the result of decreased left ventricular compliance and mitral regurgitation.

Differential Diagnosis

Systolic anterior motion of the mitral valve may occur in conditions other than hypertrophic cardiomyopathy, such as mitral valve prolapse, aortic regurgitation,[59] left ventricular aneurysm,[60] left ventricular hypertrophy,[61] and pericardial effusion, as well as in normal persons.

Asymmetric septal hypertrophy may occur in conditions other than hypertrophic cardiomyopathy, such as in the fetal state or in neonates and infants,[62] in left ventricular hypertrophy (Fig. 11–69),[63] in right ventricular hypertrophy (Fig. 11–70), in coronary artery disease,[64] and in the presence of an angled interventricular septum (Figs. 11–71, 11–72).[65] Occasionally, hypertrophic obstructive cardiomyopathy may coexist with valvular aortic stenosis (Figs. 11–73, 11–74).

Echophonocardiography

The apexcardiogram and the carotid pulse tracing can aid in the diagnosis of hypertrophic cardiomyopathy (Figs. 11–75, 11–76). With echophonocardiography, it is possible to correlate the systolic anterior motion of the mitral valve with the systolic ejection murmur and the bispherins carotid pulse (Fig. 11–77).

Restrictive Cardiomyopathies

The hallmark of the restrictive cardiomyopathies is abnormal diastolic function.[66, 67] The ventricular walls are rigid and impede adequate ventricular filling. There is normal or nearly normal systolic function. Myocardial infiltration, fibrosis, or hypertrophy is usually responsible for the abnormal function. The most common causes of restrictive cardiomyopathy include (1) cardiac amyloidosis, (2) hemochromatosis, (3) sarcoidosis, (4) endomyocardial fibrosis, (5) Löffler's endocarditis, and (6) endocardial fibroelastosis.

A number of echocardiographic findings are common to most patients with restrictive cardiomyopathies: (1) ventricular hypertrophy, (2) small left ventricular cavity, (3) abnormal motion of the posterior wall that is related to abnormal ventricular filling, and (4) pericardial effusions.

Specific echocardiographic abnormalities are also found in the different forms of restrictive cardiomyopathies, including cardiac amyloidosis, hemochromatosis, sarcoidosis, and endocardial fibroelastosis.

Cardiac Amyloidosis.[68] The echocardiographic findings that have been described in patients with cardiac amyloidosis (Figs. 11–78, 11–79) include increased septal and posterior wall thickness, thickened right ventricular wall, normal or reduced left ventricular dimensions, decreased septal and posterior wall systolic thickening, pericardial effusion, pericardial nodules, left and right atrial enlargement, increased papillary muscle thickness, thickened valves, thickened interatrial septum, and "granular sparkling" appearance of the myocardium.[69–71]

Hemochromatosis. The echocardiographic findings that have been described in patients with hemochromatosis include increased wall thickness, normal or increased left ventricular dimensions, and left atrial dilatation.[72]

Sarcoidosis.[73] In patients with sarcoidosis increased right ventricular index and right ventricular anterior wall thickness have been reported.[74]

Endocardial Fibroelastosis. Focal or diffuse areas of increased echo production arising from the endocardial interface—often several millimeters in thickness—are frequently seen in patients with fibroelastosis (Figs. 11–80 to 11–82).[75, 76] Characteristic two-dimensional echocardiographic findings include apical obliteration of one or both ventricles, bright echoes at the cavity surface, preserved ventricular function, and dilated atria with ventricles of normal size.[77]

11.6 CARDIAC INVOLVEMENT IN SYSTEMIC DISEASES

The echocardiographic findings in patients with systemic infiltrative diseases involving the heart have been reviewed by Borer.[78]

Carcinoid Heart Disease. The tricuspid valve is thickened, immobile, and frozen in a partially open position, resulting in both stenosis and insufficiency. The thickening is diffuse, extending from the base to the tips. Endocardial coating of the papillary muscles by carcinoid fibrous plaques can be seen.[79, 80] The pulmonic valve is shortened, highly reflective, and has decreased systolic motion.

Mucopolysaccharidoses. The abnormalities that occur frequently include increased wall thickness, mitral stenosis, and decreased systolic function of the left ventricle.[81]

Neurologic and Neuromuscular Diseases

Progressive (Duchenne's) Muscular Dystrophy. Fibrous replacement of the myocardium with selective scarring of the posterobasal portion of the left ventricle and posteromedial papillary muscle has been described.[82, 83] Decreased left ventricular fractional shortening has been detected with M-mode echocardiography.[84]

Friedreich's Ataxia. Cardiac hypertrophy and diffuse fibrosis are present. The signs of congestive cardiomyopathy can be seen. There may be an association with idiopathic hypertrophic subaortic stenosis.[85]

Myotonia Atrophica. The signs of congestive cardiomyopathy may be present.

Tuberous Sclerosis. Myocardial tumor masses composed of mature fat tissue have been described in patients with tuberous sclerosis.

Collagen Diseases

Scleroderma. The endocardium, myocardium, and pericardium can be involved singly or in combination.[86] The myocardium is affected more frequently with replacement of cardiac muscle by connective tissue. A congestive or a restrictive type of cardiomyopathy may be present. Pericardial effusion is common. Deformity of the mitral and aortic valves with nodularity of the cusps has been reported. The associated echocardiographic abnormalities include increased right ventricular dimension, reduced left ventricular ejection fraction, and pericardial effusion.

Periarteritis Nodosa. Patchy fibrosis of the myocardium with cardiac enlargement is frequently seen. Left ventricular hypertrophy from hypertension is also often observed. Myocardial scarring from myocardial infarction may be evident.

Lupus Erythematosus. This condition involves the endocardium, myocardium, and pericardium. The most widely known cardiac manifestations of systemic lupus erythematosus is Libman-Sacks disease. The Libman-Sacks lesions are granular verrucous growths attached to the endocardium. They may be as large as 3 to 4 mm in diameter. They can be found in any part of the endocardium but are more frequently seen in the angles of the atrioventricular valves and on the underside of the mitral valve at its base (Fig. 11–83).

Myocardial fibrosis and hypertrophy are common. The signs of congestive cardiomyopathy may be observed. Pericardial effusion is a frequent finding.

Dermatomyositis. Myocardial fibrosis and cardiomegaly may be present. Epicardial fibrosis and constrictive pericarditis have been reported.

Rheumatoid Arthritis. Valvular, myocardial, and pericardial involvement may occur in patients with rheumatoid arthritis.

The aortic and mitral valves may become fibrosed, thickened, and incompetent. Associated myocardial disease may produce the appearance of a congestive cardiomyopathy. Pericardial effusion is found frequently. It may be possible to visualize intracardiac rheumatoid nodules by echocardiography (Figs. 11–84 to 11–86).

Ankylosing spondylitis. Aortic regurgitation is the typical valvular lesion in patients with ankylosing spondylitis. The signs of congestive cardiomyopathy may be present.

Physical and Toxic Causes

Radiation. Radiation therapy directed at the thorax may damage the heart and great vessels (Figs. 11–87 to 11–89). Pericardial fibrosis occurs most commonly. Pericardial effusion and pericardial constriction are often seen.[87] Myocardial fibrosis and endocardial fibrosis can occur. The latter may produce valvular insufficiency secondary to valvular distortion. Valvular fibrosis can produce insufficiency.

Trauma. Trauma to the chest may produce cardiac contusion. Echocardiographically, a pericardial effusion and ventricular thrombi may be apparent.

Ethyl Alcohol. Alcoholic cardiomyopathy may be indistinguishable from idiopathic congestive cardiomyopathy because their echocardiographic findings are similar.[88]

Adriamycin. Echocardiography has been used in an attempt to detect preclinical left ventricular dysfunction in patients receiving Adriamycin.[89]

Anorexia Nervosa. Decreased left ventricular mass has been described in patients with anorexia nervosa.[90]

11.7 LEFT VENTRICULAR MASSES

Ports et al.[91] have reviewed the echocardiographic findings in patients with left ventricular masses.

Left Ventricular Thrombus. Left ventricular thrombus is found in several cardiac pathologic processes and is not uncommon in the presence of primary myocardial disease and coronary artery disease. Left ventricular thrombi are seen frequently during acute myocardial infarction and within left ventricular aneurysms. Echocardiographically,[92–97] left ventricular thrombi appear as echo-producing masses attached to the endocardial surface of the left ventricle (Figs. 11–90, 11–91). Often thrombi have areas of increased echo density in the borders of the left ventricle (Fig. 11–92) and an undulating or sometimes vibratory motion. A large thrombus may partially fill the cardiac apex, whose borders continue in a fairly uninterrupted mode within the left ventricular endocardium. In this situation recognition of the thrombus may be more difficult.

The best echocardiographic view in which to detect mural thrombi is the two-dimensional apical four-chamber view. This approach may demonstrate the presence of a thrombus not seen on the left parasternal views (Figs. 11–93, 11–94).

Left Ventricular Tumors. Intracardiac left ventricular tumors are rare. They may be intracavitary, in which case they appear as echo-dense masses attached to one of the ventricular walls and protruding into the left ventricular cavity, or they may be mural, in which case they are seen to involve the walls of the left ventricle and may extend into the ventricular cavity.[98–100]

Extracardiac Tumors. Most tumors that involve the left ventricle are extracardiac, arising from the anterior or posterior mediastinum (Figs. 11–95 to 11–99). Such tumors have variable echo density and may produce cardiac compression.[101] A large anterior tumor may simulate an anterior pericardial effusion. Mediastinal cysts and pericardial cysts can also displace the heart.[102]

False Tendons of the Left Ventricle. In about 1 per cent of the normal population, anomalous chordae are attached from a papillary muscle or lateral wall to the septum (Figs. 11–100, 11–101).[103–105] Occasionally, these chordae may be rather prominent and appear as a large intracardiac mass (Figs. 11–102, 11–103).

FIGURE 11–1

LEFT VENTRICLE, TWO-DIMENSIONAL AND M-MODE

Long-axis parasternal view of the left ventricle (LV) with an M-mode line in the region in which the routine left ventricular dimensions are determined. The M-mode line is immediately inferior to the tip of the mitral valve. The M-mode echocardiogram shows the right ventricle (RV), septum (S), and left ventricle. PW = posterior wall; Ao = aorta; LA = left atrium.

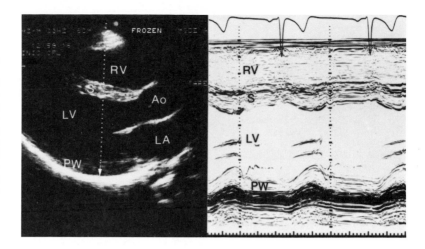

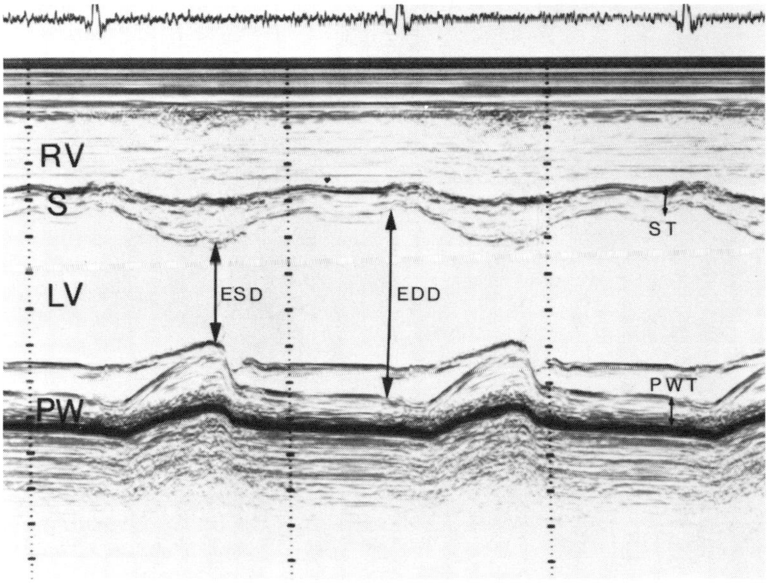

FIGURE 11–2

LEFT VENTRICLE, DIMENSIONS

The M-mode echocardiographic measurements routinely obtained include the end-diastolic (EDD) and end-systolic (ESD) diameters and the septal (ST) and posterior wall thicknesses (PWT). RV = right ventricle; S = septum; LV = left ventricle; PW = posterior wall.

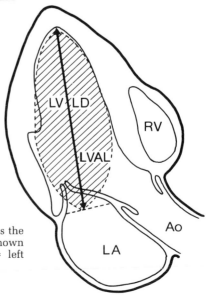

FIGURE 11–3

LONG-AXIS DIMENSION OF THE LEFT VENTRICLE

Apical long-axis view of the left ventricle. The arrow (LVLD) demonstrates the way to measure the long axis. The left ventricular area from this view is shown by the shaded ovoid (LVAL). RV = right ventricle; Ao = aorta; LA = left atrium.

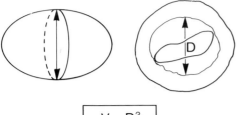

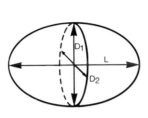

$$V = D^3$$

FIGURE 11–4
D³ METHOD, LEFT VENTRICULAR VOLUME
D is the anteroposterior diameter at the level of the tip of the mitral valve.

FIGURE 11–5
LENGTH-DIAMETER METHOD, LEFT VENTRICULAR VOLUME
D_1 is the anteroposterior diameter; D_2 is the short axis perpendicular to D_1; and L is the long axis of the left ventricle from the apical two-chamber view.

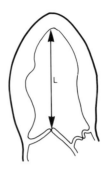

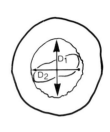

$$V = (\Pi/6)(D_1 D_2 L)$$

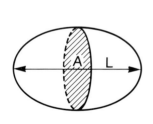

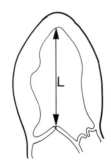

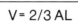

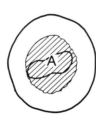

FIGURE 11–6
LENGTH-SHORT-AXIS AREA METHOD, LEFT VENTRICULAR VOLUME
A is the cross-sectional area at the level of the mitral valve, and L is the long axis of the left ventricle from the apical two-chamber view.

$$V = 2/3 \, AL$$

FIGURE 11–7
AREA-LENGTH METHOD, LEFT VENTRICULAR VOLUME
A is the area of the left ventricle from the apical two-chamber view, and L is the long axis measured from the same view.

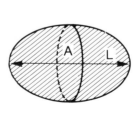

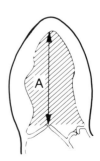

$$V = .85 \, A^2/L$$

FIGURE 11–8
"BULLET" METHOD, LEFT VENTRICULAR VOLUME
A is the area of the cross section at the level of the mitral valve, and L is the long axis measured from the apical two-chamber view.

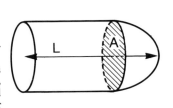
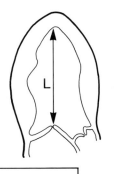
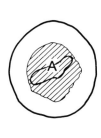

$$V = 5/6\ AL$$

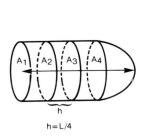

$V=$

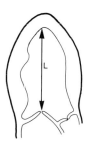

FIGURE 11–9
SIMPSON'S RULE METHOD, LEFT VENTRICULAR VOLUME
A_1, A_2, A_3, and A_4 are serial cross-sectional areas from the mitral level to the apex, and L is the long axis from the apical two-chamber view.

$h = L/4$

$$V = \left[(A_1 + A_2 + A_3)h\right] + \left[(A_4 h/2) + (\Pi/6)(h^3)\right]$$

FIGURE 11–10
LEFT VENTRICULAR MASS
By subtracting the left ventricular endocardial volume (LVVen) from the left ventricular epicardial volume (LVVep) and multiplying this number by the specific gravity of the muscle (1:055), it is possible to approximate the left ventricular mass (LVM).

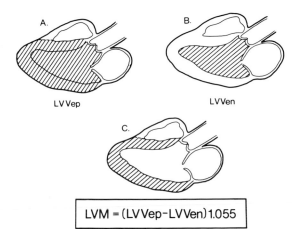

A.

B.

LV Vep

LVVen

C.

$$LVM = (LVVep - LVVen)\,1.055$$

MEDIAL ANGULATION

LATERAL ANGULATION

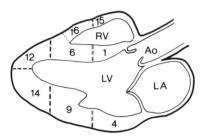
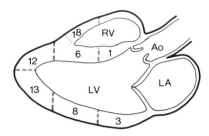

FIGURE 11–11
LONG-AXIS PARASTERNAL VIEWS
These views permit visualization of the basal (1) and middle septum (6) as well as of the inferior (9, 4) and inferolateral (8, 3) walls. The true apex (12, 14) usually cannot be recorded from this view.

MITRAL VALVE LEVEL

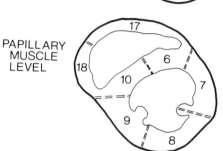

FIGURE 11–12
SHORT-AXIS PARASTERNAL VIEWS
At the mitral valve level, it is possible to visualize the basal septum (5, 1), the anterolateral wall (2, 3), and the posterobasal wall (4). At the papillary muscle level, the middle septum (10, 6) is registered, as well as the middle anterolateral (7, 8) and inferior walls (9). At the apical level, the inferoapical (14) and anteroapical (12, 13) regions are recorded.

PAPILLARY MUSCLE LEVEL

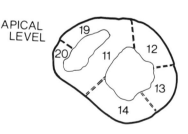

APICAL LEVEL

INFERIOR WALL

ANTERIOR WALL

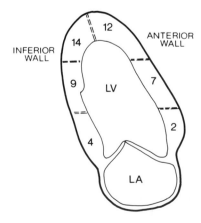

LATERAL WALL

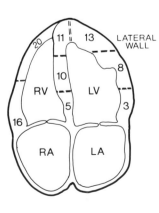

FIGURE 11–13
APICAL VIEWS
From the apical four-chamber view *(left)* it is possible to visualize the apex (11, 13), the basal (5) and middle septum (10), and the lateral wall (8, 3). From the apical two-chamber view *(right)* it is possible to visualize the apex (14, 12), and the anterior (7, 2) and inferoposterior walls (9, 4).

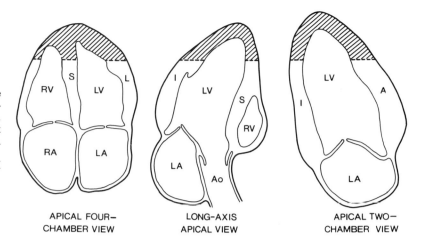

FIGURE 11–14
VENTRICULAR APEX
This area is seen best from the apical four-chamber, two-chamber, and apical long-axis views. RV = right ventricle; LV = left ventricle; RA = right atrium; LA = left atrium; S = septum; A = anterior wall; L = lateral wall; I = inferior wall; Ao = aorta.

APICAL FOUR–CHAMBER VIEW

LONG-AXIS APICAL VIEW

APICAL TWO–CHAMBER VIEW

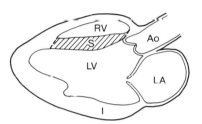

PARASTERNAL LONG-AXIS VIEW

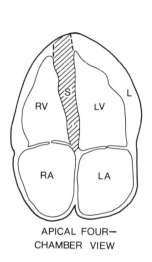

APICAL FOUR–CHAMBER VIEW

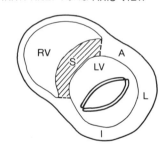

PARASTERNAL SHORT–AXIS VIEW

FIGURE 11–15
INTERVENTRICULAR SEPTUM
This area is seen best from the left parasternal long- and short-axis and apical four-chamber views. RV = right ventricle; LV = left ventricle; RA = right atrium; LA = left atrium; S = septum; L = lateral wall; I = inferior wall; Ao = aorta; A = anterior wall.

FIGURE 11–16
ANTERIOR WALL
This area is seen best from the apical two-chamber and short-axis parasternal views. RV = right ventricle; S = septum; LV = left ventricle; LA = left atrium; I = inferior wall; A = anterior wall; L = lateral wall.

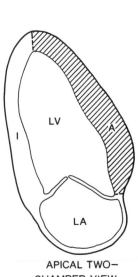

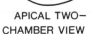

APICAL TWO–CHAMBER VIEW

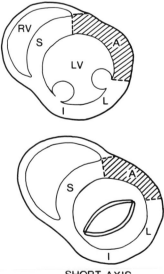

SHORT-AXIS PARASTERNAL VIEW

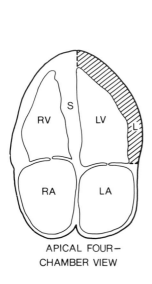

APICAL FOUR–
CHAMBER VIEW

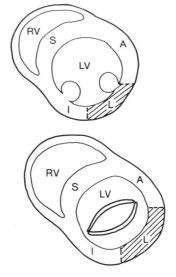

SHORT–AXIS
PARASTERNAL VIEW

FIGURE 11–17
LATERAL WALL
This area is seen best from the apical four-chamber and parasternal short-axis views. RV = right ventricle; S = septum; LV = left ventricle; RA = right atrium; LA = left atrium; L = lateral wall; A = anterior wall; I = inferior wall.

FIGURE 11–18
INFERIOR WALL
This area is seen best from the apical two-chamber and parasternal short- and long-axis views. RV = right ventricle; S = septum; LV = left ventricle; Ao = aorta; LA = left atrium; I = inferior wall; A = anterior wall; L = lateral wall.

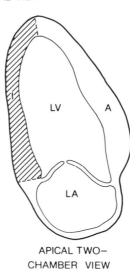

APICAL TWO–
CHAMBER VIEW

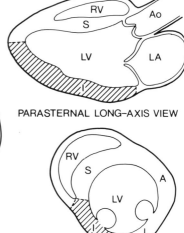

PARASTERNAL LONG–AXIS VIEW

PARASTERNAL SHORT–AXIS VIEW

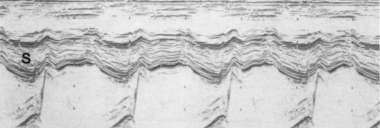
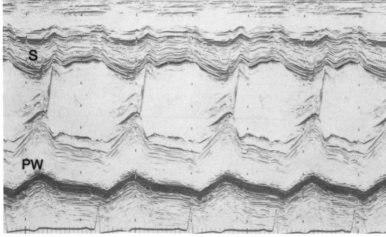

FIGURE 11–19
CONCENTRIC LEFT VENTRICULAR HYPERTROPHY
Echocardiogram of the left ventricle in a 15-year-old boy with severe aortic stenosis (120 mm Hg gradient) and left ventricular hypertrophy. The posterior wall (PW) thickness is 18 mm. The septum (S) measures 13 mm wide. The left ventricular cavity size is small. These findings are typical of concentric left ventricular hypertrophy.

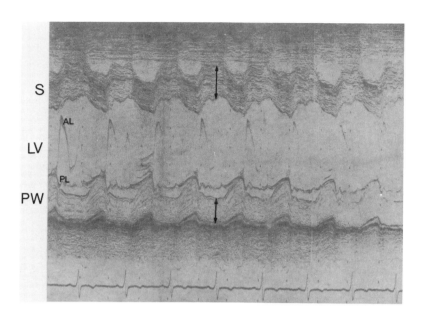

FIGURE 11–20
LEFT VENTRICULAR HYPERTROPHY
Echocardiogram recorded in a
patient with systemic hypertension with left ventricular hypertrophy and a septum (S) thicker
(18 mm) than the posterior wall
(PW) (13 mm). The outflow tract
is normal in size. There was no
systolic anterior motion of the
mitral valve to suggest hypertrophic cardiomyopathy. LV =
left ventricle; AL = anterior leaflet; PL = posterior leaflet.

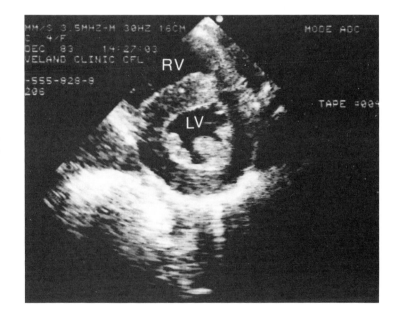

FIGURE 11–21
LEFT VENTRICULAR HYPERTROPHY
Short-axis parasternal view in a patient with severe left ventricular hypertrophy secondary to hypertension.
All ventricular walls are thickened.
The papillary muscles are quite
prominent. RV = right ventricle; LV
= left ventricle.

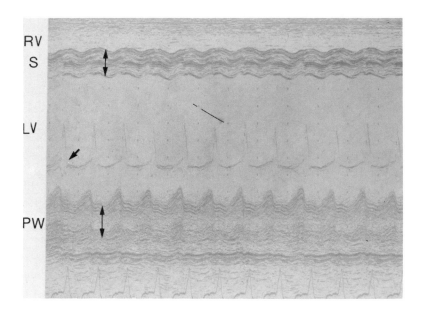

FIGURE 11-22
ECCENTRIC LEFT VENTRICULAR HY-
PERTROPHY
This view in a patient with severe long-term aortic insufficiency demonstrates a thickened
septum (S) (15 mm) and posterior wall (PW) (20 mm). There is
also marked left ventricular dilatation, which makes the left
ventricular hypertrophy appear
less marked. This type of left
ventricular hypertrophy is associated with the largest increase
in left ventricular mass. RV =
right ventricle; LV = left ventricle.

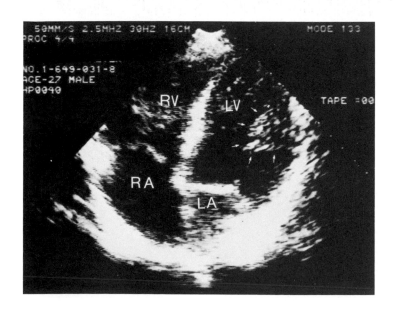

FIGURE 11-23
LARGE PAPILLARY MUSCLES, LEFT VEN-
TRICULAR HYPERTROPHY
Apical four-chamber view in a 27-
year-old man with renal failure and
severe chronic hypertension. The arrows point to a very large anterolateral papillary muscle, which fills
part of the left ventricular cavity. Care
must be taken not to confuse this
condition with a ventricular thrombus. RV = right ventricle; LV = left
ventricle; RA = right atrium; LA =
left atrium.

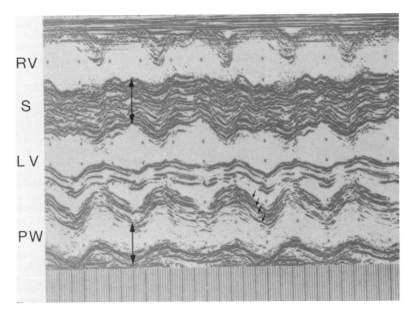

FIGURE 11–24
PROMINENT TRABECULAE CARNEAE, LEFT VENTRICULAR HYPERTROPHY
Echocardiogram of the left ventricle (LV) in a patient with long-term hypertension and severe left ventricular hypertrophy. Because of prominent trabeculae carneae, multiple parallel lines are recorded at the level of the posterior wall (PW) endocardium (small arrows). S = septum; RV = right ventricle.

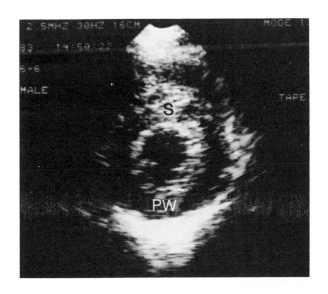

FIGURE 11–25
PROMINENT TRABECULAE CARNEAE
Short-axis left parasternal view in a patient with severe left ventricular hypertrophy. Note the prominent trabeculae carneae visible in the endocardial surface. S = septum; PW = posterior wall.

FIGURE 11–26
HYPERTENSIVE CARDIOVASCULAR DISEASE
Echocardiographic scan from the left ventricle to the aorta in a patient with severe long-term hypertension. There is marked left ventricular hypertrophy, decreased diastolic posterior wall velocity, and mild dilatation of the left atrium.

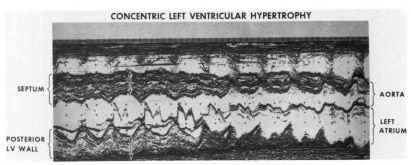

CONCENTRIC LEFT VENTRICULAR HYPERTROPHY

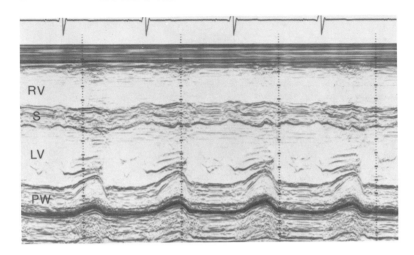

FIGURE 11–27
LEFT VENTRICULAR HYPERTROPHY IN AN ATHLETE
Left ventricular hypertrophy is seen in this view from a weight lifter who had normal blood pressure and no cardiac symptoms or findings. RV = right ventricle; S = septum; LV = left ventricle; PW = posterior wall.

FIGURE 11–28
CONGESTIVE CARDIOMYOPATHY
Left ventricular echocardiogram recorded from a 55-year-old woman with severe congestive heart failure secondary to primary myocardial disease. There is marked dilatation of the end-diastolic (9 cm) and end-systolic (7.5 cm) dimensions. RV = right ventricle; LV = left ventricle; PW = posterior wall.

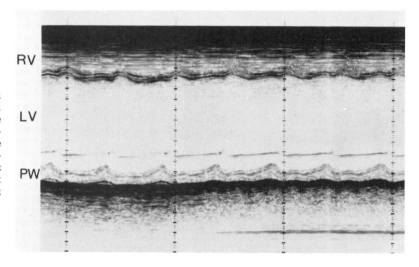

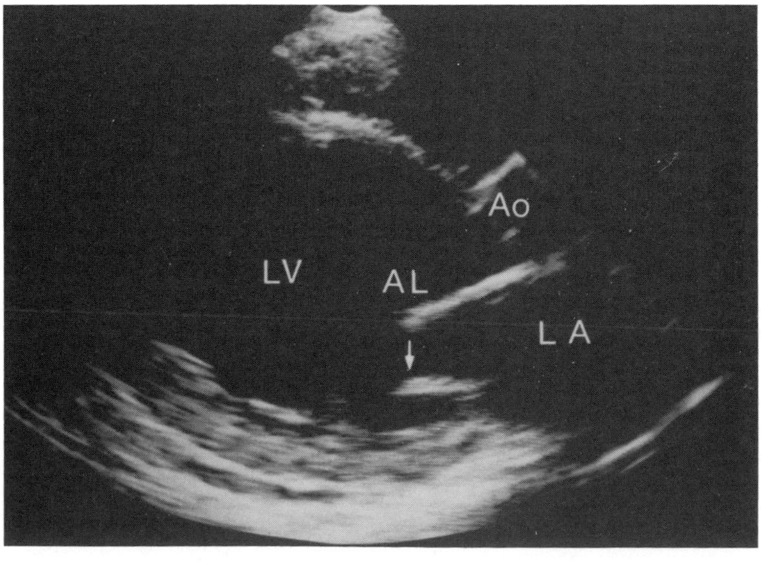

FIGURE 11–29
CONGESTIVE CARDIOMYOPATHY
Long-axis parasternal view of the left ventricle (LV) in a patient with severe congestive cardiomyopathy. There is marked left ventricular dilatation. Because of decreased cardiac output there is reduced mitral valve excursion (arrow). AL = anterior leaflet; Ao = aorta; LA = left atrium.

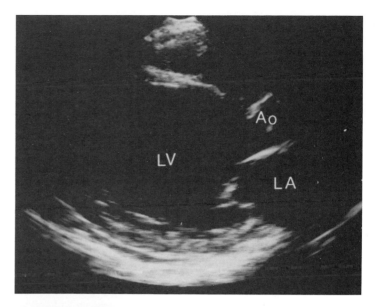

FIGURE 11–30
CONGESTIVE CARDIOMYOPATHY
Long-axis left parasternal view in the same patient as in Figure 11–29. Note the dilated left ventricle (LV) and left atrium (LA). Although this is a systolic frame, there is no apparent change in ventricular size in comparison with the view recorded in diastole (Fig. 11–29). Ao = aorta.

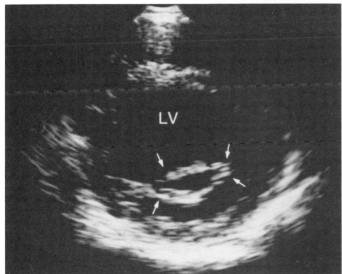

FIGURE 11–31
CONGESTIVE CARDIOMYOPATHY
Short-axis left parasternal view at the level of the mitral valve in the same patient as in Figure 11–29. Note the small mitral valve orifice size that is related to decreased cardiac output. LV = left ventricle.

FIGURE 11–32
CONGESTIVE CARDIOMYOPATHY
Apical four-chamber view in a patient with severe congestive cardiomyopathy. Note the globular dilatation of the left ventricle (LV). All other cardiac chambers are also somewhat enlarged. RV = right ventricle; RA = right atrium; LA = left atrium.

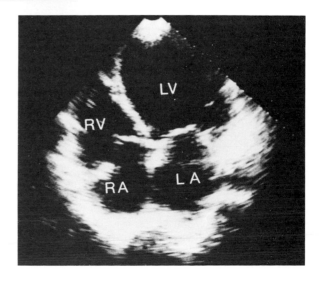

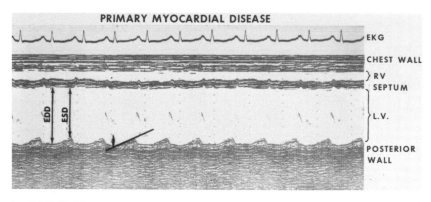

FIGURE 11–33
CONGESTIVE CARDIOMYOPATHY
Echocardiogram of the left ventricle (LV) in a patient with primary myocardial disease and severe left ventricular dysfunction. There is marked dilatation of the end-diastolic and end-systolic diameters as well as decreased systolic left ventricular function. RV = right ventricle.

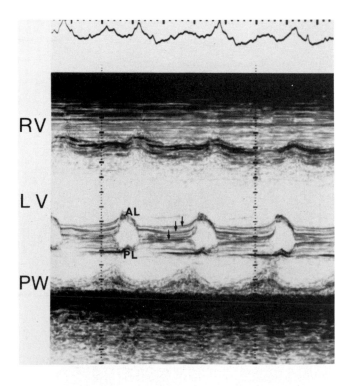

FIGURE 11–34
CONGESTIVE CARDIOMYOPATHY
Echocardiogram recorded at mitral level in a patient with primary myocardial disease, severe left ventricular dysfunction, and evidence of low cardiac output as shown by decreased mitral valve excursion and increased mitral E point to septum. Multiple systolic echoes at the level of the mitral valve are frequently observed in this condition (arrows). RV = right ventricle; LV = left ventricle; PW = posterior wall; AL = anterior leaflet; PL = posterior leaflet.

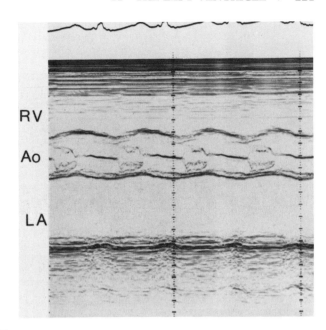

FIGURE 11–35
CONGESTIVE CARDIOMYOPATHY
Echocardiogram recorded at aortic level in the same patient as in Figure 11–34. There is decreased aortic valve excursion and decreased aortic wall amplitude—both signs of low cardiac output. RV = right ventricle; Ao = aorta; LA = left atrium.

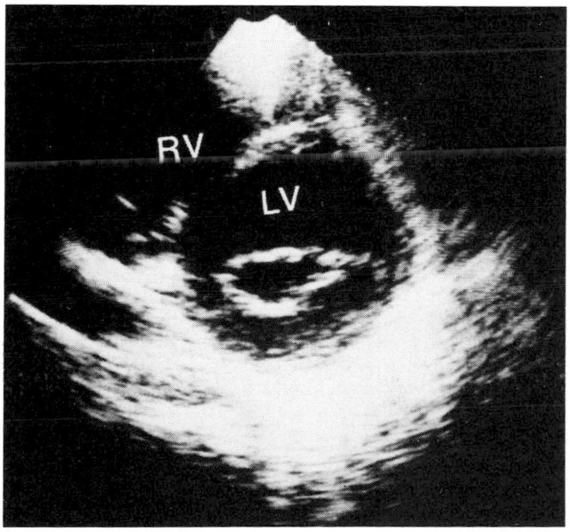

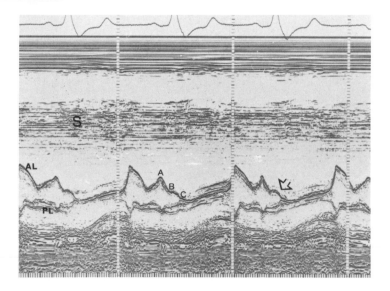

FIGURE 11–36
CONGESTIVE CARDIOMYOPATHY
Short-axis parasternal view of the left ventricle (LV) at the level of the mitral valve in a patient with severe congestive cardiomyopathy. There is marked reduction in the mitral orifice area that is caused by decreased cardiac output. RV = right ventricle.

FIGURE 11–37
INCREASED END-DIASTOLIC LEFT VENTRICULAR PRESSURE
This echocardiogram of the mitral valve shows a prominent B notch *(arrow)* in a patient with severe congestive heart failure and increased end-diastolic left ventricular pressure. AL = anterior leaflet; PL = posterior leaflet; S = septum.

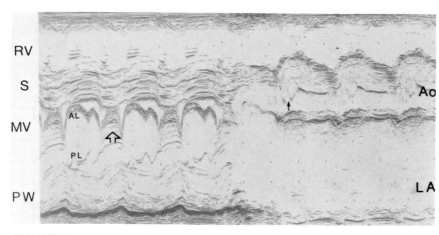

FIGURE 11–38
HYPERTROPHIC OBSTRUCTIVE CARDIOMYOPATHY
This echocardiographic scan from the left ventricle to the aorta (Ao) demonstrates most of the abnormalities seen in patients with hypertrophic cardiomyopathy. These include asymmetric septal hypertrophy, systolic anterior motion of the mitral valve (*open arrow*), mid-systolic notching of the aortic valve (*small arrow*), and large left atrium (LA). This study was obtained from a 31-year-old woman with a gradient of 70 mm Hg in the left ventricular outflow tract. RV = right ventricle; S = septum; MV = mitral valve; PW = posterior wall; AL = anterior leaflet; PL = posterior leaflet.

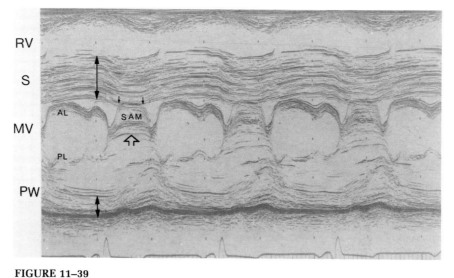

FIGURE 11–39
HYPERTROPHIC OBSTRUCTIVE CARDIOMYOPATHY
Echocardiogram recorded at the level of the left ventricle and mitral valve in the same patient as in Figure 11–38. The large arrows point to the asymmetric septal hypertrophy (septum 2.2 cm, posterior wall 1.1 cm). The open arrow points to the systolic anterior motion (SAM) of the mitral valve (MV). The small arrows point to the septal-mitral valve coaptation during systole. RV = right ventricle; S = septum; PW = posterior wall; AL = anterior leaflet; PL = posterior leaflet.

FIGURE 11–40

HYPERTROPHIC OBSTRUCTIVE CAR-
DIOMYOPATHY
These long- and short-axis parasternal views highlight the
asymmetric septal hypertrophy
and systolic anterior motion of
the mitral valve (MV) seen in a
patient with hypertrophic cardiomyopathy. RV = right ventricle; Ao = aorta; S = septum;
AL = anterior leaflet; PL = posterior leaflet; LV = left ventricle;
LA = left atrium.

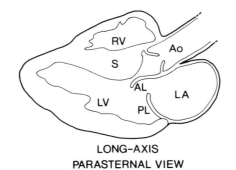

LONG-AXIS
PARASTERNAL VIEW

SHORT-AXIS
PARASTERNAL VIEW

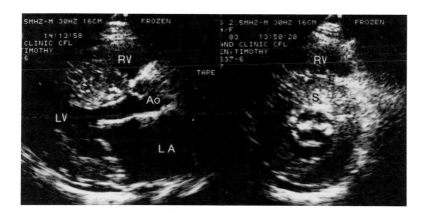

FIGURE 11–41

HYPERTROPHIC OBSTRUCTIVE CAR-
DIOMYOPATHY
Long- and short-axis views in a
37-year-old patient with obstructive cardiomyopathy (80 mm Hg
gradient). Note the thickened
septum (S), small left ventricular
cavity, and large left atrium (LA).
There is also a small pericardial
effusion. RV = right ventricle;
LV = left ventricle; Ao = aorta.

FIGURE 11–42

HYPERTROPHIC OBSTRUCTIVE CARDIOMYOPATHY
Long-axis left parasternal view in a 32-year-old
patient with hypertrophic cardiomyopathy. The
septum (S) is markedly thickened and has a
hyperrefractile left endocardial surface. The posterior wall thickness is normal *(small arrow)*.
There is mild left atrial enlargement. LV = left
ventricle; Ao = aorta; LA = left atrium.

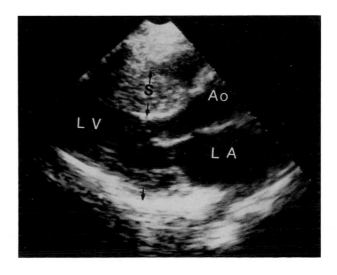

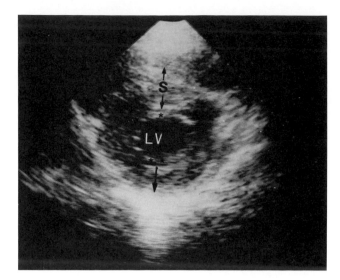

FIGURE 11–43
HYPERTROPHIC CARDIOMYOPATHY
Short-axis left parasternal view in the same patient as in Figure 11–42. This view clearly demonstrates the asymmetric septal hypertrophy. The single asterisk indicates the anterior mitral leaflet. The double asterisk marks the posterior leaflet. S = septum; LV = left ventricle.

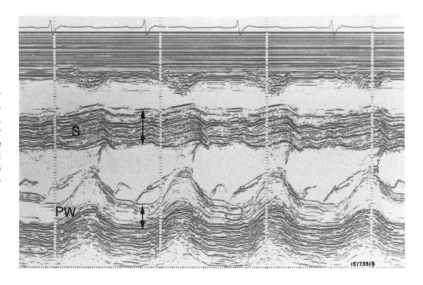

FIGURE 11–44
ASYMMETRIC SEPTAL HYPERTROPHY
Echocardiogram at the left ventricular level in a patient with hypertrophic cardiomyopathy and provokable obstruction. The septum (S) measures 2.3 cm, and the posterior wall (PW) measures 1.7 cm. The left ventricular cavity is quite small.

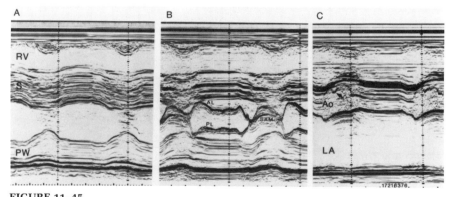

FIGURE 11–45
ASYMMETRIC SEPTAL HYPERTROPHY
Marked septal hypertrophy (3.5 cm) is seen in this patient with obstructive hypertrophic cardiomyopathy (panel A). Panel B shows the systolic anterior motion, and panel C shows midclosure of the aortic valve. RV = right ventricle; S = septum; PW = posterior wall; AL = anterior leaflet; PL = posterior leaflet; Ao = aorta; LA = left atrium.

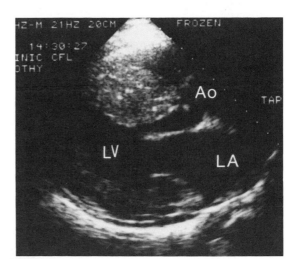

FIGURE 11–46
HYPERTROPHIC OBSTRUCTIVE CARDIOMYOPATHY
Long-axis left parasternal view in a patient with hypertrophic obstructive cardiomyopathy. Note the markedly thickened septum that has a peculiar nodular density. Ao = aorta; LV = left ventricle; LA = left atrium.

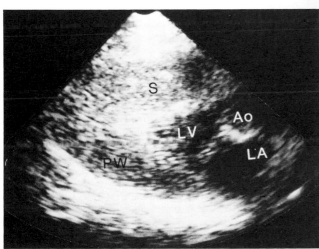

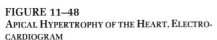

FIGURE 11–47
APICAL HYPERTROPHY OF THE HEART
Massive hypertrophy of the apex is seen in this 31-year-old man. There is marked cavity obliteration. The patient has no heart murmurs. S = septum; PW = posterior wall; LV = left ventricle; Ao = aorta; LA = left atrium.

FIGURE 11–48
APICAL HYPERTROPHY OF THE HEART, ELECTRO-CARDIOGRAM
An electrocardiogram recorded from the same patient as in Figure 11–47 shows the typical deeply inverted T waves in the lateral precordial leads.

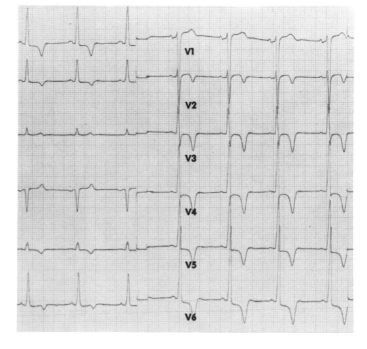

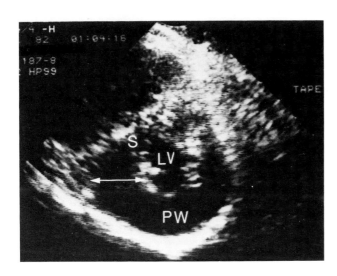

FIGURE 11–49
HYPERTROPHY IN UNUSUAL LOCATIONS, HYPER-
TROPHIC CARDIOMYOPATHY
Short-axis left parasternal view in a 42-year-
old patient with hypertrophic nonobstructive
cardiomyopathy. Note the marked thickening
of the posterior wall (PW) close to the septum
(S) (arrows). LV = left ventricle.

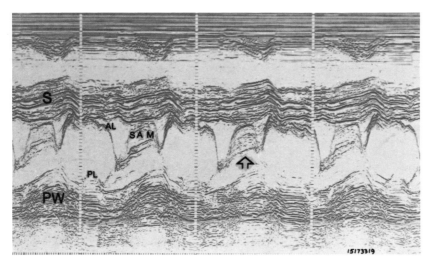

FIGURE 11–50
SYSTOLIC ANTERIOR MOTION
This echocardiogram recorded at the level of the mitral valve shows the typical
systolic anterior motion (SAM) of the mitral valve (open arrow). The SAM starts
after the point of closure of the mitral valve and ends before its opening. S =
septum; PW = posterior wall; AL = anterior leaflet; PL = posterior leaflet.

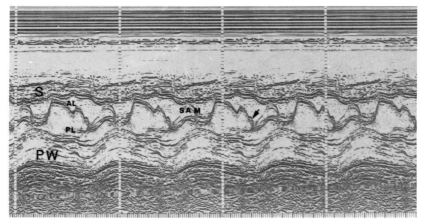

FIGURE 11–51
SYSTOLIC ANTERIOR MOTION
Mild systolic anterior motion is seen in a recording from a 34-year-old woman with a 60 mm Hg gradient in the left ventricular outflow tract. The small arrow points to a prominent B notch, which is a common finding in such patients. The asymmetric septal hypertrophy is not apparent in this view. S = septum; PW = posterior wall; AL = anterior leaflet; PL = posterior leaflet; SAM = systolic anterior motion.

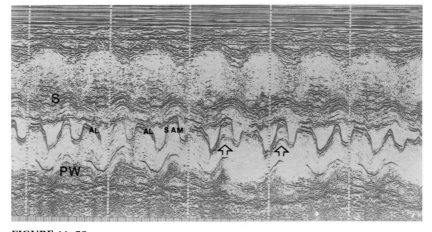

FIGURE 11–52
SYSTOLIC ANTERIOR MOTION
Variable degrees of systolic anterior motion are seen in this recording from a 77-year-old patient with hypertrophic cardiomyopathy and no gradient at rest. S = septum; PW = posterior wall; AL = anterior leaflet; SAM = systolic anterior motion.

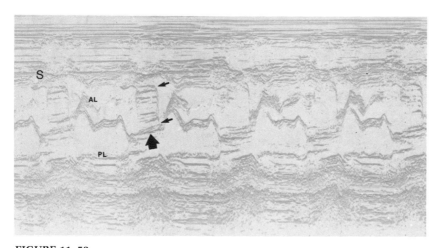

FIGURE 11–53
SYSTOLIC ANTERIOR MOTION
An unusual form of systolic anterior motion was present in a 21-year-old man with
a 30 mm Hg gradient in the left ventricular outflow tract. Note the "squared"
appearance of the systolic anterior motion (arrows). S = septum; AL = anterior
leaflet; PL = posterior leaflet.

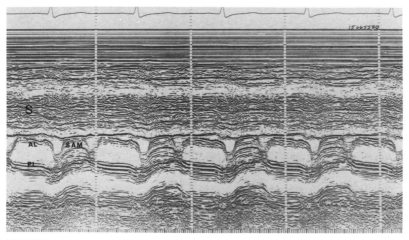

FIGURE 11–54
SYSTOLIC ANTERIOR MOTION
Marked systolic anterior motion (SAM) is seen in this recording from a 68-year-
old man. There is mitral-septal apposition during most of systole. The left
ventricular outflow tract is severely narrowed. No catheterization was performed.
S = septum; AL = anterior leaflet; PL = posterior leaflet.

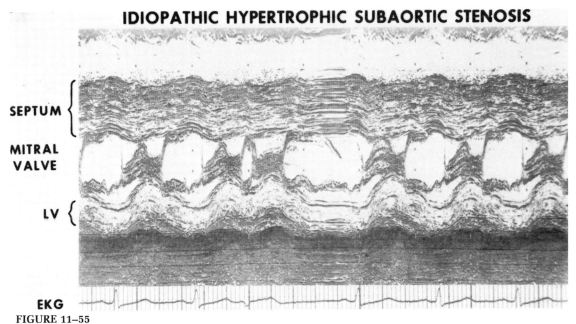

IDIOPATHIC HYPERTROPHIC SUBAORTIC STENOSIS

SEPTUM

MITRAL VALVE

LV

EKG

FIGURE 11–55
SYSTOLIC ANTERIOR MOTION AFTER PREMATURE VENTRICULAR CONTRACTION
Note the augmentation of the systolic anterior motion after the compensatory pause of a premature ventricular contraction in a patient with hypertrophic obstructive cardiomyopathy.

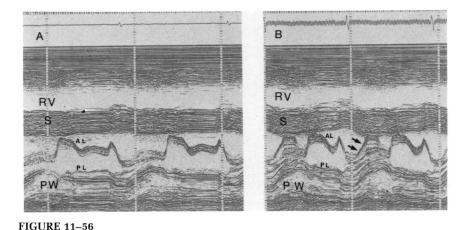

FIGURE 11–56
SYSTOLIC ANTERIOR MOTION, ADMINISTRATION OF AMYL NITRATE
Echocardiogram recorded from a 64-year-old patient with hypertrophic cardiomyopathy without obstruction at rest. Panel A shows the absence of systolic anterior motion of the mitral valve. Panel B (after amyl nitrate inhalation) shows the typical systolic anterior motion (arrows). RV = right ventricle; S = septum; PW = posterior wall; AL = anterior leaflet; PL = posterior leaflet.

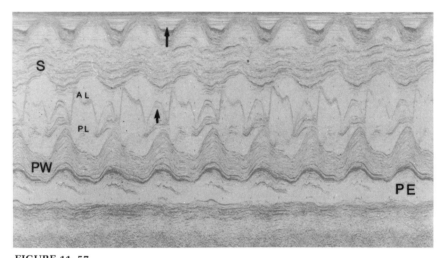

FIGURE 11–57
HYPERTROPHIC CARDIOMYOPATHY AND PERICARDIAL EFFUSION
Echocardiogram recorded in a 23-year-old man with 100 mm Hg gradient in the left ventricular outflow tract and large anterior and posterior pericardial effusion (PE). There is no swinging of the heart to explain the systolic anterior motion. S = septum; PW = posterior wall; AL = anterior leaflet; PL = posterior leaflet.

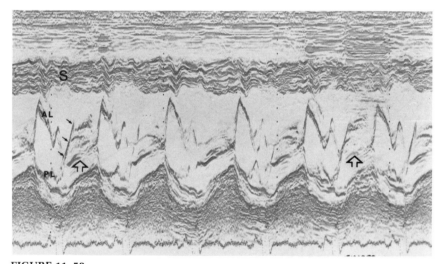

FIGURE 11–58
PSEUDOSYSTOLIC ANTERIOR MOTION
This echocardiogram at the mitral valve level shows chordae tendineae in the outflow tract (arrows) that simulate systolic anterior motion of the mitral valve. Note the normal septal thickness and the normal left ventricular outflow tract. S = septum; AL = anterior leaflet; PL = posterior leaflet.

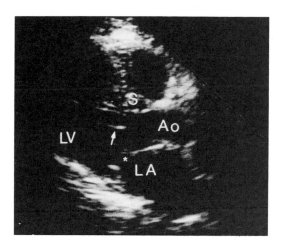

FIGURE 11–59
PSEUDOSYSTOLIC ANTERIOR MOTION
A long-axis left parasternal view recorded in the same patient as in Figure 11–58 shows a chordae tendineae in the left ventricular outflow tract *(arrow)*. Note the normal position of the mitral valve (∗). LV = left ventricle; S = septum; Ao = aorta; LA = left atrium.

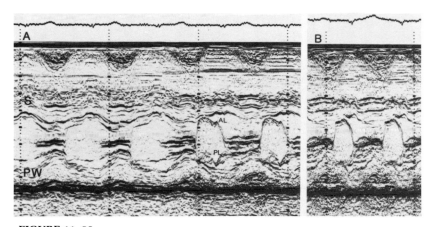

FIGURE 11–60
NONOBSTRUCTIVE HYPERTROPHIC CARDIOMYOPATHY
Echocardiograms recorded at rest *(A)* and after amyl nitrate inhalation *(B)* in a 24-year-old patient with hypertrophic cardiomyopathy. There is asymmetric septal hypertrophy but no systolic anterior motion of the mitral valve. The patient had a family history of hypertrophic cardiomyopathy but no cardiac symptoms or findings. S = septum; PW = posterior wall; AL = anterior leaflet; PL = posterior leaflet.

FIGURE 11–61
NONOBSTRUCTIVE HYPERTROPHIC CARDIOMYOPATHY
This echocardiogram recorded at the mitral valve level shows asymmetric septal hypertrophy without systolic anterior motion. S = septum; PW = posterior wall; AL = anterior leaflet; PL = posterior leaflet.

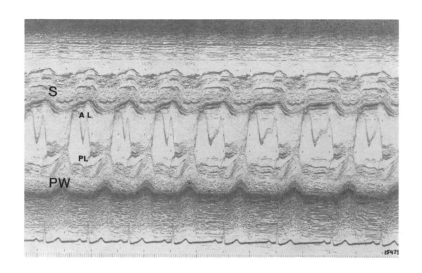

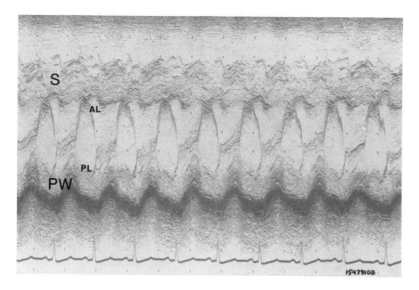

FIGURE 11–62
NONOBSTRUCTIVE HYPERTROPHIC CARDIOMYOPATHY
Echocardiogram from the same patient as in Figure 11–61 but after amyl nitrate inhalation. Note the significant increase in heart rate without systolic anterior motion of the mitral valve. S = septum; PW = posterior wall; AL = anterior leaflet; PL = posterior leaflet.

FIGURE 11–63
NONOBSTRUCTIVE HYPERTROPHIC CARDIOMYOPATHY
Long-axis left parasternal view in an 18-year-old man with a severe form of hypertrophic cardiomyopathy and no outflow tract obstruction. Note the marked hypertrophy of both the septum and the posterior wall. S = septum; PW = posterior wall; Ao = aorta; LA = left atrium.

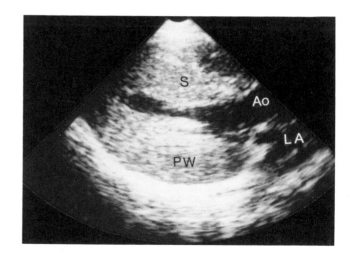

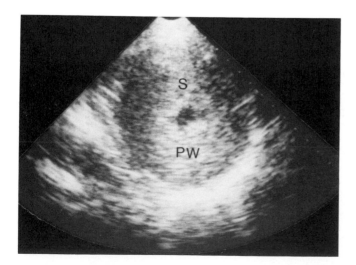

FIGURE 11–64
NONOBSTRUCTIVE HYPERTROPHIC CARDIOMYOPATHY
This short-axis parasternal view in the same patient as in Figure 11–63 shows severe left ventricular hypertrophy and cavity obliteration. S = septum; PW = posterior wall.

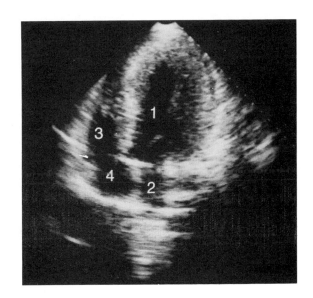

FIGURE 11–65
NONOBSTRUCTIVE HYPERTROPHIC CARDIOMYOPATHY
This apical four-chamber view in the same patient as in Figure 11–63 shows generalized left ventricular hypertrophy and a large lateral papillary muscle. (1) Left ventricle; (2) left atrium; (3) right ventricle; (4) right atrium.

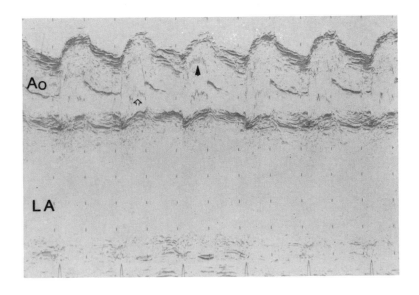

FIGURE 11–66
MID-SYSTOLIC AORTIC CLOSURE
An echocardiogram of the aortic valve in a patient with hypertrophic cardiomyopathy demonstrates mid-systolic closure of the aortic valve *(open arrow)* and systolic flutter of the right coronary cusp *(black arrow)*. There is also left atrial enlargement. Ao = aorta; LA = left atrium.

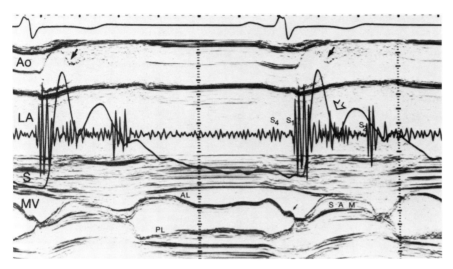

FIGURE 11–67
MID-SYSTOLIC AORTIC CLOSURE
Dual echocardiographic recording of the aorta (Ao) and mitral valve (MV). The aortic systolic semiclosure *(black arrow)* coincides with the systolic anterior motion of the mitral valve (SAM) and with the bispherins collapse of the carotid pulse *(open arow)*. LA = left atrium; S = septum; AL = anterior leaflet; PL = posterior leaflet.

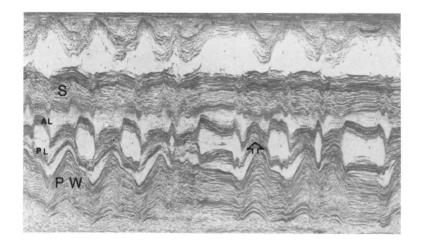

FIGURE 11–68
HYPERTROPHIC CARDIOMYOPATHY, DECREASED COMPLIANCE
Echocardiogram recorded at the mitral and left ventricular levels in a 68-year-old patient who had hypertrophic cardiomyopathy with severe septal and posterior wall hypertrophy. Note the decreased E to F slope of the mitral valve, which is a sign of diminished left ventricular compliance. S = septum; AL = anterior leaflet; PL = posterior leaflet; PW = posterior wall.

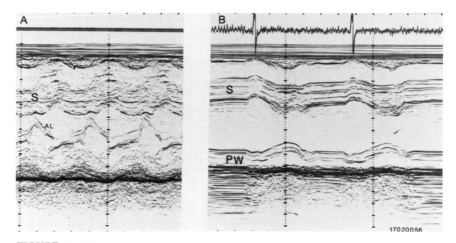

FIGURE 11–69
SEPTAL HYPERTROPHY IN LEFT VENTRICULAR HYPERTROPHY
Echocardiogram from a 35-year-old man with hypertensive cardiovascular disease. There is disproportionate septal hypertrophy. In the mitral valve there is no systolic anterior motion after amyl nitrate inhalation (panel A). S = septum; AL = anterior leaflet; PW = posterior wall.

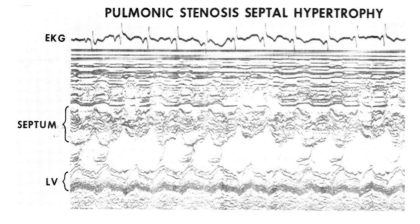

FIGURE 11–70
SEPTAL HYPERTROPHY IN RIGHT VENTRICULAR HYPERTROPHY
Echocardiogram recorded at the ventricular level in a patient with pulmonic stenosis and right ventricular hypertrophy that is manifested as disproportionate septal hypertrophy. LV = left ventricle.

FIGURE 11–71
ANGLED INTERVENTRICULAR SEPTUM
This M-mode echocardiogram shows what appears to be a massively thickened interventricular septum (S) (3.2 cm) in a 79-year-old woman. PW = posterior wall.

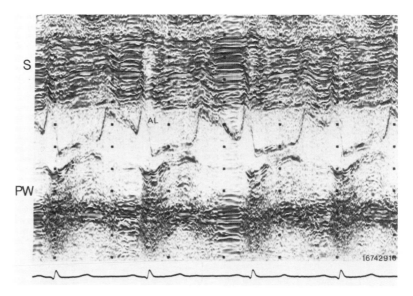

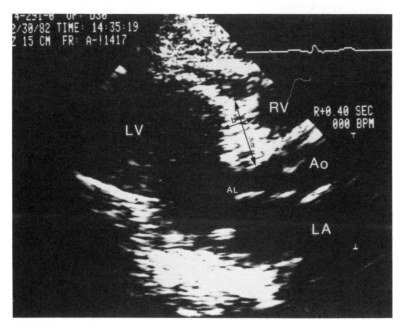

FIGURE 11–72
ANGLED INTERVENTRICULAR SEPTUM
Long-axis left parasternal view in the same patient as in Figure 11–71. Marked septal angulation makes the septum appear much thicker than it really is because the sector line runs parallel to the long axis of the basal septum. The M-mode echo goes through the septum along arrow a. The true septal thickness is arrow b. LV = left ventricle; RV = right ventricle; Ao = aorta; AL = anterior leaflet; LA = left atrium.

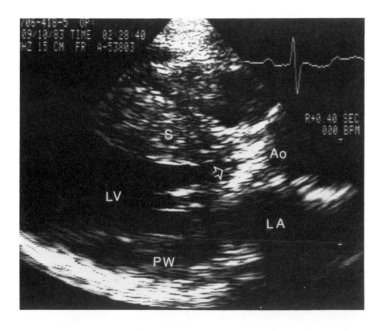

FIGURE 11–73
HYPERTROPHIC CARDIOMYOPATHY AND AORTIC STENOSIS
Long-axis left parasternal view in a patient with aortic stenosis (40 mm Hg gradient) and idiopathic hypertrophic subaortic stenosis (120 mm Hg gradient). S = septum; LV = left ventricle; PW = posterior wall; Ao = aorta; LA = left atrium.

FIGURE 11–74
HYPERTROPHIC CARDIOMYOPATHY AND AORTIC STENOSIS
Short-axis left parasternal view in the same patient as in Figure 11–73. Note the markedly thickened septum (S). PW = posterior wall.

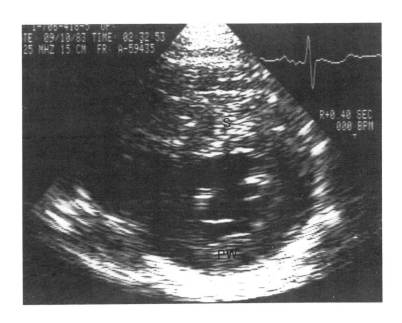

FIGURE 11–75
APEXPHONOCARDIOGRAM IN HYPERTROPHIC CARDIOMYOPATHY
The apexcardiogram (ACG) shows a prominent a wave and mid-systolic retraction. A fourth heart sound and a soft systolic ejection murmur are recorded in the phonocardiogram.

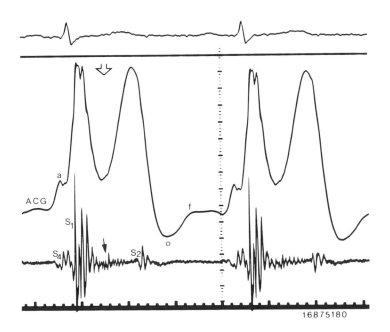

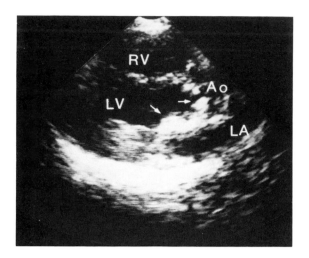

FIGURE 11–87
RADIATION CARDITIS
Echocardiogram recorded from a young female who had received several large radiation doses for treatment of Hodgkin's lymphoma. The long-axis left parasternal view demonstrates marked thickening of both the aortic and the mitral valves (arrows). RV = right ventricle; LV = left ventricle; Ao = aorta; LA = left atrium.

FIGURE 11–88
RADIATION CARDITIS
Short-axis parasternal view at the level of the mitral valve in the same patient as in Figure 11–87. The mitral valve orifice size is normal, and the anterior leaflet is markedly thickened.

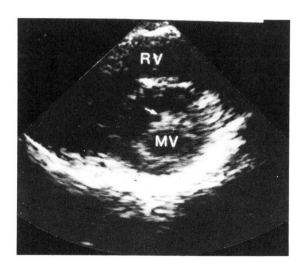

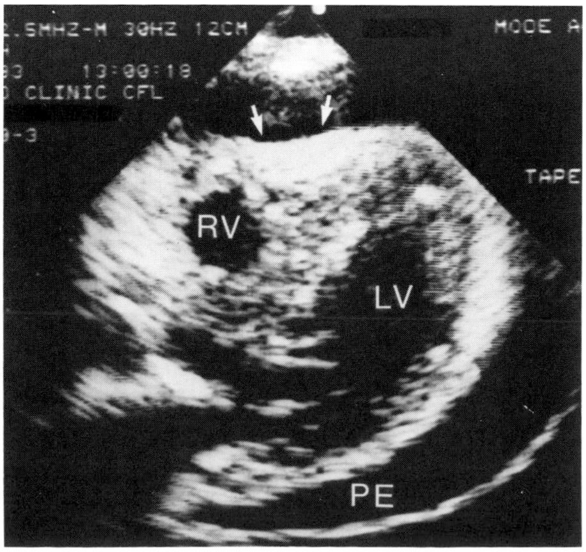

FIGURE 11–89
RADIATION CARDITIS
Apical four-chamber view in a patient with carcinoma of the breast and radiation-induced myocarditis. Note the dense fibrosis at the level of the right ventricular free wall (arrows). A large pericardial effusion (PE) is also evident. RV = right ventricle; LV = left ventricle.

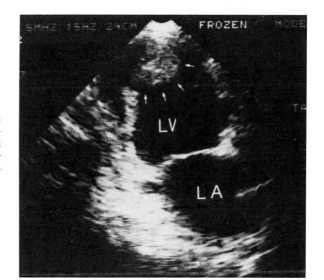

FIGURE 11–90
LEFT VENTRICULAR THROMBUS
Apical two-chamber view in a 74-year-old patient with a history of an anteroapical myocardial infarction. A large thrombus is seen in the apex (arrows). It appears as a round echo-dense mass in direct continuity with the endocardium. LV = left ventricle; LA = left atrium.

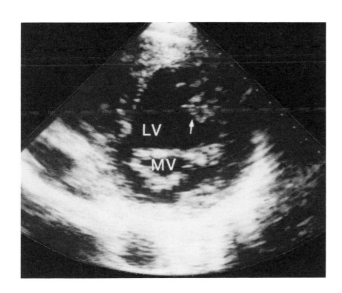

FIGURE 11–91
LEFT VENTRICULAR THROMBUS
Left parasternal view in a 75-year-old patient with a remote anterior wall myocardial infarction. A large thrombus is seen in the area of the anterior wall (arrow). LV = left ventricle; MV = mitral valve.

FIGURE 11–92
LEFT VENTRICULAR THROMBUS
Apical two-chamber view in a 53-year-old patient with a remote anteroapical infarction. An echo-dense round mass representing a large thrombus is seen in the apex (arrows). LV = left ventricle.

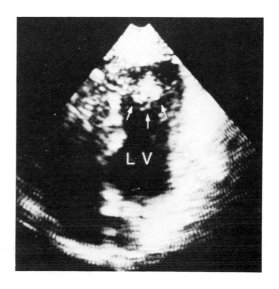

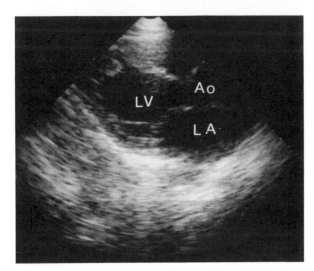

FIGURE 11–93
LEFT VENTRICULAR THROMBUS
Echocardiogram in a 31-year-old patient with congestive cardiomyopathy. A thrombus is not clearly seen in this long-axis left parasternal view. LV = left ventricle; Ao = aorta; LA = left atrium.

FIGURE 11–94
LEFT VENTRICULAR THROMBUS
Apical four-chamber view in the same patient as in Figure 11–93. A large thrombus is clearly seen at the left ventricular apex (arrows). RV = right ventricle; LV = left ventricle; RA = right atrium; LA = left atrium.

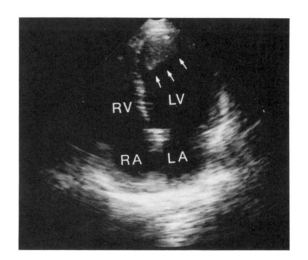

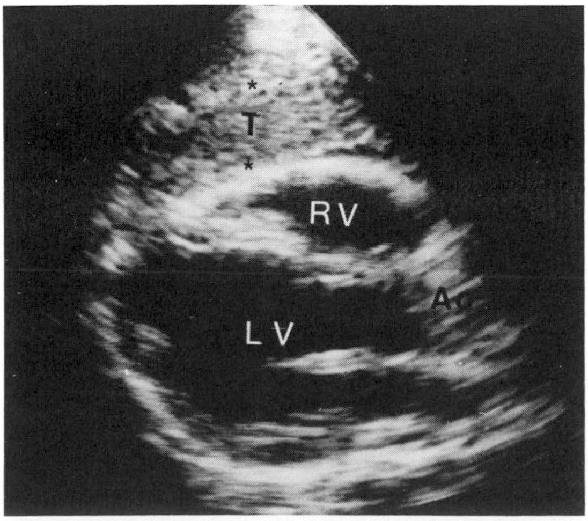

FIGURE 11–95
EXTRACARDIAC TUMOR
Echocardiogram recorded from a 19-year-old patient with a lymphosarcoma. This long-axis left parasternal view demonstrates a tumor (T) in front of the right ventricle (RV). The asterisks mark the border of the mass. LV = left ventricle; Ao = aorta.

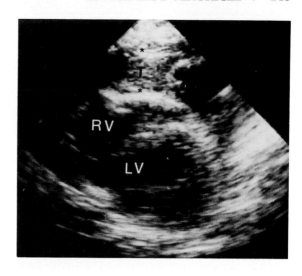

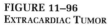

FIGURE 11–96
EXTRACARDIAC TUMOR
This short-axis left parasternal view shows the anterior mass (T) in the same patient as in Figure 11–95. RV = right ventricle; LV = left ventricle.

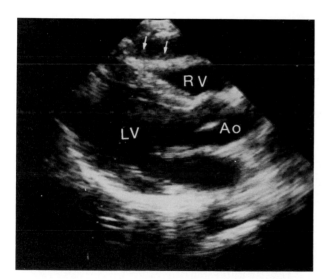

FIGURE 11–97
EXTRACARDIAC TUMOR, AFTER THERAPY
Long-axis left parasternal views from the same patient as in Figure 11–95 but after chemotherapy. Note the lysis of the tumor, with almost complete disappearance of the mass. The arrows point to an empty space where the tumor used to be. RV = right ventricle; LV = left ventricle; Ao = aorta.

FIGURE 11–98
EXTRACARDIAC TUMOR
M-mode echocardiogram recorded from an 18-year-old patient with a lymphosarcoma extending to the anterior mediastinum. Note the large, echodense area (T) in front of the right ventricle (RV) (arrow). S = septum; LV = left ventricle; T = tumor.

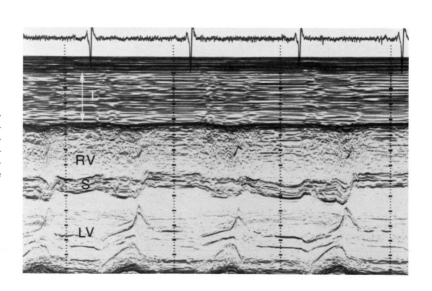

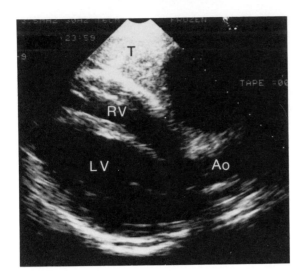

FIGURE 11–99
EXTRACARDIAC TUMOR
Long-axis left parasternal view in the same patient as in Figure 11–98. The large tumor (T) is seen to compress the right ventricle (RV). LV = left ventricle; Ao = aorta.

FIGURE 11–100
FALSE TENDON
Apical four-chamber view demonstrating a false tendon of the left ventricle (LV) *(arrows)*. The false tendon goes from the tip of the lateral papillary muscle to the middle septum. RV = right ventricle; AL = anterior leaflet; PL = posterior leaflet; LA = left atrium.

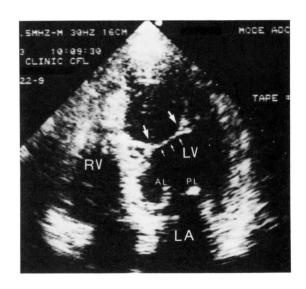

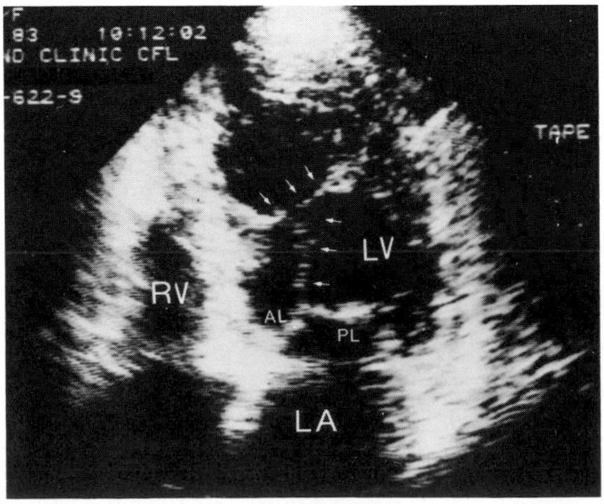

FIGURE 11–101
FALSE TENDON
Apical four-chamber view in the same patient as in Figure 11–100. In this slightly more posterior view, another false tendon can be seen to traverse the left ventricle in its longitudinal axis, from the anterior mitral leaflet (LA) to the septum. RV = right ventricle; LV = left ventricle; AL = anterior leaflet; PL = posterior leaflet.

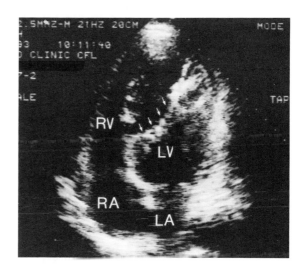

FIGURE 11–102
FALSE TENDON
Apical four-chamber view in a patient with recurrent ventricular tachycardia. A wide band is seen to traverse the left ventricle (LV) from its lateral wall to the septum (arrows). RV = right ventricle; RA = right atrium; LA = left atrium.

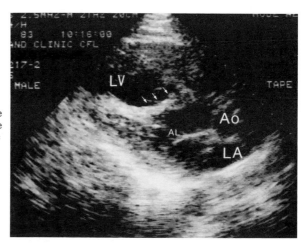

FIGURE 11–103
FALSE TENDON
Left parasternal long-axis view demonstrating a dense band of echoes from the interventricular septum to the posterior wall (arrows). LV = left ventricle; AL = anterior leaflet; Ao = aorta; LA = left atrium.

12 CORONARY ARTERY DISEASE

12.1 CORONARY ARTERY VISUALIZATION

The discovery that the left main coronary artery could be visualized by two-dimensional echocardiography stimulated several groups of investigators to evaluate the possible clinical applications of two-dimensional echocardiography in the direct diagnosis and exclusion of coronary artery occlusions.

With two-dimensional echocardiography it is possible to visualize the proximal 1 to 2 cm of the left and right coronary arteries in most patients (Fig. 12–1).

Left Coronary Artery. Two views have been used to visualize the left coronary artery by echocardiography: (1) the short-axis left parasternal view at the level of the aorta and (2) the apical four-chamber view with slight anterior angulation to include the aorta.

1. On the short-axis parasternal view (Fig. 12–2) at the level of the aorta, the left main trunk is seen as a funnel-shaped structure that originates from the left coronary sinus and continues laterally as two parallel linear echoes. Through the cardiac cycle, the left main trunk comes in and out of the echo field, so that it is usually seen during parts of systole or diastole. Usually 1 to 2 cm of the left coronary artery can be observed.

Rarely, it may be possible to visualize the bifurcation of the left main trunk into the left anterior descending artery, which courses anteriorly, and the circumflex artery, which is posteriorly directed (Fig. 12–3).[1]

2. To visualize the left main trunk from the apical view the transducer is placed in the apex in the four-chamber position with slight anterior angulation so that the aorta and pulmonary artery are imaged. Clockwise rotation of the transducer brings the ultrasonographic scan parallel to the course of the left main trunk, which is seen as two parallel lines originating from the lateral wall of the aorta at about 2 or 3 o'clock.[2]

Right Coronary Artery. The right coronary artery is more difficult to visualize than the left main trunk. It is best recorded from the parasternal short-axis view at the level of the aorta (Figure 12–4). The right coronary ostium originates from the lateral wall of the aorta at a position corresponding to about 10 o'clock. The ostium appears as two parallel lines that are directed anteriorly and to the right.

With echocardiography,[3-6] coronary artery stenosis is recognized by (1) a focal decrease in lumen size (Fig. 12–5) and (2) an increase in the focal reflectivity of the vascular walls (Fig. 12–6).

The vessel must be viewed at a location proximal and distal to the obstruction to be sure that the luminal narrowing represents a true stenotic lesion. Also, proper gain control is essential to adequately evaluate the left main trunk for the presence or absence of disease (Fig. 12–7).

Many problems remain that need to be resolved by the echocardiographic visualization of the coronary arteries before this method can become a practical clinical tool (Figs. 12–8, 12–9).

Owing to the relatively small segment of the coronary artery that can be visualized with echocardiography, the importance of having a precise anatomic diagnosis in cases of suspected coronary artery disease, and the relatively low risk of coronary arteriography, it is unlikely that, at least in the near future, echocardiography will play an important role in the diagnosis and management of patients suspected of having coronary artery stenosis.[7]

Several *congenital coronary artery anomalies* have been characterized by echocardiography:

(a) Anomalous Origin of the Left Coronary Artery from the Pulmonary Artery. The echocardiographic abnormalities described in this condition include (1) dilated and poorly contracting left ventricle, (2) dilated right coronary artery, and (3) direct visualization of the left coronary artery originating from the pulmonary artery.[8]

(b) Coronary Artery Fistulae. The dilated coronary artery appears as two dominant parallel echoes of wide lumen that originate from the aorta in the region of the involved artery.[9, 10]

During the acute febrile state of the *mucocutaneous lymph node syndrome,* a number of M-mode echocardiographic abnormalities have been described. These include decreased septal motion, pericardial effusion, and decreased left ventricular function. Two-dimensional echocardiography may reveal the presence of coronary artery aneurysm. These lesions appear as a circular echo-free space with clearly defined borders.[11, 12]

12.2 LEFT VENTRICULAR FUNCTION IN CORONARY ARTERY DISEASE

Owing to the limited area of the left ventricle that the M-mode beam interrogates, M-mode echocardiography has not proved to

be helpful in the estimation of overall ventricular function in patients with segmental wall dysfunction.

Two-dimensional echocardiography, on the other hand, has been much more helpful.[13–16] It allows a fairly good estimation of left ventricular function. However, there are some limitations. Calculations of ventricular volumes by echocardiography require an excellent recording, and this is not possible in as many as 20 to 30 per cent of patients. Outlining of the endocardial surface in end-systole and end-diastole is a difficult and tedious task. With two-dimensional echocardiography ventricular volumes generally are underestimated.

The advantage of two-dimensional echocardiography over other methods with regard to safety and the patient's comfort should stimulate further refinements to make this a more practical and precise method for the determination of left ventricular function in coronary artery disease.

The echocardiographic evaluation of systolic ejection indices and segmental left ventricular wall analysis are discussed in Chapter 11.

Patients with severely obstructed coronary arteries often have normal left ventricular wall motion at rest, and consequently no abnormalities are detected by echocardiography. New regional wall motion abnormalities occurring during exercise may be demonstrated echocardiographically. Such exercised-induced abnormalities suggest the diagnosis of coronary artery disease.[17–25] Supine and upright dynamic ergometry, as well as isometric exercise methods, can be used.

With M-mode echocardiography, the exercise-induced wall motion abnormalities that suggest the presence of ischemia include (1) a decrease in mean systolic wall thickening, (2) a decrease in maximal velocity of wall thickening, and (3) a decrease in the percentage of systolic change in the left ventricular internal dimension.

With two-dimensional echocardiography, it is possible to detect exercise-induced regional wall motion abnormalities. The views that yield the most information are the left parasternal short- and long-axis views and the apical four-chamber view.

Because of the difficulties encountered in obtaining an adequate echocardiographic recording at peak exercise and because of the ease and reliability of the exercise radionuclide techniques, exercise echocardiography is not widely used.

12.3 ACUTE MYOCARDIAL INFARCTION

M-mode echocardiography has been used to localize and quantify the degree of left ventricular asynergy in acute myocardial infarction.[26, 27] Wall motion abnormalities can be seen with two-dimensional echocardiography immediately after the onset of chest pain in patients with acute myocardial infarction.[28] These regional contraction abnormalities have a decrease in amplitude and an associated decrease in adjacent wall thickening.

Two-dimensional echocardiography may provide useful information concerning regional and global left ventricular function in persons with acute myocardial infarction.[29–33] Two-dimensional echocardiography also has been used to study the incidence of left ventricular thrombus after transmural myocardial infarction. Patients with severe apical wall motion abnormalities during acute transmural anterior myocardial infarction may be at high risk for left ventricular thrombosis.[34]

12.4 MYOCARDIAL SCAR

A myocardial scar is seen by echocardiography as a segmental area of the ventricular mass with decreased or absent motion. This area is usually thinner than the adjacent normal ventricular wall.

M-mode echocardiography can be used to recognize myocardial scar (Figs. 12–10, 12–11).[35–37] This method is limited by the small area of the left ventricle that can be visualized, which consists of the basal septum and the posterior left ventricular wall. Other areas are either impossible or impractical to view with M-mode echocardiography. Even in patients with anteroseptal infarcts, the M-mode echocardiographic appearance may be normal.[38]

The abnormalities that can be seen with M-mode echocardiography when the echo beam passes through myocardial scar tissue include (1) abnormal wall motion, which can be either decreased, absent, or paradoxic, (2) increased echo reflectivity, (3) decreased wall thickness—usually less than 7

mm in thickness or 30 per cent less than the adjacent myocardium, and (4) decreased or absent systolic thickening.[39]

Two-dimensional echocardiography permits a better appreciation of the location and size of the myocardial scar. The echo reflectivity is augmented in the scar area. The normal endocardial surface is interrupted, and the wall thickness is reduced (Fig. 12–12). The contour of the left ventricle, in contrast with that in a ventricular aneurysm, is normal. Ideally, it should be possible to demonstrate this segmental abnormality from different projections for the affected areas. A septal scar is observed best from the parasternal long-axis and short-axis views, as well as from the apical four-chamber view. An anterior scar is viewed best from the apical two-chamber projection. The short-axis parasternal view shows this wall less well. A lateral scar can be studied best from the apical four-chamber view, and an inferior scar can be studied best from the short-axis parasternal view, while the long-axis parasternal view provides less clarity. The apical scar can be seen well from any of the apical views or from a low long-axis parasternal view. Left ventricular thrombi are frequently observed in the area of myocardial scar (Figs. 12–13, 12–14).

Several reports have demonstrated a good correlation between the results of two-dimensional echocardiography and ventriculography in the localization of segmental wall abnormalities in patients with coronary artery disease.

12.5 LEFT VENTRICULAR ANEURYSM

M-mode echocardiography is of little value in the diagnosis of ventricular aneurysms. Ventricular aneurysms may be suspected in the presence of progressive chamber dilatation in a scan from the base of the left ventricle toward its apex (Fig. 12–15). M-mode echocardiography has been used to evaluate patients for whom aneurysmectomy is indicated.[40]

Two-dimensional echocardiography is far superior to M-mode echocardiography for the detection of ventricular aneurysms.[41–44] Most ventricular aneurysms involve the cardiac apex, so the best view to use to search for them is an apical view. A ventricular aneurysm appears with two-dimensional echocardiography as an area of the left ventricle with thin walls, absent endocardium, and distorted shape during systole and diastole (Fig. 12–16). There is usually a hinge point between the normal myocardium and the aneurysmal segment (Fig. 12–17). Thrombus is frequently present within the aneurysm (Fig. 12–18). Ventricular aneurysms of the inferior wall are rare and more difficult to detect by echocardiography (Fig. 12–19). Probably the best view from which to look for an aneurysm in this location is the apical two-chamber view.

12.6 LEFT VENTRICULAR PSEUDOANEURYSM

Pseudoaneurysms result from perforation of the left ventricular wall when the extravasated blood is contained by adherent parietal pericardium. A pseudoaneurysm usually has a narrow neck that connects the ventricular cavity with a larger aneurysmal sac. Pseudoaneurysms occur in any of the ventricular walls but appear to be more common in the posterior and posterolateral walls.

Two-dimensional echocardiography permits the recognition of pseudoaneurysms by the demonstration of a sudden discontinuation of the ventricular free wall, with communication through a narrow neck to a saccular or globular echo-free chamber that is external to the left ventricular cavity (Fig. 12–20).[45, 46] The maximal internal diameter is much smaller than the maximal parallel internal diameter of the aneurysmal sac.[47]

M-mode echocardiography may also permit the detection of a pseudoaneurysm (Fig. 12–21). An echo-free space that expands during systole is seen behind the free wall of the left ventricle.[48–50]

12.7 VENTRICULAR SEPTAL RUPTURE

Most septal perforations are located in the posteroapical region and are usually related to a large myocardial infarction following left anterior descending coronary artery occlusion.[51]

Findings that may be of value in the M-mode echocardiographic diagnosis of septal rupture include (1) right ventricular dilatation, (2) mid-diastolic closure of the mitral valve, and (3) abrupt posterior motion of the interventricular septum with the onset of diastole.[52, 53]

Two-dimensional echocardiography may permit direct visualization of the septal defect (Fig. 12–22), which appears as an abrupt interruption of the interventricular septum.[54–56] The perforation typically expands during systole. If the actual defect is not seen, aneurysmal bulging of the septum is highly suggestive of septal rupture. Two-dimensional echocardiography may also provide an approximation of the size of the defect as well as of its location. Left-to-right shunting can be demonstrated with negative contrast echocardiography.

12.8 PAPILLARY MUSCLE DYSFUNCTION

M-mode echocardiography is not helpful in the diagnosis of papillary muscle dysfunction, except perhaps in a negative way. If a patient has clinical evidence of mitral regurgitation and the echocardiographic appearance of the mitral valve is normal, there may be papillary muscle dysfunction. Some patients have evidence of mitral valve prolapse or flail mitral valve.[57]

Two-dimensional echocardiography is more effective in detecting papillary muscle dysfunction (Fig. 12–23).[58] This method may show evidence of papillary muscle fibrosis or calcification. Incomplete closure of the mitral valve has been described in patients with papillary muscle dysfunction. This condition can be observed most clearly from the apical four-chamber view. With systole, the affected mitral leaflet does not approach the plane of the mitral ring.

12.9 MURAL THROMBUS

Two-dimensional echocardiography is far superior to M-mode echocardiography in the detection of mural thrombus.[59–62]

A mural thrombus is seen on two-dimensional echocardiography as an abnormal intracavitary mass contiguous with the ventricular wall. The area in which this mass is located is usually a hypokinetic or akinetic region of the left ventricle. Since most of the thrombi are located in the cardiac apex, one of the apical echocardiographic views is preferred. Thrombus echo density is generally greater than that of the adjacent myocardium. An area of central echo lucency is occasionally present in large thrombi.

12.10 RIGHT VENTRICULAR INFARCTION

Right ventricular infarction may occur in patients with transmural infarction of the inferoposterior wall and of the posterior portion of the ventricular septum. Echocardiographic examination of patients with right ventricular infarct shows dilatation of the right ventricular chamber. Wall motion abnormalities of the right ventricular wall, as well as of the septum and the inferoposterior wall, may be detected.[63–66] Paradoxic septal motion and tricuspid insufficiency may also be present.

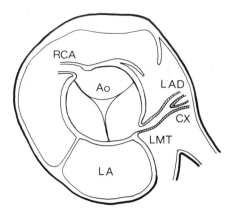

FIGURE 12–1
RIGHT AND LEFT CORONARY ARTERIES
Left parasternal short-axis view at the aortic level. The right coronary artery (RCA) is seen originating at 11 o'clock of the aortic circumference. The left main trunk (LMT) originates at about 5 o'clock and divides into the left anterior descending (LAD) and circumflex (Cx) arteries. Ao = aorta; LA = left atrium.

FIGURE 12–2
LEFT MAIN TRUNK
Left parasternal short-axis view at the great vessel level. The left main coronary artery is seen to originate from the left coronary sinus at about 5 o'clock of the aortic circumference (arrows). Ao = aorta.

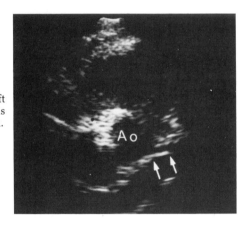

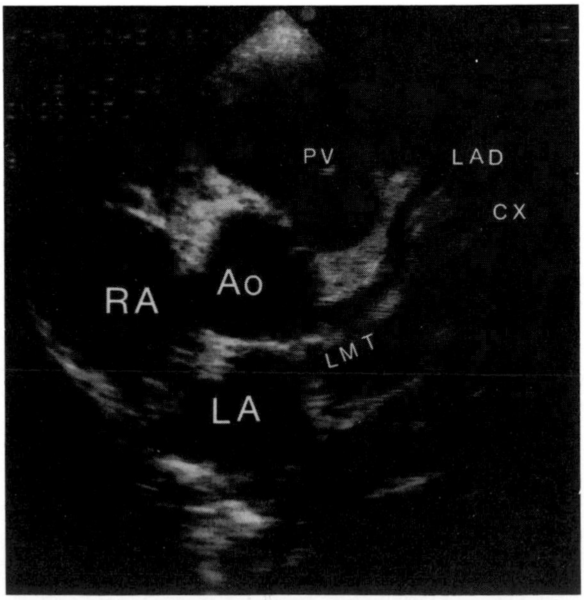

FIGURE 12–3
LEFT CORONARY ARTERY
Left parasternal short-axis view at the aortic level. The left main trunk (LMT) originates from about 5 o'clock of the aortic circumference, then divides into the left anterior descending (LAD) and circumflex (Cx) arteries. PV = pulmonic valve; Ao = aorta; LA = left atrium.

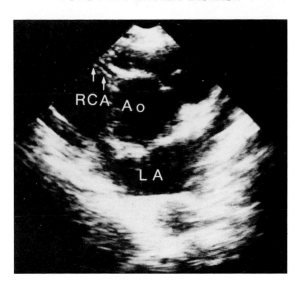

FIGURE 12–4
RIGHT CORONARY ARTERY
Short-axis left parasternal view of a normal right coronary artery (RCA) in a patient with a dilated aorta (Ao) secondary to Marfan's syndrome. The right coronary artery originates from the right coronary sinus at about 11 o'clock of the aortic circumference and is seen as two parallel lines directed anteriorly and to the right. LA = left atrium.

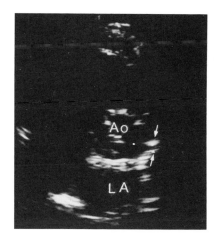

FIGURE 12–5
LEFT MAIN TRUNK STENOSIS
Short-axis left parasternal view in a patient with an 80 per cent proximal left main trunk stenosis proved at angiographic examination. Note the focal decrease in lumen size and the increased reflectivity of the vessel (*arrows*). Ao = aorta; LA = left atrium.

FIGURE 12–6
LEFT MAIN TRUNK STENOSIS
Short-axis left parasternal view and coronary arteriograph recorded in a patient with 70 per cent obstruction in the left main trunk. The arrows point to the decreased lumen as seen in the echocardiogram. Ao = aorta; LA = left atrium.

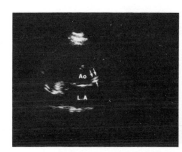
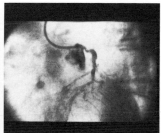

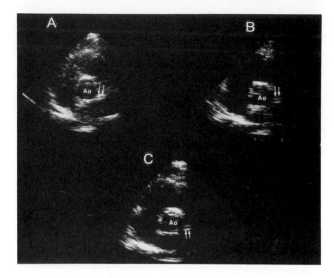

FIGURE 12–7
LEFT MAIN TRUNK STENOSIS
Short-axis left parasternal views at the aortic level with different attenuations. The obstruction is only seen in panel A, in which there is little attenuation. The view in panel C appears normal and represents a false-negative examination result. Panel B has intermediate attenuation. Ao = aorta.

FIGURE 12–8
NONVISUALIZATION OF A LEFT MAIN TRUNK LESION
Short-axis left parasternal view at the level of the aorta (Ao) in a patient with a severe left main trunk obstruction as seen in the angiogram. The obstruction is located just before the bifurcation of the main trunk and is not visualized by echocardiography.

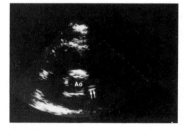 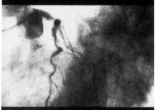

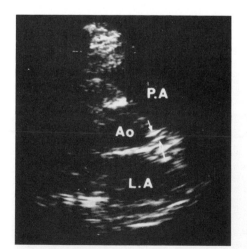

FIGURE 12–9
FALSE-POSITIVE LEFT MAIN TRUNK LESION
Short-axis left parasternal view in a patient with a normal left main trunk proved at angiography. Apparent luminal narrowing is observed by echocardiography. This appearance is most likely the result of tangential sectioning of the vessel by the sector plane. Ao = aorta; PA = pulmonary artery; LA = left atrium.

FIGURE 12–10
ANTEROSEPTAL SCAR
Echocardiogram recorded from a patient with an anteroseptal infarction at the left ventricular level. A hypokinetic septum is seen with lack of systolic thickening. The posterior wall moves normally or is even slightly hyperkinetic. LV = left ventricle.

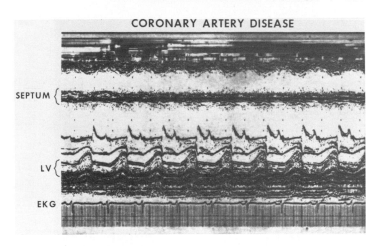

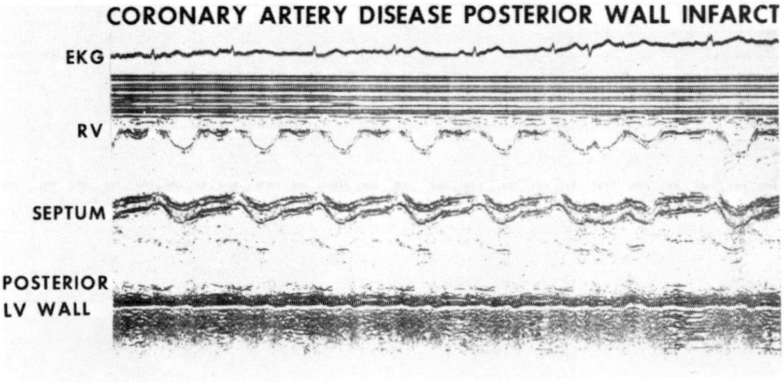

FIGURE 12–11
POSTERIOR WALL SCAR
This echocardiogram recorded at the left ventricular level demonstrates absent motion of the posterior wall in a patient with a posterior wall myocardial infarction. RV = right ventricle; LV = left ventricle.

FIGURE 12–12
MYOCARDIAL SCAR
Apical four-chamber view in a patient with an anteroapical myocardial infarction. The arrows point to scar tissue in the apex. The walls are thin. There is poor endocardial definition. There was lack of motion throughout the cardiac cycle. RV = right ventricle; LV = left ventricle; RA = right atrium; LA = left atrium.

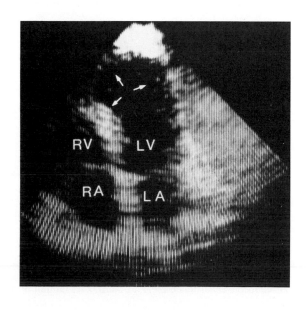

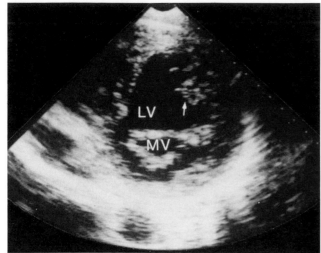

FIGURE 12–13
MYOCARDIAL SCAR, MURAL THROMBUS
Left parasternal short-axis view in a patient with an anterolateral myocardial infarction and a large mural thrombus in that area (arrow). LV = left ventricle; MV = mitral valve.

FIGURE 12–14
MYOCARDIAL SCAR, MURAL THROMBUS
Apical two-chamber view in a patient with a large anteroapical infarction and a large thrombus in the apex (arrows). LV = left ventricle; LA = left atrium.

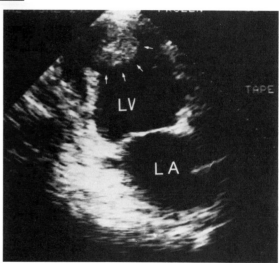

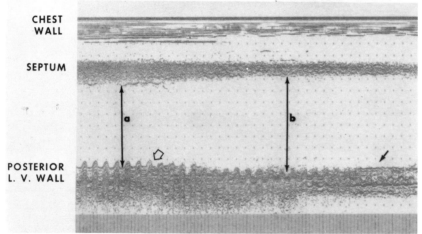

FIGURE 12–15
VENTRICULAR ANEURYSM
This echocardiogram recorded at the left ventricular (L. V.) level shows progressive dilatation of the left ventricle as the sector is directed inferiorly. At level *a* the left ventricle measures 6.5 cm, and the posterior wall has normal motion. At level *b* the left ventricle measures 8 cm, and there is no motion of the posterior wall.

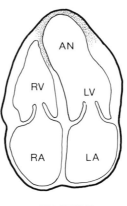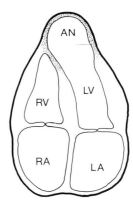

DIASTOLE   SYSTOLE

FIGURE 12–16
LEFT VENTRICULAR ANEURYSM
Diastolic and systolic frames from an apical four-chamber view in a patient with an apical aneurysm (AN). Note the distorted shape during diastole and systole. Dyskinesia makes this deformity more apparent during systole. RV = right ventricle; LV = left ventricle; RA = right atrium; LA = left atrium.

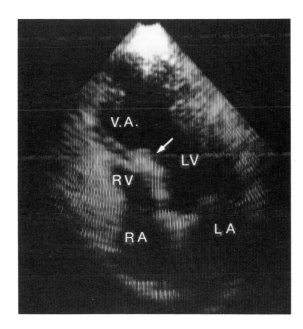

FIGURE 12–17
LEFT VENTRICULAR ANEURYSM
Apical four-chamber view in a patient with a large apical aneurysm (V.A.). Note the distorted shape of the left ventricle (LV), the thinned walls, and the hinge point (arrow). RV = right ventricle; RA = right atrium; LA = left atrium.

FIGURE 12–18
LEFT VENTRICULAR ANEURYSM, THROMBUS
Apical four-chamber view in a patient with a large apical aneurysm filled by a thrombus (arrows). LV = left ventricle.

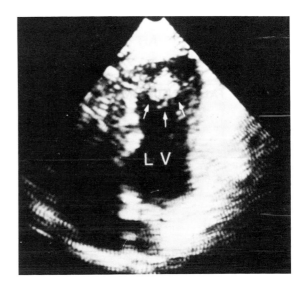

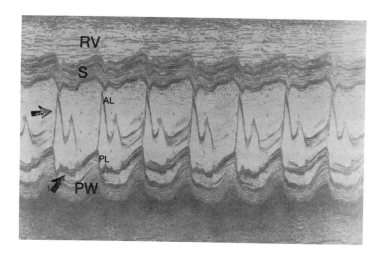

FIGURE 13–13
LEFT ATRIAL MYXOMA
Postoperative echocardiographic recording at the mitral level in the same patient as in Figure 13–9. Except for mild septal motion abnormality, the echocardiographic appearance is normal. RV = right ventricle; S = septum; AL = anterior leaflet; PL = posterior leaflet; PW = posterior wall.

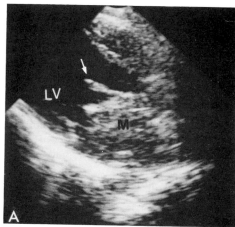

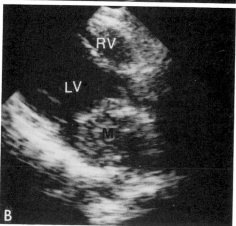

FIGURE 13–14
LEFT ATRIAL MYXOMA
Long-axis parasternal view in a patient with a large sessile myxoma (M). During the diastolic frame (D), despite the mitral valve being open (arrow), the myxoma remains in the left atrium. During systole (S), the myxoma becomes somewhat rounder. RV = right ventricle; LV = left ventricle.

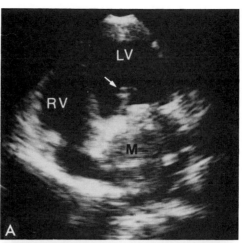

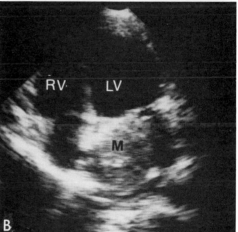

FIGURE 13–15
LEFT ATRIAL MYXOMA
Apical four-chamber views during diastole (A) and systole (B). Note the lack of tumor motion despite the opening of the mitral valve (arrow). LV = left ventricle; RV = right ventricle; M = myxoma.

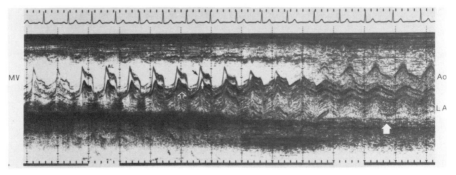

FIGURE 13–16
LEFT ATRIAL MYXOMA
Echocardiographic scan recorded in the same patient as in Figure 13–14 from the level of the mitral valve (MV) to the level of the aorta (Ao) and left atrium (LA). The myxoma occupies the left atrium during systole (arrow). During diastole, it is seen behind the mitral valve at the level of the atrioventricular groove, but it does not descend into the left ventricle. AL = anterior leaflet.

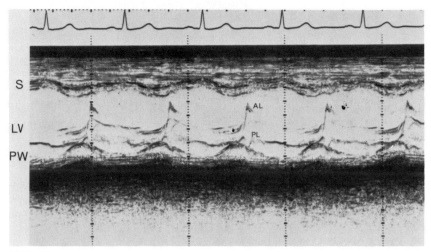

FIGURE 13–17
LEFT ATRIAL MYXOMA
Echocardiogram recorded in the same patient as in Figure 13–14 at the left ventricular
level. At this level no abnormalities are evident. S = septum; LV = left ventricle; PW
= posterior wall; AL = anterior leaflet; PL = posterior leaflet.

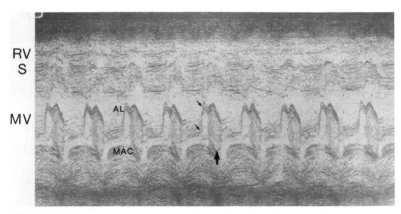

FIGURE 13–18
LEFT ATRIAL MYXOMA
An unusually long delay between the opening of the mitral valve (MV) (*small
arrows*) and the prolapse of the myxoma into the left ventricle (*black arrow*)
is apparent in this case. This delay was probably related to the elongated
shape of the tumor and its high insertion in the interatrial septum (S). RV =
right ventricle; AL = anterior leaflet; MAC = mitral annulus calcification.

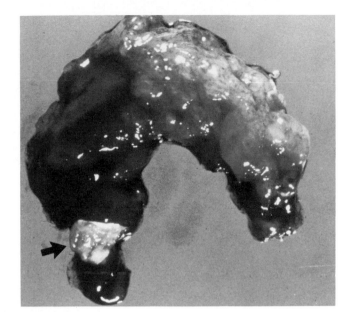

FIGURE 13–19
LEFT ATRIAL MYXOMA
Pathologic specimen from the same patient as in Figure 13–18. The arrow points to the area of insertion of the myxoma into the interatrial septum. Note the absence of a pedicle and the elongated shape and gelatinous appearance of this tumor.

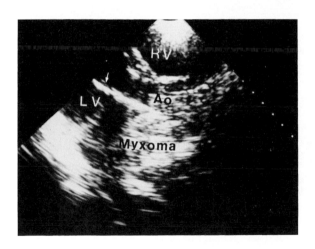

FIGURE 13–20
CALCIFIED ATRIAL MYXOMA
Long-axis left parasternal view in a patient with a large calcified myxoma. The mass is very echo-dense and sessile. Despite the mitral valve being open (arrow), the tumor does not prolapse into the left ventricle (LV). RV = right ventricle; Ao = aorta.

FIGURE 13–21
CALCIFIED ATRIAL MYXOMA
Short-axis left parasternal view at the level of the aorta (Ao) in the same patient as in Figure 13–20. Note how echo-dense the tumor is.

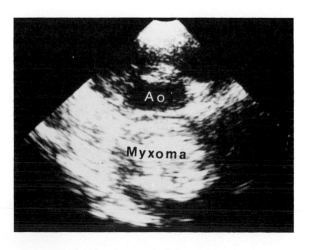

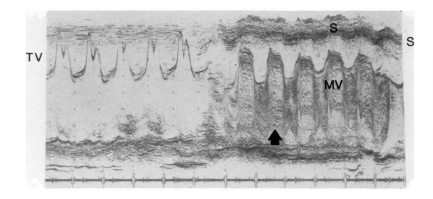

FIGURE 13–22
LEFT ATRIAL MYXOMA
Echocardiographic scan from the tricuspid valve (TV) to the mitral valve (MV) in a patient with a left atrial myxoma. This view excludes an associated right atrial myxoma. S = septum.

FIGURE 13–23
NONPROLAPSING LEFT ATRIAL MYXOMA
Echocardiographic scan from the mitral valve to the aorta (Ao). A mass of echoes is seen in the left atrium (LA) *(arrows)*. The mitral valve appears normal. The E to F slope is not reduced, and a mass of echoes is not seen behind it. This appearance is characteristic of nonprolapsing left atrial myxoma. RV = right ventricle; AL = anterior leaflet.

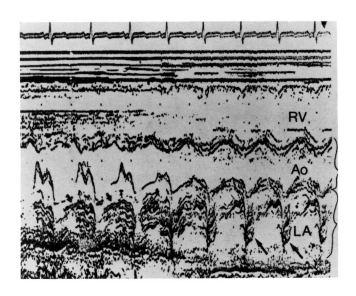

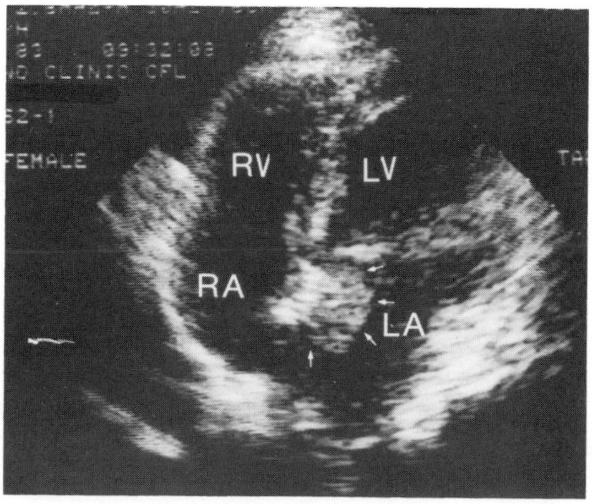

FIGURE 13–24
NONPROLAPSING MYXOMA
Apical four-chamber view in a patient with a small nonprolapsing atrial myxoma. The tumor is attached in the interatrial septum and does not prolapse into the left ventricle (LV). RV = right ventricle; RA = right atrium; LA = left atrium.

FIGURE 13–25
NONPROLAPSING ATRIAL MYXOMA
This apical four-chamber view at the time of systole demonstrates a tumor in the left atrium. The mitral valve is closed. RV = right ventricle; LV = left ventricle; RA = right atrium; M = myxoma.

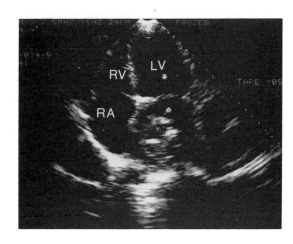

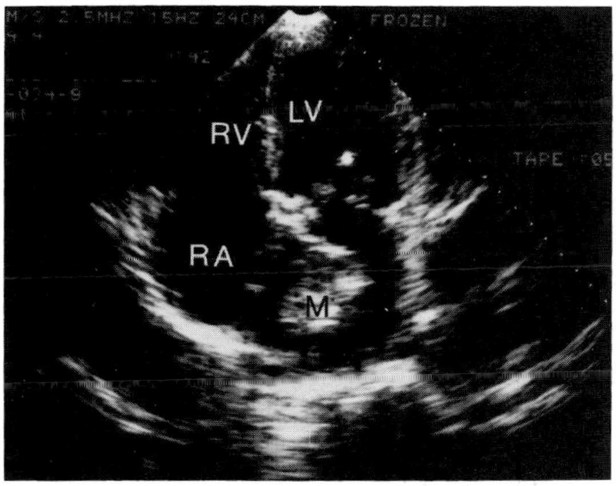

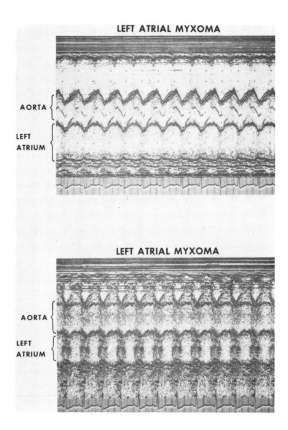

FIGURE 13–26
NONPROLAPSING ATRIAL MYXOMA
Echocardiogram recorded during diastole in the same patient as in Figure 13–25. Despite the opened mitral valve the tumor does not prolapse into the left ventricle (LV). RV = right ventricle; RA = right atrium; M = myxoma.

FIGURE 13–27
LEFT ATRIAL MYXOMA
Occasionally when a myxoma is attached high in the interatrial septum and does not prolapse into the left ventricle, the diagnosis may be missed with M-mode echocardiography, as was initially done in this case. At the level of the aortic valve the left atrium is clear, and only with higher transducer angulation does the myxoma become evident.

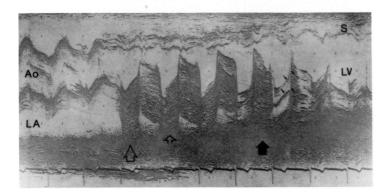

FIGURE 13–28
LEFT ATRIAL MYXOMA
Echocardiographic scan from the aorta (Ao) to the left ventricle (LV) in a patient with a myxoma attached very low in the interatrial septum (S). The myxoma is clearly seen behind the mitral valve but not at all in the left atrium (LA).

FIGURE 13–29
LEFT ATRIAL RHABDOMYOSARCOMA
Long-axis left parasternal view in a 63-year-old man who had congestive heart failure and severe mitral regurgitation. This diastolic frame shows a round irregular mass attached to the mitral valve and prolapsing into the left ventricle (LV) *(arrows)*. RV = right ventricle; Ao = aorta; LA = left atrium.

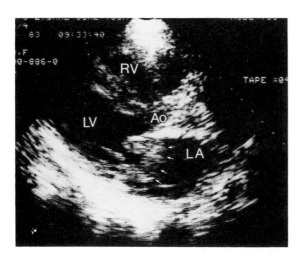

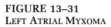

FIGURE 13–30
LEFT ATRIAL RHABDOMYOSARCOMA
Long-axis left parasternal view recorded from the same patient as in Figure 13–29. This systolic frame shows the mass of echoes partially filling the left atrium (LA). Echocardiographically, this finding is indistinguishable from a left atrial myxoma. RV = right ventricle; LV = left ventricle; Ao = aorta.

FIGURE 13–31
LEFT ATRIAL MYXOMA
A low-frequency sound occurs at the time of maximal prolapse of the tumor in the left ventricle. This is the "tumor plop" (TP), which coincides with the E point of the mitral valve (MV).

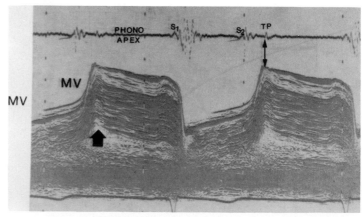

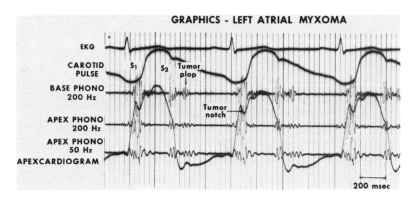

FIGURE 13–32

LEFT ATRIAL MYXOMA, GRAPHICS

The "tumor plop" coincides with the F wave of the apexcardiogram, and the "tumor notch" occurs in the upstroke of the apexcardiogram, coinciding with a loud first heart sound and is probably related to rapid decompression of the left ventricle as the tumor moves into the left atrium.

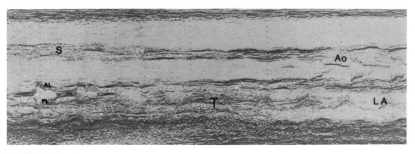

FIGURE 13–33

LEFT ATRIAL THROMBUS

Echocardiographic scan from the left ventricle to the aorta (Ao) in a 60-year-old patient with congestive cardiomyopathy. A mass of echoes (T) representing a thrombus is seen filling the lower part of the left atrium (LA). S = septum; AL = anterior leaflet; PL = posterior leaflet.

FIGURE 13–34

LEFT ATRIAL THROMBUS

Long-axis left parasternal view in a patient with mitral valve prosthesis (MP), marked enlargement of the left atrium (LA), and an echo-dense round structure adjacent to the atrioventricular groove that is suggestive of a left atrial thrombus (arrows). LV = left ventricle; RV = right ventricle; Ao = aorta.

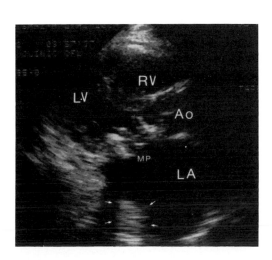

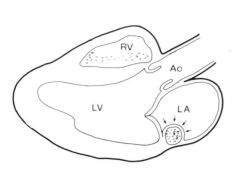
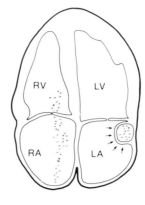

FIGURE 13–35
LEFT SUPERIOR VENA CAVA DRAINING INTO CORONARY SINUS
This diagram demonstrates micro-bubbles in a dilated coronary sinus and right heart. Such microbubbles occur after the injection of contrast material into the left arm in patients who have persistent left superior vena cava draining into the coronary sinus. RV = right ventricle; LV = left ventricle; Ao = aorta; LA = left atrium; RA = right atrium.

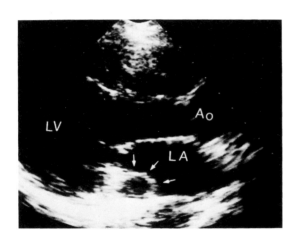

FIGURE 13–36
LEFT SUPERIOR VENA CAVA DRAINING INTO CORONARY SINUS
This long-axis left parasternal view before injection of contrast material shows a dilated coronary sinus (arrows). LV = left ventricle; Ao = aorta; LA = left atrium.

FIGURE 13–37
LEFT SUPERIOR VENA CAVA DRAINING INTO CORONARY SINUS
This long-axis left parasternal view after injection of contrast material shows the coronary sinus filled with microbubbles. LV = left ventricle; Ao = aorta; LA = left atrium.

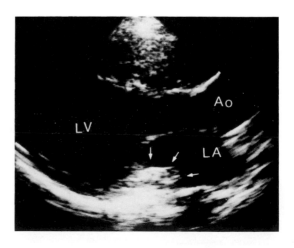

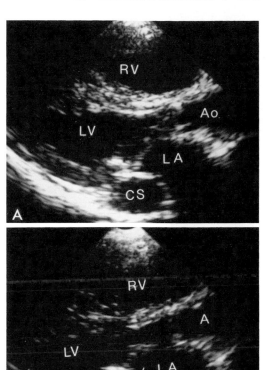

FIGURE 13–38
LEFT SUPERIOR VENA CAVA DRAINING INTO CORONARY SINUS
Long-axis left parasternal views before (A) and after (B) injection of contrast material show a dilated coronary sinus (CS) filling with microbubbles. RV = right ventricle; LV = left ventricle; Ao = aorta; LA = left atrium.

14.1 RIGHT AT:

Dilatation of the
conditions that pr
overload of the
obstruction at the
(Fig. 14–1). The
metric and exceed
± 4 to 4.2 ± 1 n
dimension and 3
to lateral dimensi

14.2 RIGHT AT

A variety of n
have been identifi
These include ri
nephroma (Figs.
omyosarcoma (Fi
bus, and vegetatic
The most comr
mas, which have
pearance similar
mas. They appea
well-defined borc
prolapse through
pending on the
stalk (Fig. 14–8).
diography provid

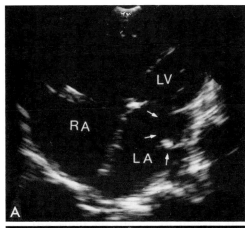

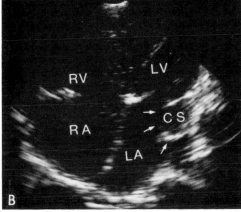

FIGURE 13–39
LEFT SUPERIOR VENA CAVA DRAINING INTO CORONARY SINUS
Apical four-chamber views before (A) and after (B) injection of contrast material show the dilated coronary sinus (CS) filling with microbubbles. LV = left ventricle; RA = right atrium; LA = left atrium; RV = right ventricle.

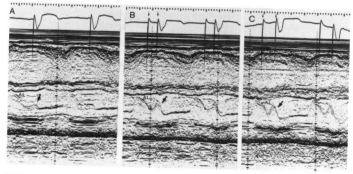

FIGURE 14–18
ATRIOVENTRICULAR SEQUENTIAL PACING
Echocardiogram recorded from a 74-year-old patient with an underlying junctional rhythm and a DDD atrioventricular sequential pacemaker. In panel A the atrial stimuli are turned off. Consequently, the a wave on the mitral valve is essentially absent. In panels B and C the pacemaker is in an atrioventricular sequential mode, with a longer PR interval (panel C). The a wave is closer to the E to F slope of the mitral valve. AL = anterior leaflet.

FIGURE 14–19
EUSTACHIAN VALVE
This apical four-chamber view demonstrates a prominent eustachian valve (arrows), which appears as a membrane across the right atrium (RA) close to the entrance of the inferior vena cava. RV = right ventricle; LV = left ventricle; LA = left atrium.

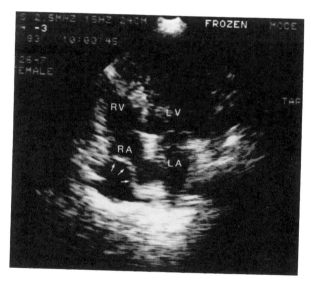

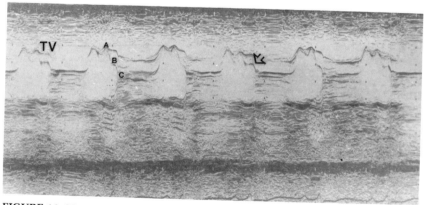

FIGURE 14–20
INCREASED END-DIASTOLIC PRESSURE OF THE RIGHT VENTRICLE
Echocardiogram of the tricuspid valve (TV) in a 26-year-old woman with scleroderma and right and left ventricular failure. The pulmonary artery pressure was 60/25 mm Hg. There is a prominent B notch in the tricuspid valve (arrow).

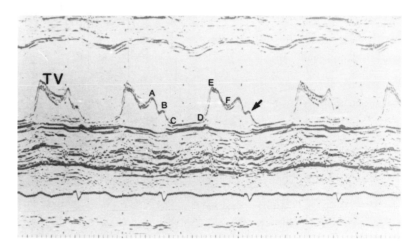

FIGURE 14–21
INCREASED END-DIASTOLIC PRES-
SURE OF THE RIGHT VENTRICLE
A prominent B notch (arrow) is
seen in the tricuspid valve (TV)
of a patient with right ventricular failure.

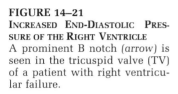

FIGURE 14–22
RIGHT VENTRICULAR HYPERTROPHY
Echocardiogram recorded from a
9-month-old girl with severe infundibular pulmonic stenosis
(105 mm Hg gradient) and severe
right ventricular and septal hypertrophy. RV = right ventricle;
S = septum; PW = posterior
wall.

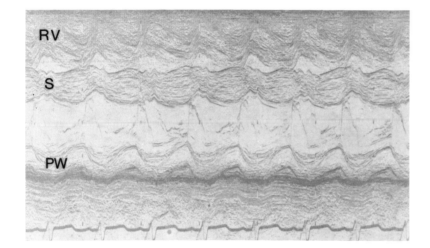

FIGURE 14–23
RHABDOMYOMA
Long- and short-axis parasternal views in a 4-month-old boy with tuberosclerosis and a
rhabdomyoma in the right ventricular outflow tract. In the long axis (A) the rhabdomyoma appears as a round mass attached to the interventricular septum. In the short
axis (B) its round shape is more apparent. LV = left ventricle; Ao = aorta; LA = left
atrium; RV = right ventricle; T = tumor.

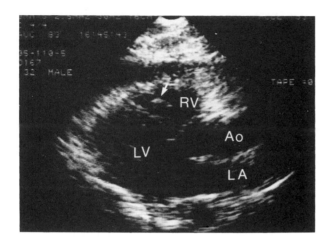

FIGURE 14–24
RIGHT VENTRICULAR THROMBUS
Long-axis parasternal view in a patient after cardiac contusion. A right ventricular thrombus is indicated by the arrows. RV = right ventricle; LV = left ventricle; Ao = aorta; LA = left atrium.

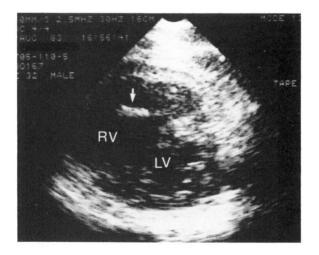

FIGURE 14–25
RIGHT VENTRICULAR THROMBUS
Short-axis left parasternal view in the same patient as in Figure 14–24. The thrombus is seen in the right ventricle (RV) close to the tricuspid valve. LV = left ventricle.

15 DISEASES OF THE PERICARDIUM

15.1 PERICARDIAL EFFUSION

Echocardiography plays an important role in the diagnosis and management of patients known or suspected to have pericardial effusion.

Normally, the pericardial space is a virtual one. That is, there is very little separation between the *visceral pericardium (epicardium)* and the *parietal pericardium*. The normal amount of pericardial fluid is believed to be less than 20 cc. This amount in general does not permit echocardiographic separation of the two pericardial layers.

A pericardial effusion produces a relatively echo-free space outside the ventricular walls.[1-4] With M-mode echocardiography, this is initially seen behind the posterior wall of the left ventricle (Fig. 15–1). With small effusions, a separation between the epicardium and the pericardium occurs only during systole. As the effusion becomes larger, this separation is in both systole and diastole. With larger effusions, the echo-free space is also seen anteriorly (Fig. 15–2).

Adequate gain control is essential to clearly define the epicardium and pericardium. Usually the strongest echo recording is that from the pericardium, so that this echo may be the only one detected with higher degrees of attenuation.

In the presence of pericardial effusion, the pericardial motion becomes attenuated, often following a flat pattern.

With two-dimensional echocardiography, the echo-free space corresponding to the pericardial effusion can be seen from many sector planes. A small effusion is more likely to be detected from the left parasternal long-axis view, in which the effusion is initially seen to accumulate behind the posterior wall (Fig. 15–3). In the short-axis view it also is apparent that a small effusion is first detected behind the posterior wall of the left ventricle (Fig. 15–4).

As the effusion enlarges, it accumulates more laterally and inferiorly. A large effusion surrounds the entire heart (Figs. 15–5, 15–6), which may be seen bouncing back and forth in the large pericardial space (Figs. 15–7, 15–8).[5] This bouncing motion of the heart can create all sorts of distortions in the motion of the valves and walls as seen by M-mode echocardiography. The most characteristic abnormality in this respect is pseudo mitral valve prolapse (Fig. 15–9).[6, 7]

Both M-mode and two-dimensional echocardiography have been used to estimate the magnitude of a pericardial effusion. The spatial orientation of two-dimensional echocardiography permits a better estimate of the amount of pericardial fluid. If the pericardial fluid is distributed evenly around the heart, it is possible to calculate the volume of the effusion using the ellipsoid volume formula and by subtracting the volume of the ventricle from the volume of the heart and effusion. This form of quantification has not proved very accurate, and most echocardiographers prefer a semiquantitative assessment of the volume of the pericardial fluid.

A small effusion generally can be detected only at a location posterior to the posterior wall, and epipericardial separation occurs only during systole. As the effusions become larger there is systolic and diastolic separation. A large effusion commonly surrounds the heart and also is present anteriorly.

Echocardiographic Differentiation of Pleural from Pericardial Effusion. A number of factors are useful in this differentiation:

1. Pericardial fluid usually does not accumulate behind the left atrium (Fig. 15–10), whereas pleural effusion does. Only rarely and with very large effusions is pericardial fluid seen behind the posterior wall of the left atrium (Fig. 15–11). A pleural effusion, if it does not accumulate behind the left atrium, stops abruptly at the level of the atrioventricular groove, whereas a pericardial effusion tapers off gradually from behind the left ventricle to the atrioventricular groove.

2. A large echo-free space seen behind the left ventricle and not anteriorly is more characteristic of pleural fluid (Fig. 15–12).

3. A pleural effusion changes somewhat in relation to respiration by becoming larger during inspiration. Pericardial effusions usually do not change in apparent size with respiration.

4. The identification of the descending aorta in the short-axis two-dimensional view at the level of the left ventricle is most helpful in differentiating pleural from pericardial effusion. A pericardial effusion appears as an echo-free space between the descending aorta and the posterior wall of the left ventricle (Fig. 15–13). A pleural effusion appears to the side of the descending aorta and does not separate it from the posterior left ventricular wall (Figs. 15–14, 15–15).[8]

In the presence of both pleural and pericardial effusions, the pericardium is seen as a laminar echo recording in between two echo-free spaces behind the posterior wall of the left ventricle (Figs. 15–16, 15–17).

False-Negative Studies. The diagnosis of pericardial effusion can be missed if particular attention is not paid to some technical details. Since the pericardial fluid is a relatively echo-free medium, inadequate attenuation may make its presence less than obvious (Fig. 15–18).

There have been some reports about echocardiography failing to indicate a clotted pericardial effusion.

Excessive enlargement of the cardiac image may place the posterior left ventricular walls in the far border of the image so that an echo-free space behind it cannot be recognized.

A loculated effusion (Figs. 15–19, 15–20) can be out of the path of the M-mode beam and be completely missed. Two-dimensional echocardiography is superior in detecting this type of effusion.

False-Positive Studies. An echo-free space located behind the posterior left ventricular wall and simulating a pericardial effusion can be seen because of the descending aorta, a large coronary sinus, or excessive medial angulation (probably in the right atrium or right ventricle). Aneurysmal dilatation and prolapse of the left atrium behind the left ventricle may also create an echo-free space at this area.[9, 10]

A pseudoaneurysm of the left ventricle in the posterior wall can also create an echo-free space in that area. In most cases, this abnormality can be adequately diagnosed by two-dimensional echocardiography.

Occasionally, pericardial fluid can accumulate behind the posterior left atrial wall and at the level of the atrioventricular groove. This accumulation may produce excessive anteroposterior motion of this wall, which in turn creates the appearance of a mass on M-mode echocardiography (Fig. 15–21).

15.2 CARDIAC TAMPONADE

The most dramatic and life-threatening form of pericardial disease is cardiac tamponade. In this condition, there is impaired left ventricular diastolic filling resulting from compression of the heart by pericardial fluid. If this condition remains unrecognized, it may be fatal. The diagnosis of cardiac tamponade is based on clinical findings. Characteristically these include elevated central venous pressure, hypotension, and pulsus paradoxus. Echocardiography plays a complementary role in the diagnosis of cardiac tamponade. The abnormalities that are frequently present are described here.

1. Pericardial Effusion. Most patients with cardiac tamponade have a large pericardial effusion with anterior and posterior collection of pericardial fluid.[11] Often the effusion is large enough so that the heart swings with the pericardial sac. *Electric alternans*, a common electrocardiographic finding in cardiac tamponade, is probably related to this bouncing motion of the heart (Fig. 15–22).

Rapid accumulation of pericardial fluid may induce cardiac tamponade so that the finding of a small pericardial effusion, as seen on echocardiography, does not rule out the possibility of tamponade.

2. Right Ventricular Compression. Patients with cardiac tamponade often have right ventricular compression (Fig. 15–23).[12] The right ventricular dimension is usually 1 cm or less. This abnormality is more obvious at the level of the body of the right ventricle. The right ventricular outflow tract is not necessarily compromised.

3. Decreased Left Ventricular Size During Inspiration. In patients with cardiac tamponade, inspiration produces dilatation of the right ventricle, shift of the interventricular septum toward the left ventricle, and compression of the left ventricle.[13]

4. Decreased Mitral E to F Slope with Inspiration. During inspiration, a decreased mitral diastolic slope and decreased mitral valve area, both suggesting decreased mitral valve flow, can be seen in patients with tamponade.

5. Posterior Motion of the Right Ventricular Wall During Diastole. In some patients with cardiac tamponade, diastolic posterior motion of the right ventricular free wall can be noted.[14,15]

6. Early Systolic "Notch" of the Right Ventricle. An early systolic "notch" can occasionally be recorded in the anterior wall of the right ventricle (Fig. 15–24).[16]

15.3 CONSTRICTIVE PERICARDITIS

Several M-mode echocardiographic abnormalities can be seen in patients with constrictive pericarditis.[17] These include thickened pericardium, "flattening" of the diastolic motion of the posterior wall, abnormal septal motion, and premature opening of the pulmonic valve.

1. Thickened Pericardium. This appears as a dense echogenic band posterior to the epicardial surface of the posterior wall (Fig. 15–25). The thickened pericardium may be seen as multiple linear echoes or as a bright homogeneous echo-dense pattern.[18]

2. "Flattening" of the Diastolic Motion of the Posterior Wall. Another frequent finding in patients with constrictive pericarditis is an abrupt slope of the early diastolic posterior wall motion. This slope can be almost perpendicular to the plane of the posterior wall in later diastole, which has a rather flat motion pattern (Fig. 15–26).

3. Abnormal Septal Motion. This abnormality consists of a brisk anterior displacement of the septum during atrial filling. In contrast to right ventricular volume overload, this displacement occurs before the beginning of the ventricular complex (QRS) on the electrocardiogram.[19, 20] This abnormality probably is caused by the inability of the posterior wall to expand during diastole.

4. Premature Opening of the Pulmonic Valve. With constrictive pericarditis a brisk downward opening motion of the pulmonic valve may be seen before ventricular or for that matter atrial systole.[21] The abnormality of the pulmonic valve is somewhat similar to that seen in patients with pulmonary hypertension and right ventricular failure, in which the increased right ventricular pressure may be transmitted to the pulmonic valve in mid-diastole and produce a wide and deep posterior displacement of the leaflet.

In the presence of constrictive pericarditis, two-dimensional echocardiography may show these features: (1) normal or decreased heart size; (2) the pericardium seen as a single or double rigid shell surrounding both ventricles and the apex (Fig. 15–27); (3) dilated inferior vena cava and hepatic veins (Fig. 15–28); (4) bulging of the interatrial and interventricular septum into the left side of the heart with inspiration; (5) hypermobile mitral and tricuspid valves; and (6) prominent ventricular diastolic filling rate.[22]

Two-dimensional echocardiography is also useful in excluding other causes of congestive heart failure such as congestive cardiomyopathy, valvular heart disease, and infiltrative cardiomyopathy.

15.4 PERICARDIAL METASTASES

Pericardial metastases are more commonly seen with carcinoma of the lung and breast, lymphoma, melanoma, and leukemia.

Echocardiographically, pericardial metastases are usually seen as highly reflective echo-dense areas, without distinct borders, that are localized on the pericardial surface. A pericardial effusion is usually present. This usually is a bloody effusion with clots that may be seen as fine undulating filaments attached to the epi- and pericardium (Fig. 15–29).

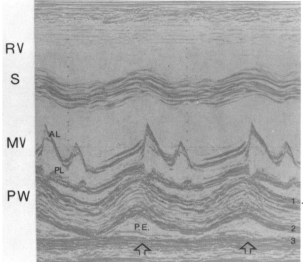

RV

S

MV

AL

PL

PW

P.E.

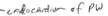

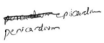

1 — endocardium of PW.

2 ~~pericardium~~ epicardium

3 pericardium

FIGURE 15–1
PERICARDIAL EFFUSION
A small pericardial effusion (P.E.) is demonstrated in this recording from a patient with renal failure. The effusion appears as an echo-free space behind the posterior left ventricular wall in between the epicardium (2) and the pericardium (3). The number 1 indicates the endocardium of the posterior wall (PW). RV = right ventricle; S = septum; MV = mitral valve; AL = anterior leaflet; PL = posterior leaflet.

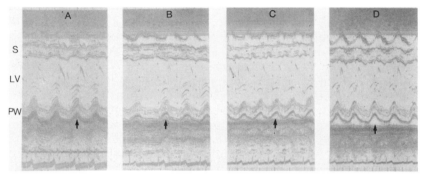

S

LV

PW

A   B   C   D

FIGURE 15–2
PERICARDIAL EFFUSION
Serial echocardiogram recorded from a subject with an enlarging pericardial effusion. Panel A shows no effusion, panel B shows minimal effusion with separation of the epicardium and pericardium, and panel C shows a small effusion with mainly systolic separation of the epicardium and pericardium. Panel D shows a moderate to large effusion with systolic and diastolic separation of the epipericardium interface and the presence of an anterior effusion. S = septum; LV = left ventricle; PW = posterior wall.

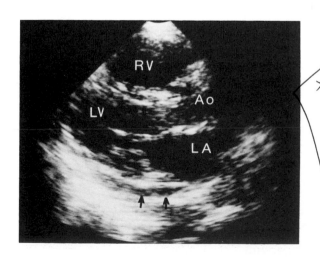

RV

Ao

LV

LA

FIGURE 15–3
SMALL PERICARDIAL EFFUSION
This long-axis left parasternal view shows a small pericardial effusion (*arrows*). Initially it accumulates posteriorly behind the posterior wall of the left ventricle (LV). RV = right ventricle; Ao = aorta; LA = left atrium.

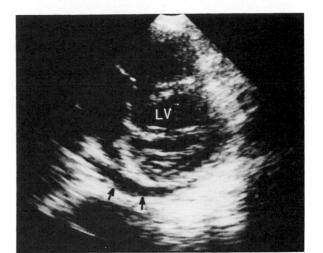

FIGURE 15–4
SMALL PERICARDIAL EFFUSION
This short-axis left parasternal view from the same patient as in Figure 15–3 shows the pericardial effusion *(arrows)* behind the posteromedial wall of the left ventricle (LV).

Short-AXS View

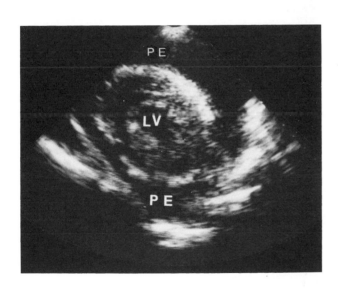

FIGURE 15–5
LARGE PERICARDIAL EFFUSION
Short-axis left parasternal view from a patient with a large pericardial effusion (PE), which surrounds the entire heart. LV = left ventricle.

FIGURE 15–6
LARGE PERICARDIAL EFFUSION
Apical four-chamber view from the same patient as in Figure 15–5. A large pericardial effusion (P.E.) can be seen surrounding the heart. RV = right ventricle; LV = left ventricle; RA = right atrium; LA = left atrium.

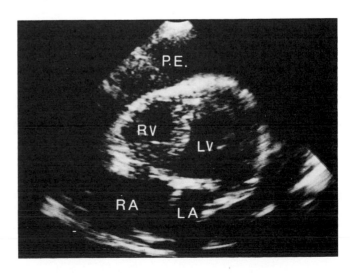

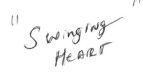

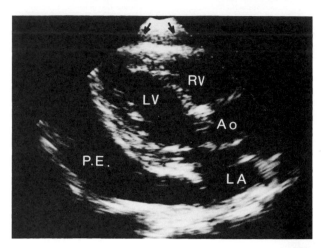

FIGURE 15–7
LARGE PERICARDIAL EFFUSION
Long-axis left parasternal view in a patient with a large pericardial effusion (P.E.) and a "swinging" heart. This frame shows the heart in its most anterior position. Only a small echo-free space is seen anteriorly (arrows). LV = left ventricle; RV = right ventricle; Ao = aorta; LA = left atrium.

FIGURE 15–8
LARGE PERICARDIAL EFFUSION
Long-axis left parasternal view from the same patient as in Figure 15–7, with the heart in its most posterior position. The anterior space is much larger in this view. P.E. = pericardial effusion; LV = left ventricle; RV = right ventricle; Ao = aorta; LA = left atrium.

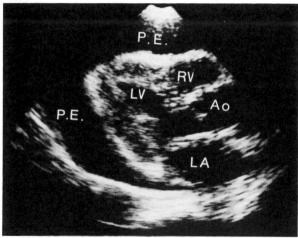

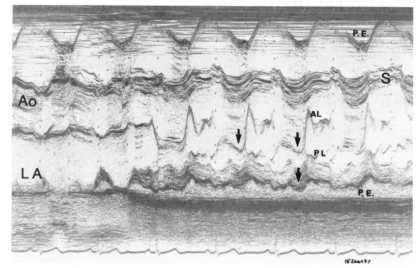

FIGURE 15–9
LARGE PERICARDIAL EFFUSION
Pseudo mitral valve prolapse. Echocardiographic "scan" from the aorta (Ao) to the left ventricle in a patient with a large pericardial effusion (P.E.). During late systole, the entire heart moves posteriorly (arrows), creating the appearance of pseudo mitral valve prolapse. This patient had a pericardial window with extraction of 400 cc of fluid and normalization of the mitral valve motion. LA = left atrium; S = septum; AL = anterior leaflet; PL = posterior leaflet.

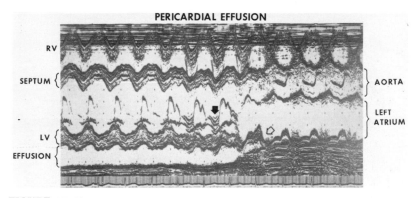

FIGURE 15–10
PERICARDIAL EFFUSION
Echocardiographic scan from the left ventricle (LV) to the aorta in a patient with
a moderate pericardial effusion. The effusion accumulates only behind the left
ventricle and stops at the level of the atrioventricular groove *(open arrow)*. The
black arrow points to pseudo mitral valve prolapse caused by swinging of the
heart with each beat. RV = right ventricle.

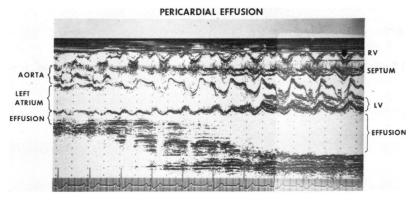

FIGURE 15–11
LARGE PERICARDIAL EFFUSION
Echocardiographic scan in a patient with rheumatic mitral valve disease and a
large pericardial effusion, which in this unusual case is seen not only behind the
left ventricle (LV) but also partially behind the left atrium. RV = right ventricle.

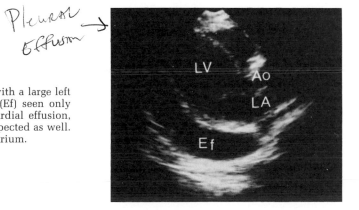

FIGURE 15–12
PLEURAL EFFUSION
Long-axis left parasternal view in a patient with a large left
pleural effusion. The large echo-free space (Ef) seen only
posteriorly suggests that this is not a pericardial effusion,
with which an anterior effusion would be expected as well.
LV = left ventricle; Ao = aorta; LA = left atrium.

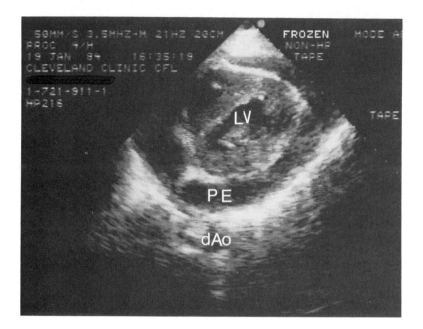

FIGURE 15–13
PERICARDIAL EFFUSION
Short-axis left parasternal view in a patient with pericardial effusion. The pericardial effusion (PE) is situated between the posterior wall of the left ventricle (LV) and the descending aorta (dAo).

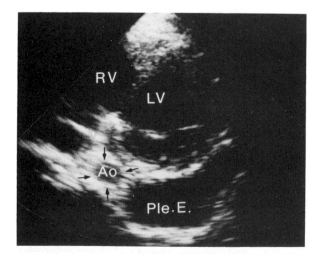

FIGURE 15–14
PLEURAL EFFUSION
Short-axis left parasternal view in a patient with recurrent pleural sarcoma and a large left pleural effusion (Ple. E.). The echo-free space behind the left ventricle corresponds to the pleural effusion, which is lateral to the decending aorta (Ao). The presence of a pericardial effusion is ruled out by the absence of a space between the descending aorta and the posterior wall of the left ventricle (LV). RV = right ventricle.

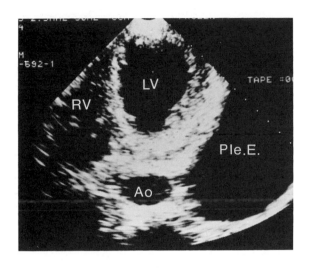

FIGURE 15–15
PLEURAL EFFUSION
Short-axis left parasternal view in a 70-year-old patient with congestive heart failure and a large left pleural effusion (Ple. E.), which is seen as an echo-free space behind and lateral to the left ventricle (LV) and not between the descending aorta (Ao) and the left ventricle, as would be seen in the presence of a pericardial effusion. RV = right ventricle.

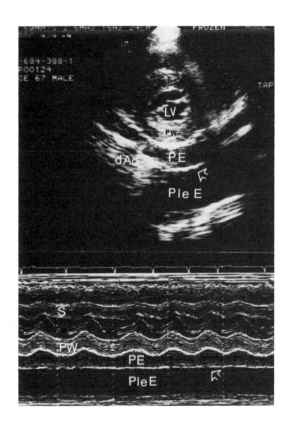

FIGURE 15–16
PLEUROPERICARDIAL EFFUSION
Short-axis left parasternal view at the left ventricular level in a 67-year-old patient with renal failure and pleural (PleE) and pericardial effusions (PE). The pericardial effusion separates the descending aorta (dAo) from the posterior wall (PW) of the left ventricle (LV), whereas the pleural effusion is lateral to the aorta. The arrow points to the pericardium, which appears as a linear echo recording. S = septum.

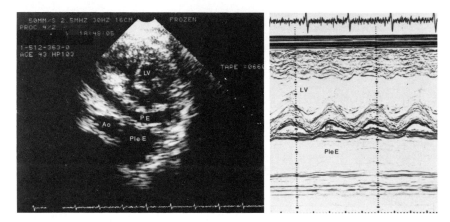

FIGURE 15–17
PLEUROPERICARDIAL EFFUSION
Short-axis left parasternal view in a patient with a pericardial effusion (PE) and a pleural effusion (PleE). The descending aorta (Ao) is posterior to the pericardial effusion and lateral to the pleural effusion. The M-mode echocardiogram was obtained from the middle of the scan. LV = left ventricle.

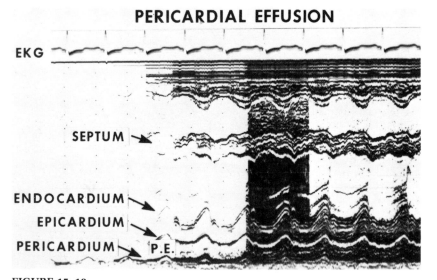

FIGURE 15–18
PERICARDIAL EFFUSION
Echocardiogram recorded at the left ventricular level in a patient with renal failure. Depending on the attenuation, the echo-free space corresponding to the pericardial effusion (P.E.) may or may not be seen.

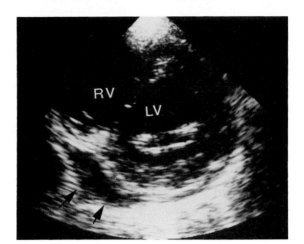

FIGURE 15–19
LOCULATED PERICARDIAL EFFUSION
Short-axis left parasternal view in a patient with a pericardial effusion loculated behind the medial aspect of the posterior left ventricular wall (arrows). An M-mode echocardiogram recorded through the middle of the left ventricle (LV) would not detect this effusion. RV = right ventricle.

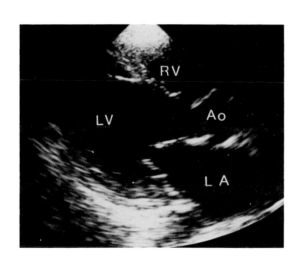

FIGURE 15–20
LOCULATED EFFUSION
Long-axis left parasternal view recorded from the same patient as in Figure 15–19. This view does not show the pericardial effusion, since the sector scan is cutting the left ventricle (LV) at an area lateral to the location of the effusion. RV = right ventricle; Ao = aorta; LA = left atrium.

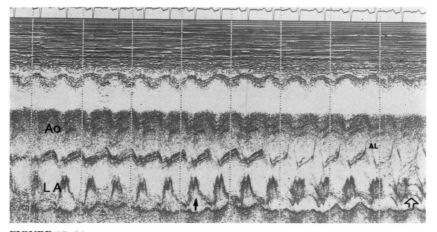

FIGURE 15–21
PERICARDIAL EFFUSION
The accumulation of fluid behind the left atrium (LA) at the level of the atrioventricular groove may produce excessive motion of the posterior left atrial wall, which on M-mode echocardiography creates the appearance of a left atrial mass (arrows). Ao = aorta; AL = anterior leaflet.

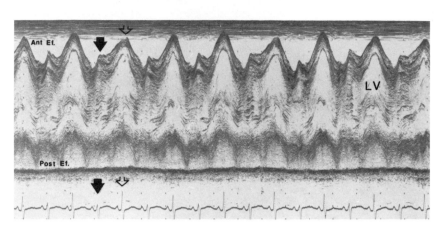

FIGURE 15–22
CARDIAC TAMPONADE
Very large anterior (Ant Ef.) and posterior (Post Ef.) pericardial effusions are evident in this recording from a patient with cardiac tamponade secondary to metastatic adenocarcinoma of the lung. Swinging of the heart and electrical alternans are present. LV = left ventricle.

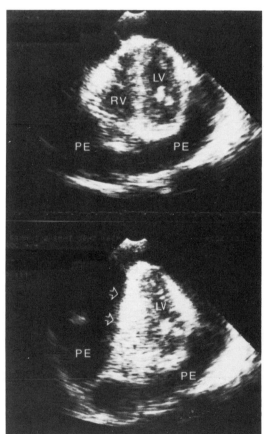

FIGURE 15–23
CARDIAC TAMPONADE
Apical four-chamber views in an 81-year-old patient with cardiac tamponade secondary to a bloody pericardial effusion (PE). A large effusion surrounds the entire heart. Marked cyclic right ventricular compression (collapse) is indicated by the open arrows. RV = right ventricle; LV = left ventricle.

RV compression
RV Collapse

FIGURE 15–24
CARDIAC TAMPONADE
A large anterior and posterior pericardial effusion (P.E.) is evident in this recording from a patient with cardiac tamponade secondary to lymphoma-induced pericardial effusion. There is exaggerated motion of the anterior right ventricular wall *(white arrow)* and significant change in right ventricular diameter with respiration. The black arrow points to a notch in the right ventricular wall, which has been cited in cardiac tamponade.

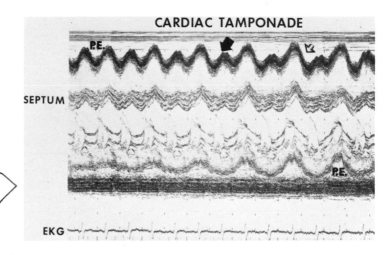

FIGURE 15–25
CONSTRICTIVE PERICARDITIS
Echocardiogram of the left ventricle in a 64-year-old patient with constrictive pericarditis. A dense band of echoes corresponding to a thickened pericardium (PER) is seen behind the posterior wall (PW). There is paradoxic septal motion *(open arrows)* and rapid early diastolic motion of the posterior wall *(small arrows).* S = septum.

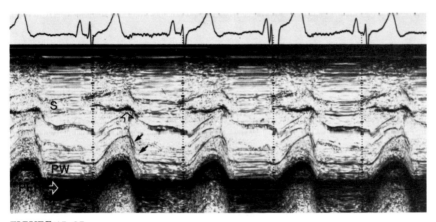

FIGURE 15–26
CONSTRICTIVE PERICARDITIS
Echocardiogram of the left ventricle in a 26-year-old patient with idiopathic constrictive pericarditis. The open arrow points to a flat diastolic motion of the posterior wall (PW), which follows a very rapid early diastolic slope *(black arrow).* RV = right ventricle; S = septum; LV = left ventricle.

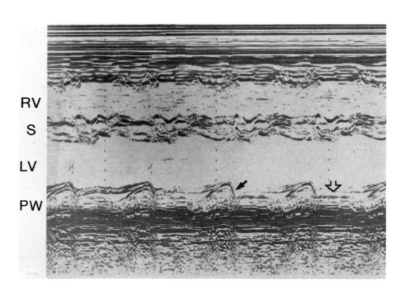

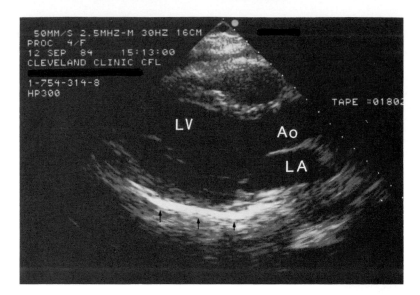

FIGURE 15–27
CONSTRICTIVE PERICARDITIS
This long-axis left parasternal view in a patient with constrictive pericarditis demonstrates a dense "shell" behind the posterior left ventricular wall. LV = left ventricle; Ao = aorta; LA = left atrium.

FIGURE 15–28
CONSTRICTIVE PERICARDITIS
Subcostal echocardiogram in a patient with constrictive pericarditis and dilated inferior vena cava (IVC) and hepatic vein (HV).

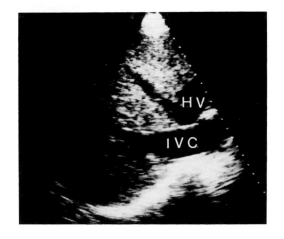

FIGURE 15–29
HEMORRHAGIC PERICARDIAL EFFUSION
Short-axis left parasternal view in a patient with a large bloody pericardial effusion (PE). The arrows point to undulating structures that are presumably clots or adherences within the pericardial sac. LV = left ventricle.

16 CONGENITAL HEART DISEASE

16.1 DEDUCTIVE ECHOCARDIOGRAPHY

The correct echocardiographic diagnosis of patients with congenital heart disease depends on the accurate definition of intracardiac anatomy and great vessel relation.[1]

Adequate echocardiographic evaluation of patients with complex congenital heart disease requires a systematic approach for assessing the relationship between the great arteries to the ventricles, the interventricular septum, the atrioventricular valves, the semilunar valves, and the atrium. By identifying the individual parts of the heart, the total cardiac anatomy can be reconstructed. Some general principles that serve to help the echocardiographer in properly identifying the different cardiac structures are described.

A. Atria

The atria follow the position of the lungs and abdominal viscera.[2] In the chest x-ray, if the stomach air bubble appears on the left, the left atrium is in the proper place; if the stomach air bubble is on the right, the left atrium is on the right side of the heart. The positions of the stomach and liver in the abdominal cavity can also be ascertained by echocardiography (Fig. 16–1).

The inferior vena cava, which can be vis-ualized with two-dimensional subxiphoid echocardiography, always drains into the right atrium.

B. Atrioventricular Valves

The insertion of the tricuspid valve in the interventricular septum is 5 to 10 mm closer to the apex than is the mitral valve (Fig. 16–2). This anatomic fact readily permits the correct identification of the atrioventricular valves and consequently of the ventricles, which always follow the position of the valves.

Another possible way of differentiating the mitral from the tricuspid valve is by identifying a trileaflet valve that is tricuspid or a bileaflet valve that is mitral. This can be done from a short-axis parasternal view (Figs. 16–3, 16–4) or from the subxiphoid short-axis view.

C. Ventricles

Identification of the ventricles depends on the recognition of the atrioventricular valves. The mitral valve is always in the anatomic left ventricle. The tricuspid valve is always in the anatomic right ventricle. There are two papillary muscles in the left ventricle. They are of equal size and arise from the medial and lateral walls. The right ventricle has three papillary muscles that vary in size and site of origin.[3] In addition, the right ventricle has the moderator band (Fig. 16–5). This muscular structure stretches from the lower interventricular septum to the anterior right ventricular wall.

D. Great Vessels

If the great vessels cross at the origin, the anterior vessel is invariably the pulmonary artery. If the great vessels are transposed and one is anterior to the other, the anterior vessel is usually the aorta. If the vessels are transposed and lie beside one another, it is necessary to follow their course to identify them. The vessel that courses superiorly and gives rise to the arteries of the neck is the aorta. The vessel that courses posteriorly into the thorax and then bifurcates is the pulmonary artery. Because of its bifurcation it also appears to end first. Recognizing the coronary arteries can help to identify the aorta as the great vessel from which they originate.

E. Semilunar Valves

1. The semilunar valves are always in their corresponding great vessel. So, if the aorta is identified, the aortic valve can be found within it. Likewise, the pulmonary artery contains the pulmonic valve.

2. Since the systemic resistance is higher than the pulmonary resistance, the ejection time of the aortic valve is shorter than that of the pulmonic valve. This fact can be used to differentiate the aortic from the pulmonic valve, except in the presence of severe pulmonary hypertension, in which the ejection time may be equal in both valves.

16.2 CARDIAC MALPOSITIONS[4]

Situs Solitus. This is the normal position of the heart. In this position the descending aorta, left atrium, apex, and stomach are all on the left.

Situs Inversus (Dextrocardia). The descending aorta, left atrium, apex, and stomach are all on the right.

Dextroversion. The descending aorta, left atrium, and stomach are on the left, and the apex is on the right.

Levoversion. The descending aorta, left atrium, and stomach are on the right, but the apex is on the left.

Mesocardia. The descending aorta, left atrium, and stomach are to the right, and the apex is in the midline.

Corrected Transposition.[5] In this condition, the venous blood returns to the heart from the inferior and superior venae cavae into the right atrium, passes to an anatomic left ventricle through a mitral valve, and exits to the pulmonary artery. The pulmonary veins drain arterialized blood into the left atrium, which is connected to an anatomic right ventricle with the tricuspid valve in it. The blood is then expelled into the aorta. There is ventricular inversion with preservation of normal physiology. The diagnosis of this condition is aided by the use of contrast echocardiography. A peripheral injection of echocardiographic contrast material shows the microcavitations to appear in the right atrium and then to pass into the left ventricle, which functions as a venous ventricle. The left ventricle can be recognized as having the mitral valve, which is further away from the apex than is the tricuspid valve (Figs. 16–6, 16–7).

16.3 ABNORMALITIES OF THE INTERATRIAL SEPTUM

A. Atrial Septal Defect

There are three main types of atrial septal defect (Fig. 16–8).

1. *Ostium Secundum.* This is by far the most common type, representing approximately 70 per cent of all types of defects in the interatrial septum. It is located in the area of the foramen ovale. This type of defect is a true deficiency in the interatrial septum and should not be confused with a patent foramen ovale.

2. *Ostium Primum.* These defects are less common, representing approximately 20 per cent of the atrial septal defects. They are located lower in the interatrial septum and are considered a partial form of the common atrioventricular canal (*incomplete atrioventricular canal*).

3. *Sinus Venosus Defects.* These represent only about 2 to 3 per cent of all defects. They are located in the junction of the interatrial septum and the superior vena cava and are often associated with anomalous venous return.

An unusual location for an atrial septal defect is in the coronary sinus orifice.

All forms of atrial septal defect have the echocardiographic features of right ventricular volume overload (Fig. 16–9), including (1) right ventricular dilatation, (2) paradoxic septal motion, and (3) increased tricuspid valve opening excursion.[6–9]

ECHOCARDIOGRAPHIC FEATURES

Besides these general factors, each form of atrial septal defect has some specific echocardiographic features, as discussed next.[10]

Ostium Secundum. Direct visualization of the atrial septal defect can be achieved from any of several sector plane views (Fig. 16–10). Since from the subcostal view the interatrial septum lies perpendicular to the sector plane, this view provides the best imaging window. The defect is seen as a dropout of echoes in the middle of the interatrial septum. The borders of the defect are usually more echogenic, producing a broadening effect in the margins. This effect helps to differentiate a true defect from an echo dropout in the area of a normal fossa ovalis.

Contrast echocardiography is particularly helpful in the detection of right-to-left shunts at the atrial level. With two-dimensional echocardiography, the echocardiographic contrast material, when injected into a peripheral vein, can be seen to arrive in the right atrium and then to pass partially through the atrial septal defect into the left atrium (Figs. 16–11, 16–12). With M-mode echocardiography with the transducer directed toward the mitral valve, the echocardiographic contrast material is seen first in the right ventricle and then entering the left ventricle through the mitral valve funnel.

Even in the absence of significant right-to-left shunt at the atrial level, contrast echocardiography can help by the demonstration of the negative contrast effect. This consists of the observation of a jet of blood coming through the interatrial septum from the left atrium and "washing out" part of the contrast material in the right atrium (Fig. 16–13).

It is also possible to visualize a few echocardiographic contrast bubbles to pass from the right to the left atrium in the presence of an atrial septal defect with predominant left-to-right shunt. In the presence of significant echocardiographic dropout at the level of the interatrial septum, contrast echocardiography may serve to confirm the integrity

of this structure by demarcation of a medial boundary with contrast material (Fig. 16–14).

Ostium Primum Atrial Septal Defect. In this condition the interatrial septum is deficient in its inferior portion (Fig. 16–15). This is a mild form of the *endocardial cushion defect malformation* or so-called *partial atrioventricular canal.*

Both the mitral and tricuspid valves insert at the same level. The atrial septum just superior to the point of leaflet insertion is absent.

There is usually a mitral valve cleft, and the opening of the mitral valve is toward the left ventricular outflow tract, which is narrowed.

The best views in which to demonstrate an ostium primum atrial septal defect by echocardiography are the apical four-chamber and subcostal views. The characteristic echocardiographic abnormalities of an ostium primum defect include mitral-tricuspid alignment, deficient low interatrial septum, and cleft mitral valve. Further information related to this subject is to be found in the later discussion of endocardial cushion defect.

Sinus Venosus. Direct visualization of the sinus venosus type of atrial septal defect has been reported.

The view that best demonstrates this abnormality is the subcostal position with a diligent examination of the superior region of the interatrial septum. An area of echo dropout is seen superior to the fossa ovalis, in close proximity to the entrance of the superior vena cava into the right atrium.

B. Common Atrium

Common atrium consists of complete or virtual absence of the atrial septum. There are two atrial appendages but one common atrial chamber. Elements of the endocardial cushion malformation sometimes coexist, especially a cleft mitral valve.

Echocardiographically a common atrium can be best seen from the apical four-chamber (Fig. 16–16) and four-chamber subcostal views, in which there are no echoes at all between the atria. A single large atrial chamber is visualized above the ventricles.

C. Patent Foramen Ovale

Patent foramen ovale can be demonstrated with contrast echocardiography. During the

Valsalva maneuver, some microbubbles may be seen passing from the right to the left atrium.

D. Atrial Septal Aneurysm

Aneurysm of the interatrial septum may occur in association with an atrial septal defect in the presence of right ventricular inflow or outflow obstruction, or aneurysm may occur as an isolated abnormality. Aneurysms usually involve the area of the fossa ovalis.

With M-mode echocardiography, linear echoes in the right atrium behind the tricuspid valve suggest the presence of an aneurysm of the interatrial septum. These findings are not specific. With two-dimensional echocardiography, septal aneurysms appear as localized thin pouches of the atrial septum that bulge toward both the right and the left atrium with a saillike motion (Fig. 16–17). Contrast echocardiography can help in further delineating the aneurysm, which appears as a filling defect in the atrial cavity toward which it bulges (Fig. 16–18).

16.4 ABNORMALITIES OF THE INTERVENTRICULAR SEPTUM

A. Ventricular Septal Defects

Ventricular septal defect can be classified as supracristal, membranous, muscular, atrioventricular canal, or conotruncal.

Supracristal Ventricular Septal Defect. This defect lies above the crista ventricularis. It is situated immediately beneath the pulmonary orifice so that the valve forms part of the superior margin of the septal defect (Fig. 16–19).

Echocardiographically, this defect can be visualized from the long-axis parasternal view with slight leftward angulation; from the short-axis parasternal view at the level of the aorta, at which the defect is seen as an echo dropout at approximately 1 to 2 o'clock of the aortic circumference; or from the subcostal short-axis view, in which the defect is seen at a location just inferior to the pulmonic valve and opposite to the parietal band of the crista ventricularis.

Membranous Ventricular Septal Defect. These are the most common defects of clinical significance, although small muscular ventricular defects probably have a higher overall incidence. This defect lies below and posterior to the crista, in close continuity with the septal leaflet of the tricuspid valve. The defect is found just below the aortic valve close to the commissure forming the right and noncoronary cusps or at about the 11 o'clock position of the aortic circumference (Fig. 16–20).

Membranous ventricular septal defects can be seen from the long-axis parasternal view with slight rightward angulation. In this view an echo dropout is seen at the level of the membranous septum just beneath the aorta. In the short-axis parasternal view at the level of the aorta, the defect is apparent immediately beneath the aorta at about 11 o'clock of the aortic circumference. From an apical four-chamber view the defect may be imaged in the membranous septum at a location just inferior to the insertion of the septal tricuspid leaflet. Similar findings are encountered from the subcostal four-chamber view. The subcostal short-axis view serves to differentiate this type of defect from the supracristal type. A membranous defect in this view is seen in an anteroinferior position in relation to the aorta, at about the 12 o'clock position, whereas the supracristal defect is at about the 3 to the 4 o'clock position in this view.

Muscular Ventricular Septal Defect. Small ventricular septal defects in the area of the muscular septum are very common in infants. Such defects usually have no clinical significance. Over 90 per cent of these close spontaneously and are usually too small (less than 2 mm) to be imaged by echocardiography. Large muscular septal defects are more rare but also have greater clinical significance. They may be single or multiple or they may appear as a relatively thin muscular septum with sievelike fenestrations. They may be located quite inferiorly in the interventricular septum, sometimes beneath the moderator band, so that its identification is rather difficult.

This type of defect can be imaged best from the apical four-chamber view and the subcostal four-chamber view, in which the defect can be recognized in the middle or inferior part of the septum. These defects also can be seen from short-axis parasternal views, and if the defect is not in the lower third of the septum it can also be detected from the long-axis parasternal view (Fig. 16–21).

Atrioventricular Canal Ventricular Septal Defects. Occasionally an isolated ventricular septal defect may be found in the posterior inlet septum, at a location posterior to the tricuspid valve, between this valve and the mitral valve. Such a defect is in the position that it would occupy if it were part of a complete endocardial cushion defect. This phenomenon is further discussed under atrioventricular canal defects.

Conotruncal Ventricular Septal Defects. This type of defect is seen in Fallot's tetralogy.

Normal echocardiographic findings are common among patients with small ventricular septal defects. In patients with large ventricular septal defects, these abnormalities can be seen: (1) left ventricular dilatation, (2) left atrial dilatation, and (3) hyperkinetic left ventricular contractility.[11–13]

Contrast echocardiography may help in detecting a shunt at ventricular level. This technique is particularly helpful with right-to-left shunts. In M-mode echocardiography, with the beam directed toward the mitral valve, echocardiographic contrast material injected into a peripheral vein appears first in the right ventricle and then in the left ventricle in the outflow tract area. This is in front of the anterior leaflet of the mitral valve. The mitral valve funnel is free of echocardiographic contrast material (Fig. 16–22). With two-dimensional echocardiography, the passage of contrast material directly through the defect can be observed (Figs. 16–23 to 16–25).

B. Ventricular Septal Aneurysms

Ventricular septal aneurysms usually involve the membranous ventricular septum. Echocardiographically, they appear as outgrowths originating in the septum and protruding into the right ventricle.[14–16] They can be seen from the apical four-chamber view (Fig. 16–26).

16.5 ENDOCARDIAL CUSHION DEFECTS

The endocardial cushion forms part of the central portion of the heart at which the atria and the ventricle come together. It contributes to the development of the septal leaflet of the tricuspid valve, the anterior mitral leaflet, and convergence of the atrial and ventricular septa. Endocardial cushion defects include varying combinations of these four contiguous parts of the heart. Four categories of endocardial cushion defects are defined.

1. Partial or Incomplete Endocardial Cushion Defect. This consists of an ostium primum septal defect usually with a cleft mitral valve.

2. Inlet Ventricular Septal Defect. This ventricular septal defect is situated in the endocardial cushion part of the interventricular septum.

3. Isolated Mitral or Tricuspid Clefts

4. Complete Endocardial Cushion Defect. This type consists of a defect in the lower part of the atrial septum (ostium primum), together with clefts in the anterior mitral and septal tricuspid leaflets and a defect in the interventricular septum.

According to the degree of leaflet abnormality and the area in which chordae tendineae anchor the common atrioventricular valve, the complete endocardial cushion defects are classified as one of three types (Fig. 16–27):

A. RASTELLI TYPE A. This is the most common form and is characterized by atrial and ventricular septal defects with clefts in the mitral and tricuspid valves and anchorings of either mitral valve or tricuspid valve, or both, to the crest of the ventricular septal defect on the ipsilateral side.

B. RASTELLI TYPE B. In this type of defect, chords from the mitral apparatus cross the ventricular septal defect and are anchored to a papillary muscle in the right side of the septum.

C. RASTELLI TYPE C. In this disorder, there is a free-floating poorly formed leaflet that is anchored in the right and left ventricle but not in the interventricular septum.

This section describes the echocardiographic findings in complete endocardial cushion defect and cleft mitral valve.[17–20]

The echocardiographic diagnosis of complete endocardial cushion defect depends on the demonstration of right ventricular volume overload, narrowed left ventricular outflow tract, direct visualization of the endocardial cushion defect, tricuspid-mitral alignment, and cleft mitral valve.

1. RIGHT VENTRICULAR VOLUME OVERLOAD. Right ventricular dilatation and abnormal septal motion are usually present (Fig. 16–28). Significant mitral insufficiency secondary to a cleft mitral valve may normalize septal motion.

2. NARROWED LEFT VENTRICULAR OUTFLOW TRACT. The distance from the mitral valve during systole to the interventricular septum is decreased (Fig. 16–29). During diastole, there is prolonged mitral-septal apposition. This is related to the abnormal attachment of the anterior leaflet to the septum. The opening of the anterior leaflet is abnormal, moving toward the outflow tract and frequently appearing to go through the septum (Figs. 16–30, 16–31). The subxiphoid view is probably the best plane for visualization of the narrowed left ventricular outflow tract. This view demonstrates the "goose neck deformity" in the same form that is seen on the frontal plane angiogram. The long-axis left parasternal view also permits visualization of the abnormal mitral motion into the outflow tract (Figs. 16–32 to 16–34).

3. DIRECT VISUALIZATION OF THE ENDOCARDIAL CUSHION DEFECT. With an M-mode echocardiographic scan, fragmentation with segments of absence of interventricular septal echoes can be demonstrated (Figs. 16–30, 16–31).

With two-dimensional echocardiography, the ventricular and atrial components of the defect can be visualized. The best view to use is the apical four-chamber projection (Figs. 16–35, 16–36). From the long-axis parasternal view, it is also possible to view the endocardial cushion defect, particularly its ventricular septal component. This view also permits visualization of the mitral valve moving through the defect.

4. TRICUSPID-MITRAL ALIGNMENT. In patients with endocardial cushion defects, there is tricuspid-mitral alignment. This phenomenon can be best demonstrated from the apical four-chamber view in which the septal leaflet of the tricuspid valve is seen at the same level as the mitral valve and not closer to the apex, as seen in normal individuals (Fig. 16–37).

5. CLEFT MITRAL VALVE. The best projection to study this abnormality is the short-axis left parasternal view at the level of the mitral valve. The diastolic appearance of the mitral valve is changed from the normal ovoid or "fish mouth" appearance to a more triangular opening, with separation of the anterior leaflet into two parts (the mitral valve actually becomes "tricuspid") (Fig. 16–38). The cleft is usually eccentric toward the medial commissure. The extent of the cross section in which the diastolic separation of the anterior leaflet appears varies depending on the size of the cleft. In patients with a complete cleft, the separation is seen from the top to the base of the valve. In patients with incomplete clefts, the separation is observed only toward the tip of the valve. During systole, the two parts of the anterior leaflet meet at the center and form an echo-dense area, which may be seen to overlap to some degree (Fig. 16–39). The accessory chordae are seen as thick linear echoes between the ridges of both parts of the anterior leaflet and the septum. After surgical repair of the cleft, the anterior leaflet of the mitral valve is not seen to separate during diastole. With M-mode echocardiography a cleft mitral valve frequently appears with a cloud of echoes behind it (Fig. 16–40) and sometimes has a fine diastolic flutter (Fig. 16–41). The signs of left ventricular volume overload are common (Fig. 16–42).

The apical four-chamber view allows detection of both atrial and ventricular septal leaflets with the common atrioventricular valve between the defects. This view also allows differentiation of the Rastelli type of endocardial cushion defect on the basis of atrioventricular valve morphology and chordae tendineae attachments.

16.6 STRADDLING ATRIOVENTRICULAR VALVES

These abnormalities consist of ventriculoatrial malalignment in which a leaflet crosses into the contralateral ventricle through a ventricular septal defect. The suspensory apparatus of the valve usually remains within the ventricle on its own side. The atrial septum and the crux of the heart are shifted with reference to the ventricular septum so that some overlap occurs.[21–23] Tricuspid valves usually straddle ventricular septal defects of the endocardial cushion defect type. Mitral valve straddling is less common and occurs in association with more anterior or superior muscular ventricular septal defects.

16.7 ANOMALOUS PULMONARY VENOUS RETURN

Classification

Abnormal pulmonary venous return can be classified as anomalous pulmonary venous drainage or anomalous pulmonary venous connection.

1. Anomalous Pulmonary Venous Drainage. The pulmonary veins are connected to the left atrium, but one or more veins are directed so that their flow passes preferentially into the right atrium through an atrial septal defect.

2. Anomalous Pulmonary Venous Connection

A. PARTIAL. One or two of the pulmonary veins enter either the right atrium or a systemic vein directly. They typically involve the veins from the right lung and more frequently enter the superior vena cava. Partial anomalous pulmonary venous connection almost invariably coexists with an atrial septal defect.

B. TOTAL. The four pulmonary veins either enter the right atrium directly or more often form a common pulmonary venous chamber that lies posterior to the left atrium. From there a separate ventricular channel connects this confluence of veins to either the coronary sinus, the left innominate vein (through a vertical vein), or the portal vein.

Echocardiographic Abnormalities

The echocardiographic abnormalities that can be seen in patients with anomalous venous return include right ventricular volume overload, direct visualization of the pulmonary veins, and visualization of the common pulmonary venous chamber.[24–27]

1. Right Ventricular Volume Overload. All forms of anomalous pulmonary venous return have echocardiographic findings of right ventricular volume overload with a dilated right ventricle and paradoxic septal motion.

2. Direct Visualization of the Pulmonary Veins. Direct visualization of the pulmonary veins is more helpful to exclude anomalous venous connection than to determine the diagnosis.

3. Visualization of the Common Pulmonary Venous Chamber. In patients with total anomalous venous connections, direct demonstration of the common pulmonary venous chamber behind the left atrium is possible with M-mode and two-dimensional echocardiography (Fig. 16–43). This chamber appears as an echo-free space behind the left atrium. The apical four-chamber and subxiphoid views are best suited for demonstration of this abnormality.

16.8 PATENT DUCTUS ARTERIOSUS

The pulmonary orifice of the ductus is located immediately to the left of the bifurcation of the pulmonary trunk. The aortic end of the ductus usually lies just below the origin of the left subclavian artery. It is usually largest at its aortic insertion. After birth, there is an initial stage of functional closure in which there is minimal or no shunt. Anatomic closure usually occurs by the fourth to eighth week. If the ductus does not close and its caliber is large, there is a shunt from the aorta to the pulmonary artery. This shunt produces left atrial enlargement and left ventricular volume overload, since the left heart has to handle both the normal pulmonary venous return and the shunted blood.

Echocardiographic Findings

The echocardiographic findings in patients with patent ductus arteriosus include left atrial enlargement, left ventricular volume overload, direct visualization of the ductus, and verification of left-to-right shunt by injection of contrast material.[28–31]

1. Left Atrial Enlargement. This can be best characterized by the ratio of the left atrial dimension divided by the dimension of the aorta (Fig. 16–44). This ratio is 0.7 to 0.85 in normal individuals and approximately 1.2 in patients with large left-to-right shunt at the level of the ductus.

2. Left Ventricular Volume Overload. Dilatation of the left ventricle with increased septal and posterior wall motion is frequently found in patients with patent ductus (Fig. 16–44).

3. Direct Visualization of the Ductus. It may be possible to directly view a patent ductus with two-dimensional echocardiography. The projection that appears most useful for this purpose is the short-axis left parasternal view. The descending aorta is seen below the pulmonary artery, and the patent ductus is seen as an echo-free communication between them (Fig. 16–45).

4. Contrast Echocardiography. Aortic contrast medium injections from umbilical artery catheters can be useful for verifying left-to-right shunt through a patent ductus arteriosus.

16.9 LEFT VENTRICULAR INFLOW OBSTRUCTION

Congenital inflow obstruction to the left ventricle can occur at the level of the mitral valve or proximal to it. The most common causes of such obstruction include congenital mitral stenosis, "parachute" mitral valve, cor triatriatum, and mitral atresia.

1. Congenital Mitral Stenosis. This condition can be the result of a supravalvular ring, annular hypoplasia, abnormalities of the leaflets, chordae tendineae, or papillary muscles, or a combination of these conditions.

M-mode echocardiography[32–34] demonstrates decreased E to F slope of the mitral valve, diastolic anterior motion of the posterior leaflet, and frequently diastolic flutter of both anterior and posterior leaflets in the absence of aortic insufficiency.

Two-dimensional echocardiography permits the evaluation of the mitral ring size, which is often small. Visualization of the mitral valve orifice size is not as reliable as in acquired mitral stenosis. This is because the effective orifice lies between the chordae and the papillary muscles and cannot be visualized clearly by two-dimensional echocardiography.

2. "Parachute" Mitral Valve. There may be a wide spectrum of papillary muscle abnormalities that in some cases are very close to each other or fused. A single papillary muscle may exist without the anterolateral muscle. This condition is characteristic of the "parachute" mitral valve.

3. Cor Triatriatum. This anomaly is characterized by drainage of the pulmonary veins into an accessory left atrial chamber that lies at an area proximal to the true left atrium (Fig. 16–46).[35, 36] The dilated chamber communicates with the left ventricle through the mitral valve and contains the left atrial appendage and the fossa ovalis. The malformation is often associated with an atrial septal defect.

The best projection with which to study the abnormality is the apical four-chamber view in which the left atrium is seen to be divided by a membrane in the middle.

4. Mitral Atresia. This anomaly is characterized by a "blind" dimple in the floor of the left atrium. Mitral valvular tissue is usually not recognizable. The condition is often associated with aortic atresia and is part of the hypoplastic heart syndrome.

Echocardiographically, there is no identifiable mitral valve tissue. Dense echoes are recorded only in the mitral region. The left ventricle is diminutive.

16.10 CONGENITAL AORTIC STENOSIS

Echocardiography can be very useful in determining the site of left ventricular outflow tract obstruction,[37, 38] and permits the differentiation of several conditions (Fig. 16–47), including:
1. Valvular aortic stenosis
2. Bicuspid aortic valve
3. Subvalvular aortic stenosis
   Discrete membranous aortic stenosis
   Diffuse fibromuscular subvalvular obstruction
   Tunnel subaortic stenosis
4. Supravalvular aortic stenosis

1. Congenital Valvular Aortic Stenosis

The echocardiographic diagnosis of congenital aortic stenosis is based on the demonstration of reduced aortic valve orifice size, decreased leaflet separation, and domed aortic valves.[39–42]

Reduced Aortic Valve Orifice. With two-dimensional echocardiography, it may be possible to view the aortic valve orifice in cross section by obtaining an image from the short-axis left parasternal view. With significant stenosis this orifice is appreciably reduced in size. Care must be taken to record the actual orifice. A good correlation between the size of this orifice and the aortic valve area calculated during catheterization has been found.

Decreased Leaflet Separation. Because of the usual domed configuration of the congenitally stenotic valve, the M-mode echocardiogram may not show a decreased leaflet excursion (Fig. 16–48) unless its beam passes directly through the top of the dome. Because of this, M-mode echocardiography has not been very useful in the diagnosis of congenital aortic stenosis.

With two-dimensional echocardiography, on the other hand, it is possible to measure the leaflet separation at the top of the dome (Fig. 16–49). This measurement, if corrected for aortic size, yields a fairly good correlation with aortic gradient. It is also possible to follow the results of valvuloplasty by this method (Fig. 16–50).

Domed Aortic Valves. The presence of "doming" is a very helpful criterion for the diagnosis of aortic stenosis. This condition can be appreciated best in the long-axis left parasternal view, in which during systole the leaflets are fully separated at their base but are close together at their tips (Fig. 16–51). Frequently, doming of only one leaflet can be visualized, but this is sufficient to make the appropriate diagnosis (Fig. 16–52). Reverse doming of the leaflets can be seen during diastole, in which the leaflets are seen to move toward the left ventricular outflow tract (Fig. 16–53).

2. Bicuspid Aortic Valve

It has been estimated that the bicuspid aortic valve occurs in approximately 2 per cent of the population. A bicuspid aortic valve can be functionally normal, stenotic, or incompetent.

The two cusps can be oriented so that one is anterior and the other is posterior, with the commissure at 9 o'clock and 3 o'clock of the aortic circumference, or they can be right and left, with the commissures at 12 and 6 o'clock, respectively (Fig. 16–54). A raphe is often present in the anterior or in the right cusps.

The echocardiographic diagnosis of bicuspid valve is based on the demonstration of two cusps and two commissures.[43–47] This is best registered in the short-axis parasternal view (Figs. 16–55, 16–56). The leaflets are somewhat redundant, so they may be seen to prolapse somewhat during diastole into the left ventricular outflow tract. This also produces multiple linear echoes during diastole in the M-mode echocardiogram (Fig. 16–57). Often one leaflet is larger than the other, and they have a somewhat oblique orientation within the aorta. This produces *eccentric closure*, which can be appreciated in the long-axis left parasternal view or with M-mode echocardiography (Figs. 16–58,

16–59). The degree of eccentricity can be expressed quantitatively by calculating the eccentricity index according to the formula

$$ET = \frac{1}{2} \frac{A}{a}$$

where A is the aortic root diameter, and a is the distance from the line of aortic cusp coaptation to the nearest aortic wall, with both measured at the onset of diastole.

It should be remembered that excessive angulation of the transducer can create a pseudo eccentric closure (Fig. 16–60) that is the same as that noted with left atrial enlargement.

A small raphe can be confused with an extra commissure, and a bicuspid valve can be confused with a tricuspid valve (Fig. 16–61). Sometimes it is not possible to image the aortic valve with adequate detail to be able to distinguish the number of leaflets.

Simultaneously recorded echocardiograms and phonocardiograms of patients with bicuspid aortic valve show the coincidence of the ejection click with the opening of the aortic valve (Fig. 16–62).

3. Subvalvular Aortic Stenosis

The dynamic forms of subvalvular aortic stenosis—hypertrophic obstructive cardiomyopathies—are described in the section on cardiomyopathies. The discussion presented here relates to the fixed forms of subvalvular aortic stenosis, of which there are three main groups: discrete membranous subvalvular aortic stenosis, diffuse fibromuscular subvalvular aortic stenosis, and tunnel aortic stenosis.

a. Discrete Membranous Subvalvular Aortic Stenosis. This condition involves a thick discrete fibrous membrane that is located immediately beneath the aortic valve and that obstructs an otherwise normal left ventricular outflow tract. The membrane may eventually produce aortic valve damage. This form of stenosis can be imaged best from the apical or subcostal left ventricular outflow tract views. It may be only partially imaged from the long-axis left parasternal view.[48, 49]

The inner margins of the membrane are more echo-dense and easier to image. However, often it is possible to visualize the full extent of the membrane, which appears as a fine line beneath the aortic valve and moving in the direction of flow during systole and prolapsing towards the left ventricle during diastole. M-mode echocardiography provides some nonspecific findings for the detection of the abnormality. These include (1) systolic mid closure of the aortic valve, (2) excessive aortic valve fluttering, (3) a band of echo-producing tissue in the outflow tract, which can occasionally be recorded (Fig. 16–63), (4) left ventricular hypertrophy, and (5) systolic anterior motion of the mitral valve, which occasionally can be seen in patients with fixed subvalvular stenosis.

b. Diffuse Fibromuscular Subvalvular Aortic Stenosis. This form consists of a thick fibromuscular ring involving the anterior and posterior margins of the left ventricular outflow tract. These rings are at a location somewhat more distal to the aortic valve (approximately 1 cm or more below it) than is the discrete membrane in the membranous form. The diffuse long segment of hypoplasia of the subvalvular left ventricular outflow tract can be easily imaged from the apical and subcostal left ventricular outflow tract views and from the long-axis left parasternal view.

There is anterior displacement of tissue from the junction between the anterior mitral leaflet and the aorta as well as protrusion of tissue from the interventricular septum.

c. Tunnel Aortic Stenosis. This is an extreme form of fibromuscular subvalvular stenosis in which the left ventricular outflow tract is severely narrowed. Echocardiographically, this appears as an extreme form of fibromuscular stenosis. The authors have seen a patient with bicuspid aortic stenosis in whom a ring of calcium extended into the left ventricular outflow tract and simulated tunnel subaortic stenosis (Figs. 16–64, 16–65).

4. Supravalvular Aortic Stenosis

There are three types of supravalvular aortic stenosis.

1. Membranous Type. This form involves a fibrous diaphragm containing a perforation localized immediately above the aortic valve. This abnormality can be best imaged from the long-axis left parasternal view. Echocardiographically, the membrane appears as a discrete thin linear echo extending inward from the aortic walls and narrowing the lumen in a localized segment.

2. Hourglass Deformity. This form con-

sists of localized segmental hourglass-shaped narrowing immediately above the aortic sinuses. The caliber of the poststenotic aorta is normal or reduced but not dilated. This pattern is often a feature of a syndrome with associated infantile hypercalcemia, elfinlike facies, peripheral pulmonic stenosis, and stenosis of other arteries in the body. There is a more extensive and diffuse area of narrowing of the ascending aorta. Both the aortic lumen and the aortic diameter are narrowed.[50, 51] This abnormality can also be detected with M-mode echocardiography,[52] in which gradual reduction of the aortic root diameter is seen as the supravalvular region of the ascending aorta is scanned (Fig. 16–66).

3. Hypoplasia of the Aorta. This form is characterized by uniform narrowing of the entire ascending aorta beginning near the origin of the coronary arteries (Fig. 16–67).

16.11 COARCTATION OF THE AORTA

Coarctation of the aorta is produced by a localized deformity of the media that is manifested by a curtainlike infolding that eccentrically narrows the aortic lumen. Externally the aorta exhibits an indentation or localized concavity. The coarctation is usually located immediately beyond the origin of the left subclavian artery, just distal to the ligamentum arteriosum. Occasionally the coarctation is located before the ligamentum arteriosum; this is the "preductal" variety (Fig. 16–68).

The term *pseudocoarctation* has been used to designate an abnormality characterized by tucking at the site of the ligamentum arteriosum but without narrowing of the aortic lumen.

Coarctation is often associated with bicuspid aortic valve, patent ductus arteriosus, and ventricular septal defect.[53]

Coarctation of the aorta can be visualized best with two-dimensional suprasternal scanning.[54–56] It appears as a localized decrease in the diameter of the aortic lumen, with the area of maximal narrowing distal to the origin of the left subclavian artery.

There is often focal thickening in the area of coarctation. This condition produces an area of greater echo reflectivity. The aortic pulsations proximal to the coarctation are characteristically increased in intensity. Distal to the obstruction, the aorta is dilated again, but the pulsations are damped.

16.12 PULMONIC STENOSIS

Congenital obstruction to right ventricular outflow can be classified as valvular, subvalvular, or supravalvular pulmonic stenosis (Fig. 16–69).

1. Valvular Pulmonic Stenosis. This is the most common form and is characterized by a conical or dome-shaped zone with a narrow outlet at its apex. Three raphes extend from the central orifice to the walls of the pulmonary artery. Poststenotic dilatation of the pulmonary artery is usually present. The characteristic echocardiographic finding of pulmonic stenosis is doming of the valve.[57] This can be viewed best from the short-axis left parasternal view when the stenotic and somewhat thickened pulmonic valve curves away from the pulmonary artery during systole. Frequently only the posterior pulmonic valve can be seen.

With M-mode echocardiography, an exaggerated pulmonic valve *a* wave can be seen (Fig. 16–70). False-positive and false-negative findings do exist (Fig. 16–71), but the presence of doming of the pulmonic valve plus a large *a* wave on the M-mode pulmonic echocardiogram are usually associated with hemodynamically significant pulmonic stenosis. Septal hypertrophy and right ventricular hypertrophy are usually present in association with significant pulmonic stenosis (Fig. 16–72). In the presence of valvular pulmonic stenosis, a phonocardiogram may demonstrate an ejection click that characteristically increases in intensity with expiration (Fig. 16–73).

2. Subvalvular Pulmonic Stenosis. This condition is generally associated with a ventricular septal defect and is the result of either a localized narrowing at the entrance of the outflow tract *(infundibular)* or more rarely the result of hypertrophy of the vulvar muscle or abnormal muscle groups *(subinfundibular).* This abnormality is also visualized best from the short-axis left parasternal view. There is an increased amount of echo production from the anterior and posterior parts of the infundibulum with narrowing of the outflow tract in this region. Distal to this obstruction the pulmonic valve is seen in an area of normal diameter. This condition can be an isolated abnormality or

more frequently occurs as part of Fallot's tetralogy.

With M-mode echocardiography large-amplitude high-frequency fluttering of the pulmonic valve is a characteristic finding of patients with subvalvular pulmonic stenosis.

3. Supravalvular Pulmonic Stenosis. This condition is the result of narrowing of either the pulmonary trunk or its branches. This abnormality can be imaged best from the left parasternal border or from the subcostal right ventricular outflow tract. Increased echo production is seen immediately distal to the pulmonic valve, with reduction and narrowing of the lumen.[58]

16.13 EBSTEIN'S ANOMALY

The anatomic abnormality in Ebstein's anomaly consists of displacement of fused and malformed portions of the tricuspid valvular tissue into the right ventricular cavity (Fig. 16–74). The leaflets are attached in part to the tricuspid annulus and in part below it. The right ventricle above the displaced tricuspid valve is quite thin and has the anatomic appearance of right atrial wall. The septal and posterior leaflets are more affected and deformed than the anterior leaflet.

Ebstein's anomaly is frequently associated with an interatrial septal defect. Functionally there may be tricuspid stenosis or more frequently tricuspid insufficiency with right ventricular volume overload.

The best echocardiographic view in which to visualize this abnormality is the apical four-chamber view. The septal leaflet of the tricuspid valve inserts into the interventricular septum far closer to the apex than the corresponding mitral valve (Fig. 16–75).[58–61] Normally the distance between the insertion points in the septum of the tricuspid and mitral valves is only a few millimeters. With Ebstein's anomaly this separation increases considerably, ranging from 1.4 to 3.2 cm. The apical four-chamber view also permits identification of the tricuspid annulus, which remains in its normal position, and of the size of the atrialized ventricle, which is the area between the displaced tricuspid valve and the tricuspid annulus.

The long-axis left parasternal view shows an enlarged right ventricle with a flattened left ventricle. The anterior leaflet, which is long and redundant, is seen to move widely in a saillike fashion (Fig. 16–76).

On M-mode echocardiography the most characteristic finding is delayed tricuspid closure (Figs. 16–77 to 16–79).[62] The anterior leaflet has increased excursion during diastole and is often recorded simultaneously with the mitral valve, which is seen to close sooner. If closure of the tricuspid valve occurs 50 msec after closure of the mitral valve, the diagnosis of Ebstein's anomaly is very likely. The E to F slope of the anterior tricuspid valve is often reduced.

16.14 TRICUSPID ATRESIA

In tricuspid atresia, tricuspid valve tissue cannot be identified. A small imperforate dimple is found in the floor of the right atrium, but no communication exists between the right atrium and the right ventricle. There is always an interatrial septal defect and usually a ventricular septal defect (Fig. 16–80). Other abnormalities frequently associated with tricuspid atresia are transposition of the great vessels and pulmonic stenosis.

The most common form of tricuspid atresia is the variety that occurs with pulmonic stenosis—normally related great vessels and small ventricular septal defect. The left ventricle is usually large.

Tricuspid atresia is best imaged with two-dimensional echocardiography from the apical and subcostal four-chamber views. A dense band of echoes is seen at the level of the tricuspid ring, but no tricuspid leaflets are identified (Fig. 16–81). A large atrial septal defect is frequently seen. The right ventricle is small and communicates with a small left ventricle through a ventricular septal defect.

CONOTRUNCAL ABNORMALITIES

The echocardiographic findings in patients with conotruncal abnormalities have been the subject of several review articles.[63–66] The material in this section is outlined according to the following classification:

  A. Conditions with aortic override
    1. Fallot's Tetralogy
    2. Pulmonary atresia with ventricular septal defect
    3. Persistent truncus arteriosus
  B. Transposition of the great arteries
  C. Double outlet right ventricle

16.15 FALLOT'S TETRALOGY

The four abnormalities encountered in Fallot's tetralogy are pulmonic stenosis, ventricular septal defect, dextroposition of the aorta, and right ventricular hypertrophy (Fig. 16–82). Of these, two elements are of prime importance—the ventricular septal defect and the pulmonic stenosis. In classic Fallot's tetralogy, a large ventricular septal defect is situated beneath the mouth of the aorta and inferiorly to the crista supraventricularis. This condition is the so-called *conotruncal ventricular septal defect*. The pulmonic stenosis can be located at any of the four different sites in this order of frequency: infundibulum, pulmonary valve, pulmonary trunk, and subinfundibular zone. The coexistence of valvular and infundibular stenosis is frequent. Dextroposition of the aorta with variable degrees of septal override is frequently but not invariably present. Right ventricular hypertrophy is a secondary result of the outflow tract obstruction. A right aortic arch occurs in 20 to 30 per cent of patients with Fallot's tetralogy.

Echocardiography can be very helpful in the evaluation of patients with Fallot's tetralogy. With the long-axis left parasternal view (Fig. 16–83), it is possible to demonstrate the conotruncal ventricular septal defect and the aortic override. Dilatation of the aorta is also apparent from this view. Mitral-aortic continuity can be demonstrated in this projection. The right ventricular cavity appears enlarged and hypertrophied.

The short-axis parasternal view (Fig. 16–84) at the base of the heart shows the hypoplastic right ventricular outflow, a dilated aortic root, and the presence of a pulmonic valve, which may be stenosed.

With M-mode echocardiography, a scan from the aorta to the left ventricle shows a dilated aortic root, aortic override (Fig. 16–85), and a ventricular septal defect evident as a disruption of the continuity between the aorta and the interventricular septum. Higher transducer position may give the impression of aortic override in a normal subject (Fig. 16–86).

Two-dimensional echocardiography has also been used to evaluate the results of corrective surgery in patients with Fallot's tetralogy. This technique allows for the evaluation of the integrity of the ventricular septal defect patch (Fig. 16–87) as well as for the evaluation of the right ventricular outflow tract after myomectomy (Fig. 16–88).

16.16 PULMONARY ATRESIA WITH VENTRICULAR SEPTAL DEFECT

Pulmonary atresia can be viewed as the ultimate expression of pulmonary stenosis, and therefore this abnormality represents the severest form of Fallot's tetralogy. The right ventricular infundibulum terminates in a cul-de-sac at the level of the atresic pulmonic valve. Often the infundibulum and pulmonary artery are hypoplastic as well.

This abnormality has also been designated *pseudotruncus arteriosus* because its physiopathology is similar to that of truncus arteriosus, although embryologically they are different. In pulmonary atresia, in contrast to truncus arteriosus, there is an aorticopulmonary septum.

Pulmonary atresia with ventricular septal defect cannot be differentiated echocardiographically from truncus arteriosus.

16.17 PERSISTENT TRUNCUS ARTERIOSUS

Persistent truncus arteriosus can be classified according to these four categories:

Type I. The pulmonary arteries arise from the posterior or left lateral wall of the trunk with a short main pulmonary artery.

Type II. The pulmonary arteries arise from the back wall with separate origins but are quite close to each other.

Type III. The pulmonary arteries are on the lateral side of the trunk and are quite small.

Type IV. No pulmonary arteries arise from the trunk. The pulmonary circulation originates from the bronchial arteries.

Echocardiography provides important information about patients with truncus arteriosus. In the long-axis left parasternal view (Fig. 16–89), truncus arteriosus is very similar and may be indistinguishable from Fallot's tetralogy. A large great vessel is seen to override the interventricular septum from which it is separated by a ventricular septal defect. A great vessel measuring 4 cm or more is more likely to be a truncus arteriosus than an aorta. In the short-axis view (Fig. 16–89) only one large great vessel is seen with no pulmonary artery around it. Lack of demonstration of a pulmonic valve favors the diagnosis of truncus arteriosus over Fallot's tetralogy. With suprasternal two-dimensional echocardiography, it may be possible to visualize the origin of the pulmonary artery from the truncus arteriosus and hence determine the type of truncus arteriosus under study. With M-mode echocardiography, it is possible to evaluate the presence of an incompetent truncus arteriosus by the demonstration of mitral, tricuspid, and interventricular septal fluttering during diastole (Figs. 16–90, 16–91).

16.18 TRANSPOSITION OF THE GREAT ARTERIES

In dextroposition of the great arteries (Fig. 16–92) or simple transposition the aorta arises to the right and anteriorly from the right ventricle and the pulmonary artery from the left and posteriorly from the left ventricle, at which it maintains continuity with the mitral valve. Connections between the systemic and pulmonary circulation are essential for survival and are in the form of a ventricular septal defect, an atrial septal defect, a patent ductus, or large bronchial arteries.

Both M-mode and two-dimensional echocardiography have been used to evaluate patients with transposition of the great arteries.[67–70] With the parasternal long-axis view it may be possible to identify the courses of the anterior aortic artery and the posterior pulmonary artery. These arteries are often imaged simultaneously, with one below the other. The pulmonary artery courses posteriorly and may be seen to bifurcate. The short-axis view at the base of the heart shows both great vessels in their short axes. That is, the pulmonary artery is not seen to wind around the aorta. The posterior vessel can be identified as the pulmonary artery by demonstration of its bifurcation.

With M-mode echocardiography, both great vessels and semilunar valves are recorded simultaneously (Fig. 16–93). The one with the shortest ejection time is the pulmonic valve unless there is equalization of pulmonary and systemic pressures.

16.19 DOUBLE OUTLET RIGHT VENTRICLE

In this condition both the pulmonary artery and the aorta arise from the right ventricle. A ventricular septal defect provides the left ventricle with its only outlet. The great vessels lie side by side, or the pulmonary artery is situated slightly posteriorly. A subpulmonary conus separates the pulmonic valve from the mitral valve (Fig. 16–94).

The long-axis parasternal view shows the parallel course of both great arteries originating from the anterior right ventricle. The pulmonary artery is the posterior vessel and can be recognized by its posterior angulation toward the lung and its bifurcation. A ventricular septal defect is easily seen in this projection and represents the only left ventricular outflow tract site. A mass of echoes representing the subpulmonary conus is seen to separate the mitral valve from the pulmonary artery.[71]

16.20 SINGLE VENTRICLE

This condition consists of congenital anomalies in which there are two atria but only one ventricle. There are usually two atrioventricular valves, but occasionally a common atrioventricular valve is present. The common ventricle is a morphologic left ventricle with a small outlet chamber that represents the infundibular portion of the right ventricle. The great vessels are almost always transposed.

The echocardiographic diagnosis of single ventricle is based on the demonstration of the absence of an interventricular septum (Fig. 16–95).[72–76] This finding can be imaged best from the apical and subcostal views. Transposition of the great arteries, usually an associated abnormality, can be demonstrated best in short-axis views at the base of the heart. With M-mode echocardiography, it is possible to simultaneously record the tricuspid and mitral valves without a ventricular septum in between.

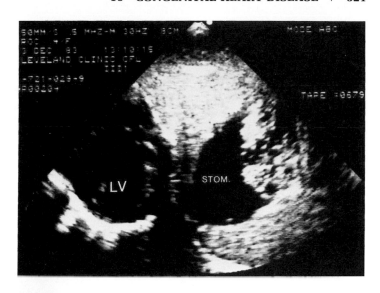

FIGURE 16–1
POSITION OF ABDOMINAL VISCERA
This right subcostal view in a patient with mirror image dextrocardia demonstrates the presence of the stomach (STOM.) on the right upper quadrant of the abdomen. The left ventricle (LV) is seen in cross section.

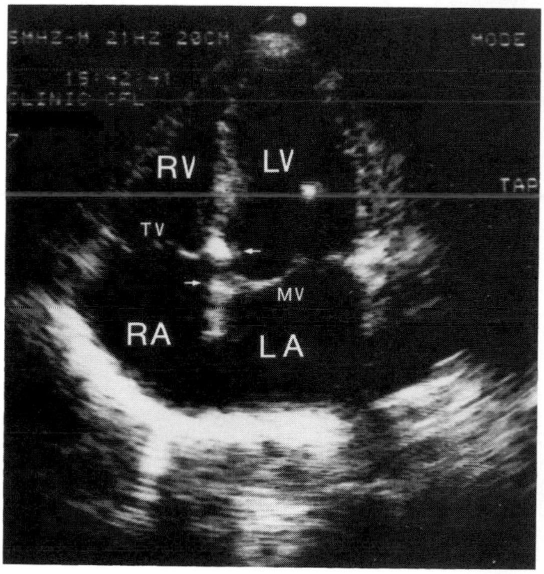

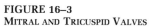

FIGURE 16–2
MITRAL AND TRICUSPID INSERTION IN THE SEPTUM
This apical four-chamber view clearly demonstrates the insertion of the tricuspid valve (TV) closer to the apex *(arrows)*. RA = right ventricle; LV = left ventricle; RA = right atrium; LA = left atrium; MV = mitral valve.

FIGURE 16–3
MITRAL AND TRICUSPID VALVES
Left parasternal view in a patient with an atrial septal defect. The right ventricle is dilated. The tricuspid (TV) and mitral (MV) valves are seen in the short-axis view.

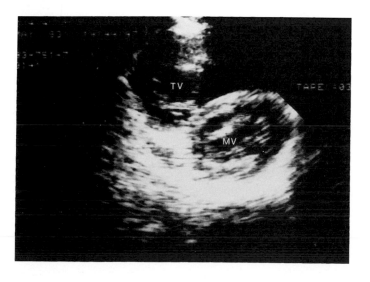

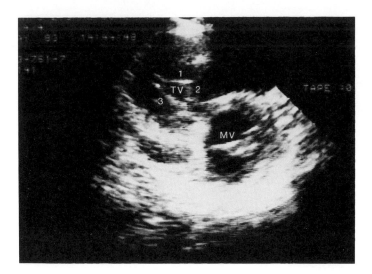

FIGURE 16–4
MITRAL AND TRICUSPID VALVES
Short-axis view in same patient as in Figure 16–3 during early systole. The mitral valve (MV) is closed, and the tricuspid valve (TV) is closing. The presence of three leaflets in the tricuspid valve is clearly demonstrated.

FIGURE 16–5
MODERATOR BAND
Apical four-chamber view in a patient with atrial septal defect with a dilated right ventricle. The moderator band is clearly seen toward the apex of the right ventricle (RV) as an echo-dense band parallel to the tricuspid valve plane *(arrow)*. LV = left ventricle; RA = right atrium; LA = left atrium.

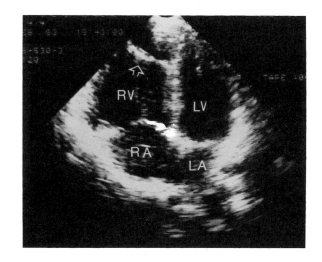

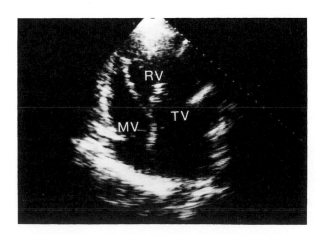

FIGURE 16–6
CORRECTED TRANSPOSITION OF THE GREAT VESSELS
This apical four-chamber view demonstrates the mitral valve (MV) further away from the apex than is the tricuspid valve (TV). This positioning serves to identify the right and left ventricles as being inverted. RV = right ventricle.

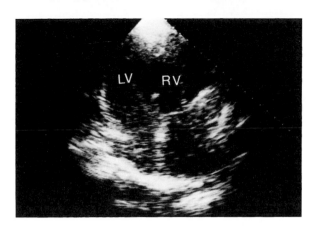

FIGURE 16–7
CORRECTED TRANSPOSITION OF THE GREAT VESSELS
Contrast echocardiogram recorded from the same patient as in Figure 16–6. It can be seen that the anatomic left ventricle (LV) receives the venous circulation (microbubbles from the injection). This finding serves to confirm the diagnosis. RV = right ventricle.

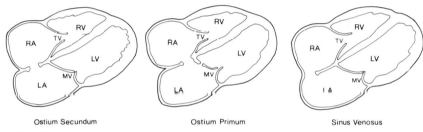

Ostium Secundum   Ostium Primum   Sinus Venosus

FIGURE 16–8
ATRIAL SEPTAL DEFECTS, CLASSIFICATION
The three main types of atrial septal defects are ostium secundum, ostium primum, and sinus venosus. RV = right ventricle; TV = tricuspid valve; RA = right atrium; LA = left atrium; MV = mitral valve; LV = left ventricle.

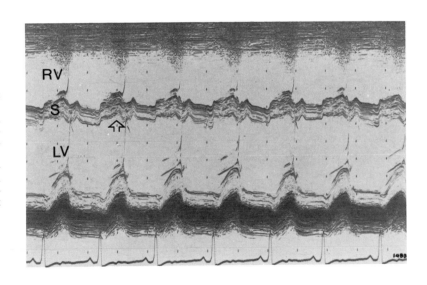

FIGURE 16–9
RIGHT VENTRICULAR VOLUME OVERLOAD
Echocardiogram recorded from a 19-year-old patient with an ostium secundum atrial septal defect and a 4 to 1 QP/QS ratio. There is right ventricular enlargement and paradoxic septal motion (arrow). RV = right ventricle; S = septum; LV = left ventricle.

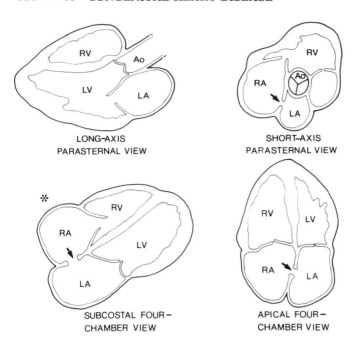

LONG-AXIS
PARASTERNAL VIEW

SHORT-AXIS
PARASTERNAL VIEW

SUBCOSTAL FOUR–
CHAMBER VIEW

APICAL FOUR–
CHAMBER VIEW

FIGURE 16–10
OSTIUM SECUNDUM ATRIAL SEPTAL DEFECT
Direct visualization of the atrial septal defect can be achieved from any of several sector plane views, as shown in this diagram. The subcostal window (*) permits the best visualization of the interatrial septum and therefore is the preferred view in which to identify an atrial septal defect. RV = right ventricle; LV = left ventricle; Ao = aorta; LA = left atrium; RA = right atrium.

FIGURE 16–11
RIGHT-TO-LEFT SHUNT AT ATRIAL LEVEL
Apical two-chamber view in a patient with a large right-to-left shunt at the atrial level. This frame recorded before the injection of contrast material shows no abnormality. LV = left ventricle; LA = left atrium.

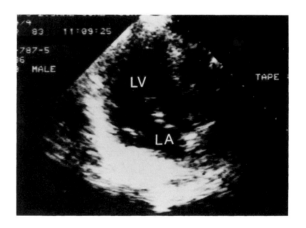

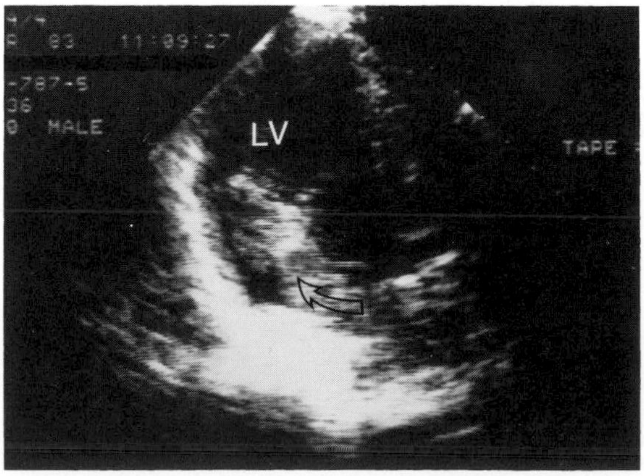

FIGURE 16–12
RIGHT-TO-LEFT SHUNT AT ATRIAL LEVEL
Echocardiogram recorded from the same patient as in Figure 16–11 after the injection of contrast material into a peripheral vein. The bubbles fill the left atrium and part of the left ventricle (LV) to demonstrate a right-to-left shunt at the atrial level.

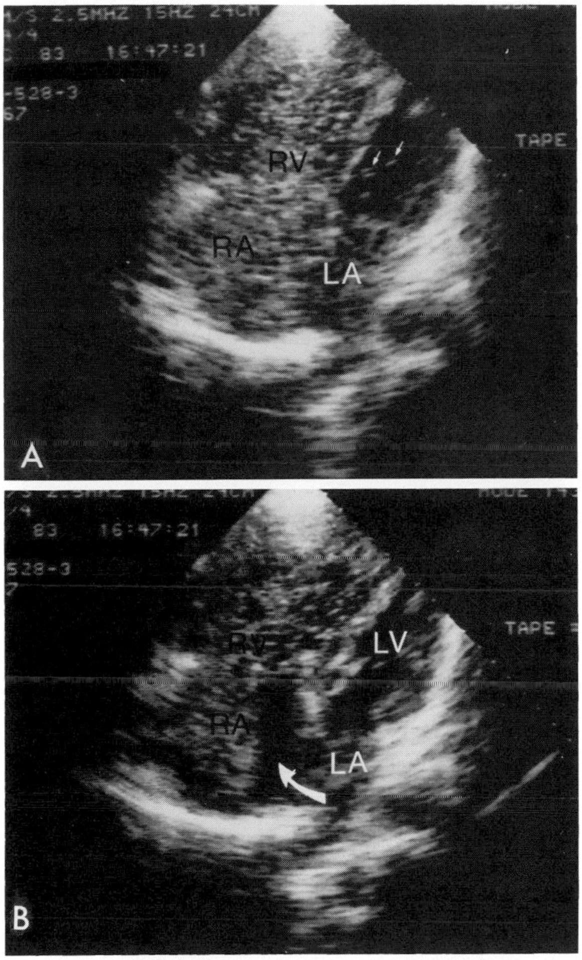

FIGURE 16–13
ATRIAL SEPTAL DEFECT, NEGATIVE CONTRAST EFFECT
Contrast two-dimensional echocardiograms recorded from a 59-year-old patient with a secundum atrial septal defect with a QP/QS ratio of 2.3 to 1. Panel *A* shows the contrast material arriving in the right atrium (RA) and right ventricle (RV). Panel *B* shows a washout effect *(arrow)* that is produced by a jet of blood coming from the left atrium (LA) to the right atrium. A few bubbles pass to the left side of the heart *(arrows in top panel)*. LV = left ventricle.

FIGURE 16–14
CONTRAST ECHOCARDIOGRAPHY
In a patient with polycythemia of unknown origin contrast echocardiography demonstrates the integrity of the interatrial septum. Before the injection of contrast material, significant dropout of echoes at the level of the interatrial septum suggested the possibility of a septal defect. LV = left ventricle; RV = right ventricle; RA = right atrium; LA = left atrium.

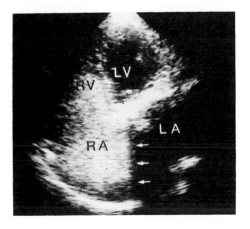

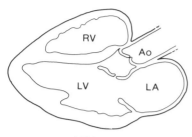

LONG–AXIS
PARASTERNAL VIEW

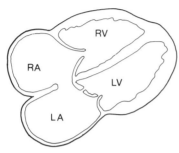

SUBCOSTAL FOUR–
CHAMBER VIEW

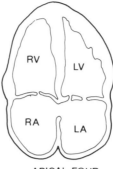

APICAL FOUR–
CHAMBER VIEW

FIGURE 16–15
OSTIUM PRIMUM ATRIAL SEPTAL DEFECT
The long-axis view best demonstrates the abnormal motion of the cleft mitral valve toward the outflow tract. The apical four-chamber and the subcostal four-chamber views demonstrate absence of atrial septum at a location immediately superior to the atrioventricular valves. The best view with which to demonstrate this is the subcostal one. RV = right ventricle; LV = left ventricle; Ao = aorta; LA = left atrium; RA = right atrium.

FIGURE 16–16
COMMON ATRIUM
This apical four-chamber view demonstrates the absence of an interatrial septum. A large single chamber is seen above the ventricles (CA). RV = right ventricle; LV = left ventricle.

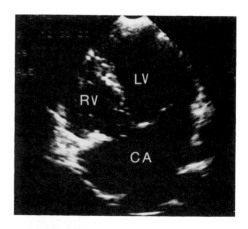

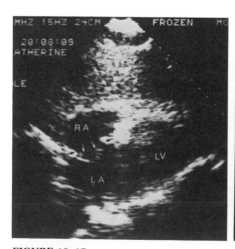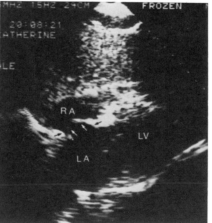

FIGURE 16–17
ATRIAL SEPTAL ANEURYSM
Subcostal four-chamber views in a patient with an aneurysm of the interatrial septum. This appears as a localized thin pouchlike area of the interatrial septum, which has a saillike motion *(white arrows)*. The black arrows point to the plane of the interatrial septum. RA = right atrium; LA = left atrium; LV = left ventricle.

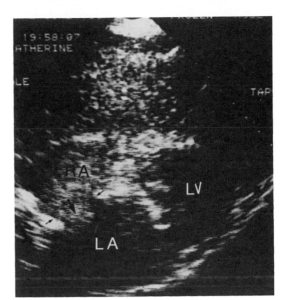

FIGURE 16–18
ATRIAL SEPTAL ANEURYSM
Subcostal four-chamber view recorded from the same patient as in Figure 16–17 after the injection of contrast material into a peripheral vein. The small arrows point to the plane of the interatrial septum. The large arrow shows the contrast material filling the pouchlike area created by the aneurysm. RA = right atrium; LA = left atrium; LV = left ventricle.

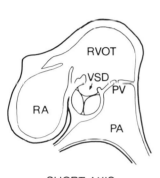

SHORT-AXIS
PARASTERNAL VIEW

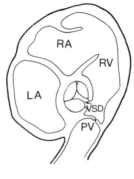

SUBCOSTAL
SHORT-AXIS

FIGURE 16–19
SUPRACRISTAL VENTRICULAR SEPTAL DEFECT
Parasternal short-axis and subcostal short-axis views demonstrate the close proximity of the ventricular septal defect (VSD) with the pulmonic (PV) and aortic valves. RVOT = right ventricular outflow tract; RA = right atrium; PA = pulmonary artery; LA = left atrium; RV = right ventricle.

FIGURE 16–20
MEMBRANOUS VENTRICULAR SEPTAL DEFECT
This type of defect can be visualized from several planes, as shown in this diagram by the arrows. This defect lies immediately below the aortic valve, and occasionally tricuspid valve tissue may be seen across it. RV = right ventricle; LV = left ventricle; Ao = aorta; LA = left atrium; RA = right atrium.

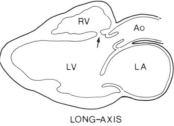

LONG-AXIS
PARASTERNAL VIEW

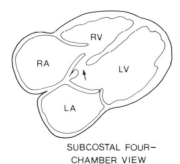

SUBCOSTAL FOUR-
CHAMBER VIEW

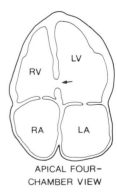

APICAL FOUR-
CHAMBER VIEW

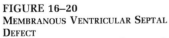

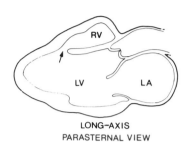

LONG–AXIS
PARASTERNAL VIEW

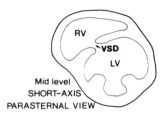

Mid level
SHORT–AXIS
PARASTERNAL VIEW

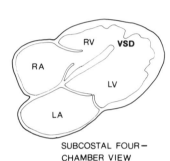

SUBCOSTAL FOUR–
CHAMBER VIEW

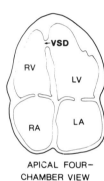

APICAL FOUR–
CHAMBER VIEW

FIGURE 16–21
MUSCULAR VENTRICULAR SEPTAL DEFECT
This type of defect may be localized quite inferiorly in the interventricular septum, as demonstrated by this diagram. The defect has to be fairly large to be visualized by echocardiography. RV = right ventricle; LV = left ventricle; RA = right atrium; VSD = ventricular septal defect.

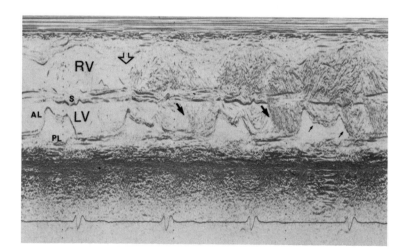

FIGURE 16–22
VENTRICULAR SEPTAL DEFECT,
CONTRAST INJECTION
Echocardiogram at the mitral valve level in a 30-year-old woman with multiple low-lying ventricular septal defects and systemic pulmonary hypertension. A significant right-to-left shunt is demonstrated by a peripheral injection of contrast material. The microbubbles are first seen in the right ventricle (RV) and then in the outflow tract of the left ventricle (LV). The mitral funnel is clear. S = septum; AL = anterior leaflet; PL = posterior leaflet.

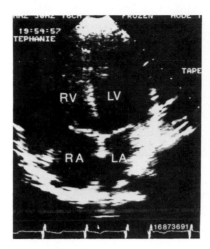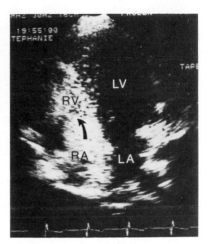

FIGURE 16–23
VENTRICULAR SEPTAL DEFECT, CONTRAST INJECTION
Apical four-chamber view in a 17-year-old woman with membranous ventricular septal defect, pulmonary hypertension (88 mm Hg), and a bidirectional shunt with a QP/QS ratio of 1.2:1. The frame to the left was recorded before the contrast material arrived at the right heart. There are echo dropouts at the level of the membranous septum and at the level of the fossa ovalis. The frame to the right shows the contrast material entering the right heart. RV = right ventricle; LV = left ventricle; RA = right atrium; LA = left atrium.

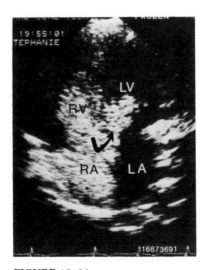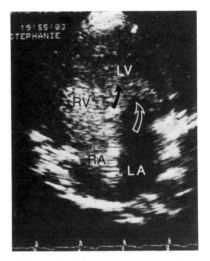

FIGURE 16–24
VENTRICULAR SEPTAL DEFECT, CONTRAST INJECTION
Apical four-chamber view in the same patient as in Figure 16–23. The echocardiographic contrast material, after arriving at the right ventricle (RV), passes to the left ventricle (LV) through a high ventricular septal defect. The interatrial septum is intact. RA = right atrium; LA = left atrium.

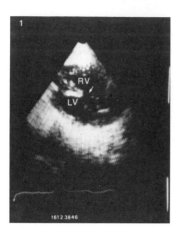
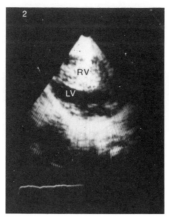
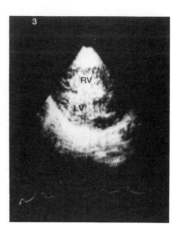

FIGURE 16–25
VENTRICULAR SEPTAL DEFECT, CONTRAST INJECTION
Long-axis left parasternal views in a patient with a large ventricular septal defect and
right-to-left shunt. Frame 1 was recorded before the arrival of contrast material into
the heart. The ventricular septal defect is indicated by the small arrow. In frame 2 the
contrast material fills the right ventricle (RV), and in frame 3 it fills the left ventricle
(LV) after passage through the ventricular septal defect.

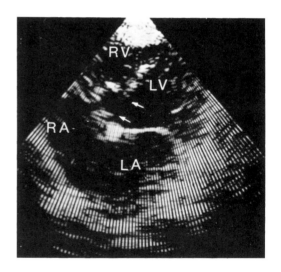

FIGURE 16–26
VENTRICULAR SEPTAL ANEURYSM
Apical four-chamber view in a 51-year-old man with a
small ventricular septal defect and a large septal aneurysm
protruding into the right ventricle (RV) (arrows). LV = left
ventricle; RA = right atrium; LA = left atrium.

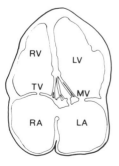
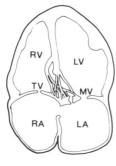
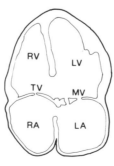

RASTELLI TYPE A   RASTELLI TYPE B   RASTELLI TYPE C

FIGURE 16–27
ENDOCARDIAL CUSHION DEFECTS, CLAS-
SIFICATION
The Rastelli classification of endocardial cushion defects includes three
types: Type A: anchoring of the chordae in the crest of the ventricular
septum; Type B: papillary muscle in
the right septum with chordae to the
mitral valve; Type C: free-floating
leaflets. RV = right ventricle; LV =
left ventricle; TV = tricuspid valve;
MV = mitral valve; RA = right
atrium; LA = left atrium.

ENDOCARDIAL CUSHION DEFECT

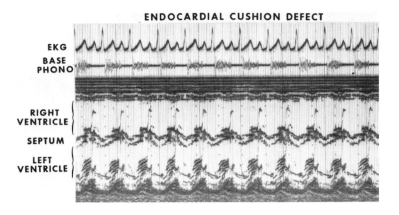

FIGURE 16–28
ENDOCARDIAL CUSHION DEFECT
This study at the ventricular level in a patient with endocardial cushion defect shows the characteristic features of right ventricular volume overload, which include a dilated right ventricle and paradoxic septal motion.

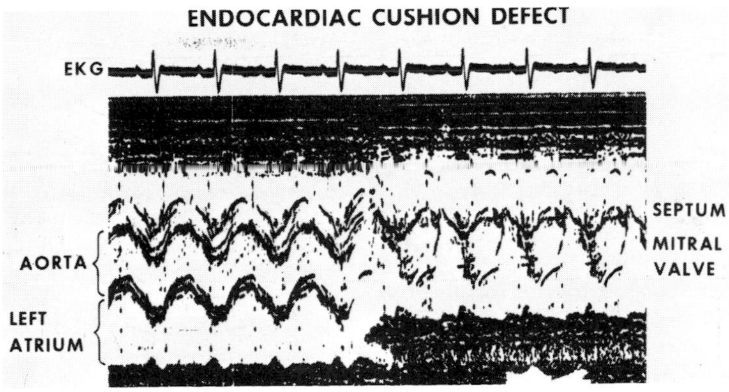

ENDOCARDIAC CUSHION DEFECT

FIGURE 16–29
ENDOCARDIAL CUSHION DEFECT
This echocardiographic scan from the aorta to the mitral valve in a patient with an endocardial cushion defect demonstrates the small size of the left ventricular outflow tract and diastolic apposition of the mitral valve with the septum.

FIGURE 16–30
ENDOCARDIAL CUSHION DEFECT
This echocardiogram was recorded at the valve level and shows continuity of the mitral (MV) and tricuspid valves (TV) through the interventricular septum. This view was recorded in a 20-year-old patient with Down's syndrome and complete endocardial cushion defect. RV = right ventricle; LV = left ventricle.

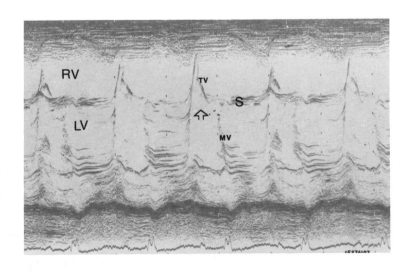

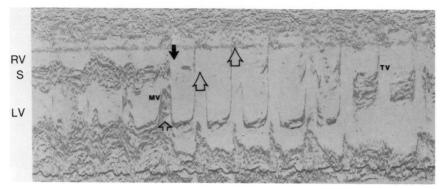

FIGURE 16–31
ENDOCARDIAL CUSHION DEFECT
This study is from a 6-month-old child with Down's syndrome and a complete endocardial cushion defect. There are echo dropouts at the level of the ventricular septum *(black arrow)* and apparent mitral-tricuspid continuity as the probe is directed from left to right *(open arrows)*. RV = right ventricle; S = septum; LV = left ventricle; MV = mitral valve; TV = tricuspid valve.

FIGURE 16–32
ENDOCARDIAL CUSHION DEFECT
Two-dimensional long-axis diagram representing the left parasternal view in a patient with endocardial cushion defect. The abnormal positions of the mitral valve (MV), the mitral cleft, and the proximity of the mitral and tricuspid (TV) valves through a ventricular septal defect should be noted. RV = right ventricle; LV = left ventricle; Ao = aorta; LA = left atrium.

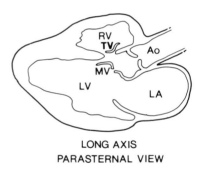

LONG AXIS
PARASTERNAL VIEW

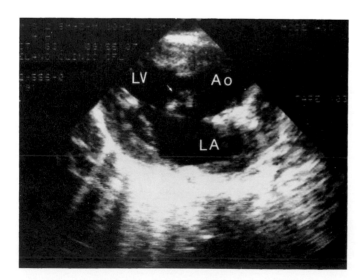

FIGURE 16–33
ENDOCARDIAL CUSHION DEFECT
Long-axis left parasternal view in a patient with atrioventricular canal defect. The abnormal position of the anterior mitral leaflet in the left ventricular outflow tract should be noted. LV = left ventricle; Ao = aorta; LA = left atrium.

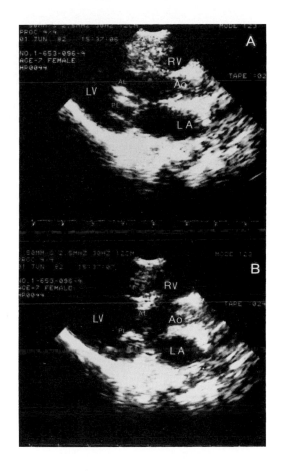

FIGURE 16–34
ENDOCARDIAL CUSHION DEFECT
Systolic (A) and diastolic (B) frames from a long-axis left
parasternal view in a 7-year-old patient with atrioventricular
canal defect. There is abnormal motion of the anterior mitral
valve leaflet (AL) toward the outflow tract during diastole.
RV = right ventricle; LV = left ventricle; Ao = aorta; LA
= left atrium; PL = posterior leaflet.

FIGURE 16–35
ENDOCARDIAL CUSHION DEFECT
Apical four-chamber view in a 2-month-old
baby with a large endocardial cushion defect. The arrow points to the ventricular
septal defect. RV = right ventricle; LV =
left ventricle; RA = right atrium.

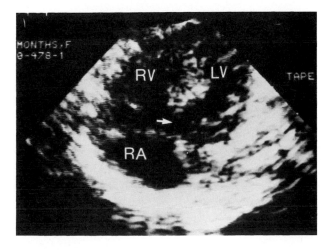

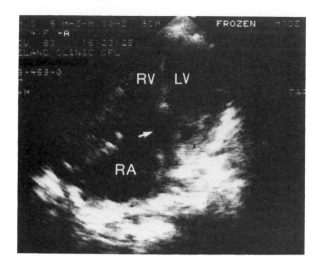

FIGURE 16-36
ENDOCARDIAL CUSHION DEFECT
Apical four-chamber view in a patient with a large endocardial cushion defect. There is a total absence of tissue in the area of the endocardial cushion. RV = right ventricle; LV = left ventricle; RA = right atrium.

FIGURE 16-37
ENDOCARDIAL CUSHION DEFECT, MITRAL TRICUSPID ALIGNMENT
Apical four-chamber view demonstrating mitral-tricuspid alignment. Both leaflets appear at the same level as a continuous line in the middle of the endocardial cushion defect. RV = right ventricle; LV = left ventricle; RA = right atrium; LA = left atrium. The asterisks point to the cushion defect.

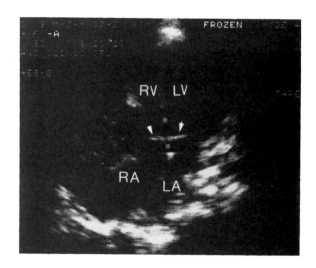

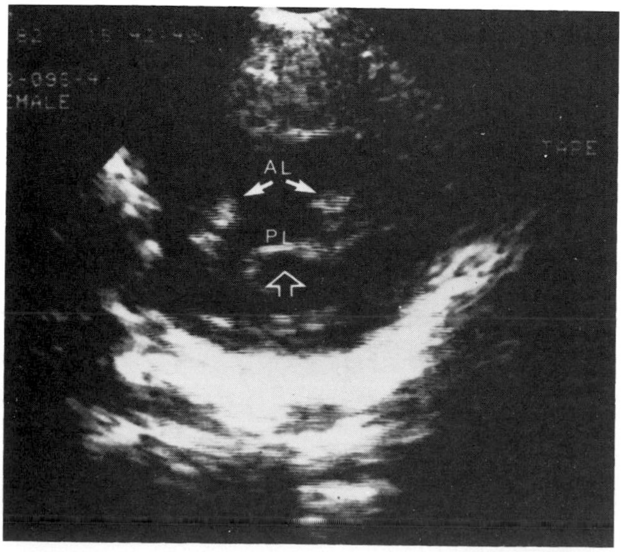

FIGURE 16-38
CLEFT MITRAL VALVE
Left parasternal view in a patient with endocardial cushion defect and a cleft mitral valve. The anterior leaflet (AL) is partitioned in the center to form two leaflets (arrows). The normal posterior leaflet (PL) is indicated by the open arrow.

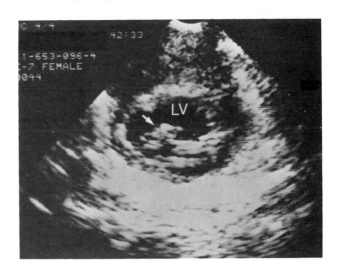

FIGURE 16–39
CLEFT MITRAL VALVE
Short-axis left parasternal view in a 7-year-old girl with Down's syndrome and mitral regurgitation secondary to a cleft mitral valve. This systolic frame shows the two parts of the anterior leaflet overlapping and forming an echodense structure toward the middle commissure (*arrow*). LV = left ventricle.

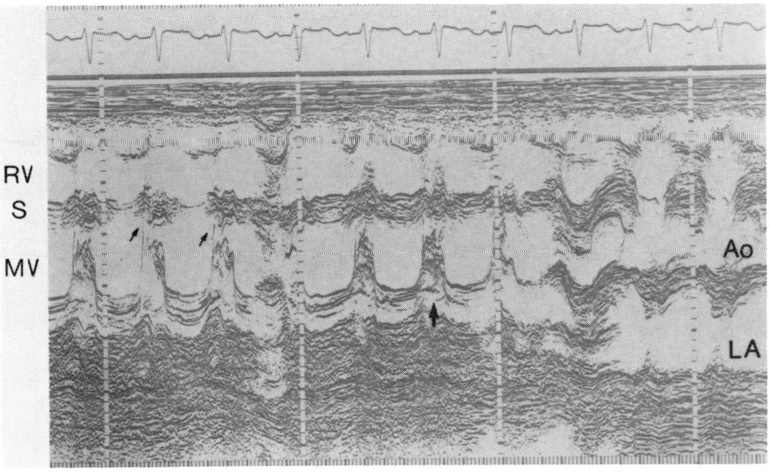

FIGURE 16–40
CLEFT MITRAL VALVE
Echocardiographic scan from the mitral valve to the aorta in a baby with endocardial cushion defect and cleft mitral valve. There is a "cloud" of echoes behind the anterior mitral leaflet, which is probably related to the abnormal motion of the valve and to tissue ingrown at the leaflet level. RV = right ventricle; S = septum; MV = mitral valve; Ao = aorta; LA = left atrium.

FIGURE 16–41
CLEFT MITRAL VALVE
Echocardiogram of the mitral valve in a 10-year-old girl with an atrioventricular canal ventricular septal defect and a cleft mitral valve. The arrow points to fine diastolic flutter in part of the anterior mitral leaflet. The patient did not have aortic insufficiency, and the flutter is probably related to turbulence created by the ventricular septal defect around the cleft mitral valve. S = septum; LV = left ventricle; PW = posterior wall; AL = anterior leaflet.

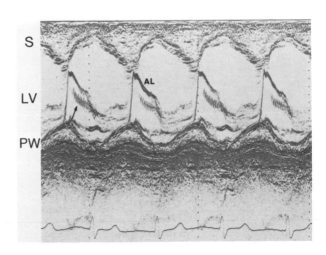

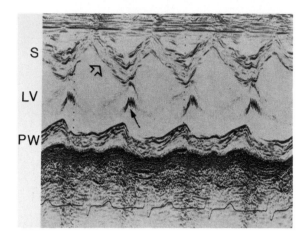

FIGURE 16–42
CLEFT MITRAL VALVE, LEFT VENTRICULAR VOLUME OVERLOAD
Echocardiogram recorded at the left ventricular level in the same patient as in Figure 16–41. Marked left ventricular volume overload is demonstrated by the markedly increased septal motion and left ventricular dilatation. S = septum; LV = left ventricle; PW = posterior wall.

FIGURE 16–43
TOTAL ANOMALOUS PULMONARY VENOUS CONNECTION
This apical four-chamber view demonstrates the pulmonary veins draining into a common pulmonary vein (CPV) behind the left atrium (LA), from which area it drains into the right atrium (RA). RV = right ventricle; LV = left ventricle.

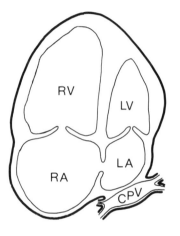

PATENT DUCTUS ARTERIOSUS

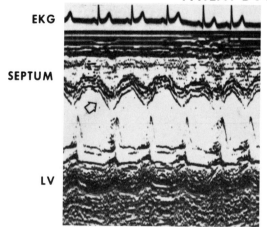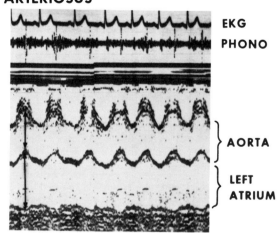

FIGURE 16–44
PATENT DUCTUS ARTERIOSUS
This echocardiogram recorded at the level of the left ventricle (LV) and aorta and left atrium in a patient with a patent ductus arteriosus demonstrates left atrial enlargement and left ventricular volume overload.

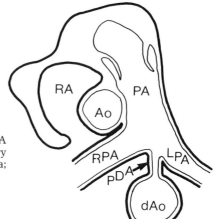

FIGURE 16–45
PATENT DUCTUS ARTERIOSUS
Left parasternal view at the level of the pulmonary artery bifurcation. A persistent ductus arteriosus (PDA) is seen to connect the pulmonary artery (PA) with the descending aorta (dAo). RA = right atrium; Ao = aorta; RPA = right pulmonary artery; LPA = left pulmonary artery.

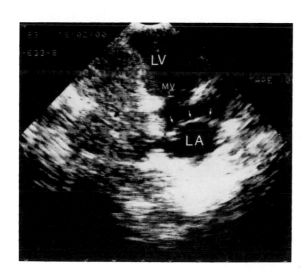

FIGURE 16–46
COR TRIATRIATUM
Apical two-chamber view in a patient with cor triatriatum. A membrane (arrows) divides the left atrium (LA). The mitral valve (MV) is seen closer to the left ventricle (LV).

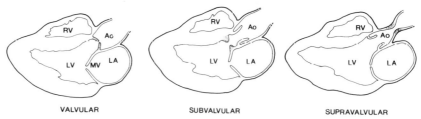

VALVULAR   SUBVALVULAR   SUPRAVALVULAR

FIGURE 16–47
AORTIC STENOSIS, CLASSIFICATION
This diagram demonstrates the three types of congenital aortic stenosis: valvular, subvalvular, and supravalvular. RV = right ventricle; LV = left ventricle; Ao = aorta; MV = mitral valve; LA = left atrium.

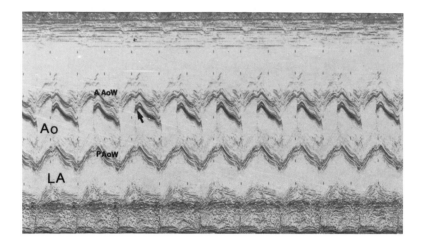

FIGURE 16–48
CONGENITAL AORTIC STENOSIS
Echocardiogram of the aortic valve in a 15-year-old boy with severe aortic stenosis (120 mm Hg gradient). Despite the severe degree of stenosis the leaflet excursion is normal. Ao = aorta; LA = left atrium; AAoW = anterior aortic wall; PAoW = posterior aortic wall.

FIGURE 16–49
CONGENITAL AORTIC STENOSIS
This long-axis parasternal view in a patient with congenital aortic stenosis demonstrates decreased leaflet separation at the tip of the doming valve. LV = left ventricle; Ao = aorta.

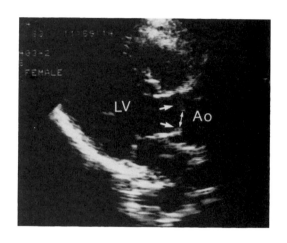

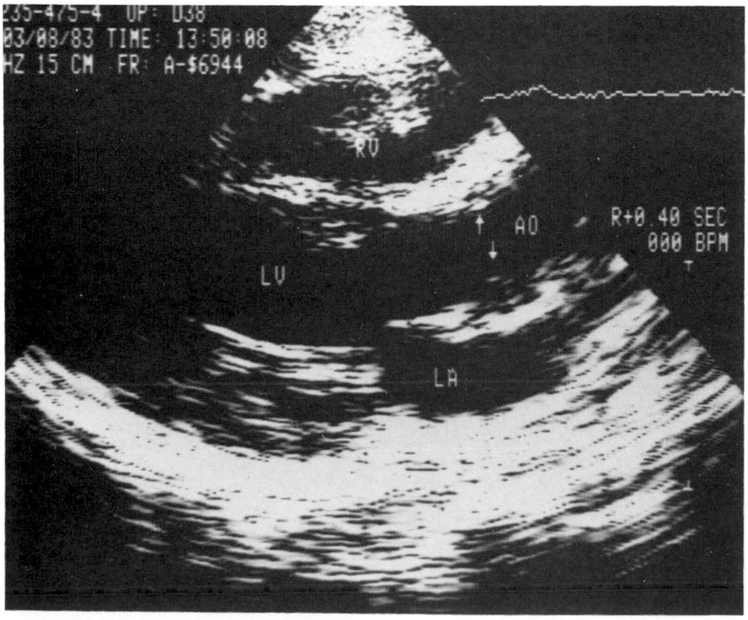

FIGURE 16–50
CONGENITAL AORTIC STENOSIS, AFTER VALVULOTOMY
Long-axis left parasternal view in a 16-year-old boy with congenital aortic stenosis (preoperative gradient 116 mm Hg) after successful valvuloplasty (postoperative gradient 15 mm Hg). There is normal leaflet separation during systole (arrows). RV = right ventricle; LV = left ventricle; Ao = aorta; LA = left atrium.

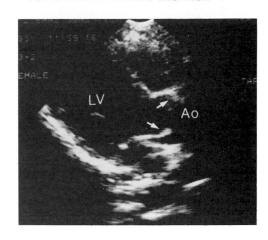

FIGURE 16–51
BICUSPID AORTIC VALVE
Long-axis left parasternal view in a 17-year-old patient with bicuspid aortic valve, aortic stenosis, and insufficiency. The arrows point to doming of the leaflets. LV = left ventricle; Ao = aorta.

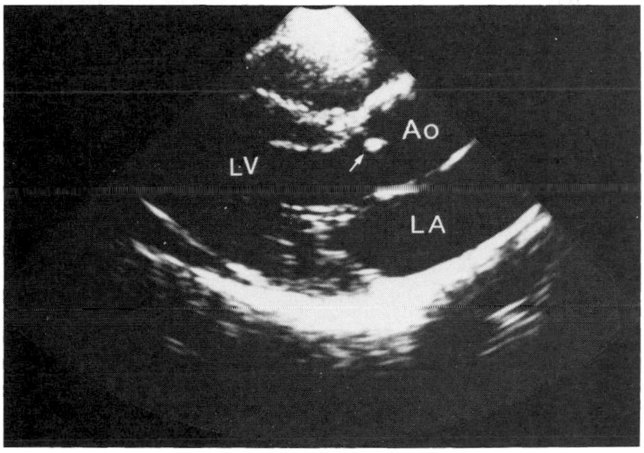

FIGURE 16–52
CONGENITAL AORTIC STENOSIS
Long-axis left parasternal view in a 22-year-old man with mild doming of the anterior aortic valve leaflet (arrow). There is nodular thickening at the tip of the valve, which is a frequent finding in patients with congenital aortic stenosis. LV = left ventricle; Ao = aorta; LA = left atrium.

FIGURE 16–53
BICUSPID AORTIC VALVE
Long-axis left parasternal view in a patient with bicuspid aortic valve and significant "reverse doming" of the leaflets (arrows). This diastolic frame shows the aortic valve bowing toward the left ventricular outflow tract. RV = right ventricle; LV = left ventricle; Ao = aorta; AL = anterior leaflet; LA = left atrium.

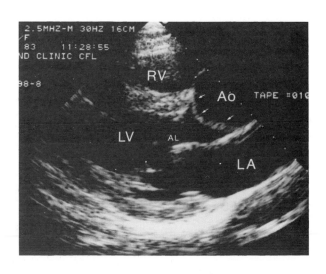

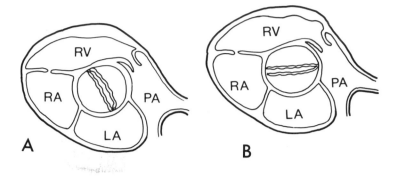

FIGURE 16–54
BICUSPID AORTIC VALVE
Short-axis views at the aortic level demonstrate the two common orientations of the bicuspid aortic valve. In diagram A the orientation is more vertical; in diagram B it is more horizontal. RV = right ventricle; RA = right atrium; LA = left atrium; PA = pulmonary artery.

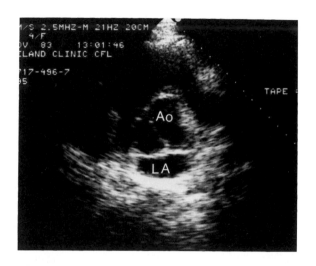

FIGURE 16–55
BICUSPID AORTIC VALVE
Left parasternal short-axis view at the level of the aorta (Ao) in a patient with bicuspid aortic valve. Two leaflets are seen with a single commissure traversing from 10 to 6 o'clock of the aortic circumference. LA = left atrium.

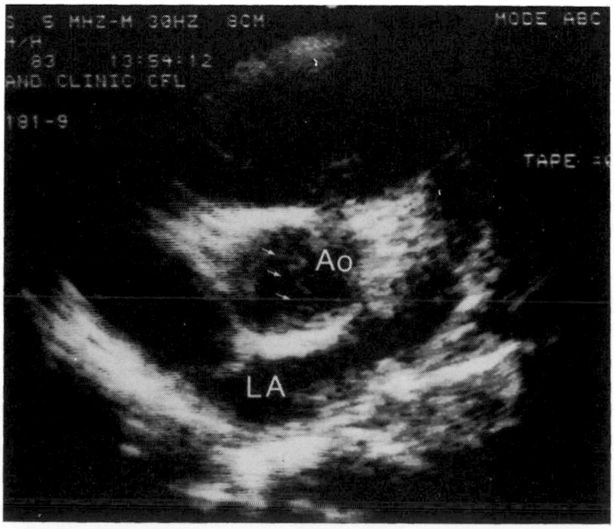

FIGURE 16–56
BICUSPID AORTIC VALVE
This left parasternal short-axis view at the aortic level shows a single middle commissure traversing from 12 to 6 o'clock of the aortic circumference. The arrows point to the irregular commissure, which is the result of large and redundant leaflets. Ao = aorta; LA = left atrium.

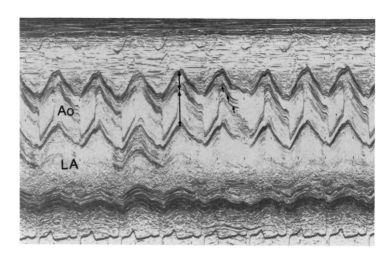

FIGURE 16–57
BICUSPID AORTIC VALVE
Echocardiogram recorded in a 12-year-old boy with Hunter's syndrome and bicuspid aortic valve. There are eccentric closure of the aortic valve *(large arrows)* and multiple diastolic linear echoes *(small arrows)*. Ao = aorta; LA = left atrium.

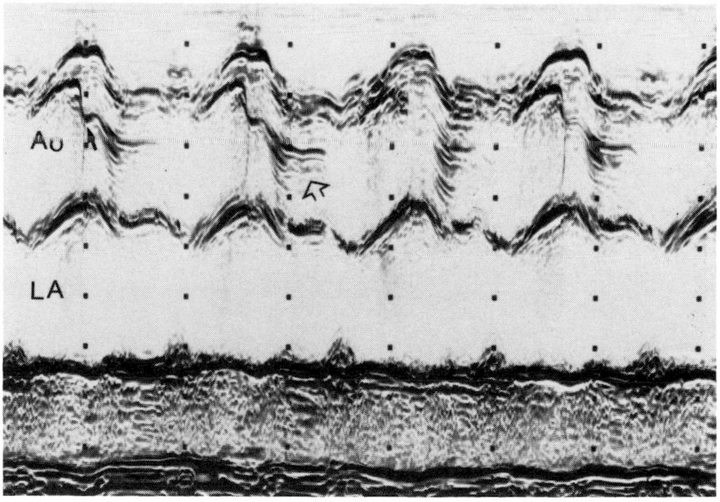

FIGURE 16–58
BICUSPID AORTIC VALVE
Eccentric aortic valve closure *(small arrow)* and multiple diastolic linear echoes *(large arrow)* are seen in this view from a patient with bicuspid aortic valve. Ao = aorta; LA = left atrium.

FIGURE 16–59
BICUSPID AORTIC VALVE, ECCENTRIC CLOSURE
Echocardiogram recorded at the aortic valve level in a patient with bicuspid aortic valve. Eccentric closure of the leaflets can be seen.

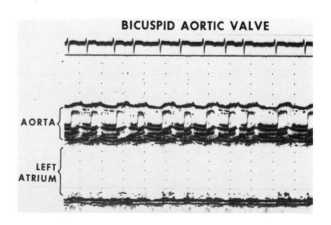

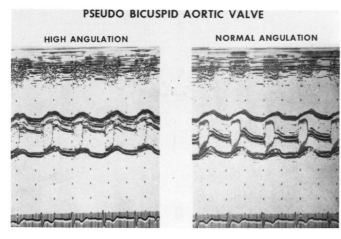

PSEUDO BICUSPID AORTIC VALVE

HIGH ANGULATION   NORMAL ANGULATION

FIGURE 16–60
PSEUDO BICUSPID AORTIC VALVE
These echocardiograms demonstrate how high transducer position may produce eccentric closure of aortic valve, which may be confused with eccentric closure of the bicuspid aortic valve. The appearance of the aortic valve is normal with normal transducer angulation.

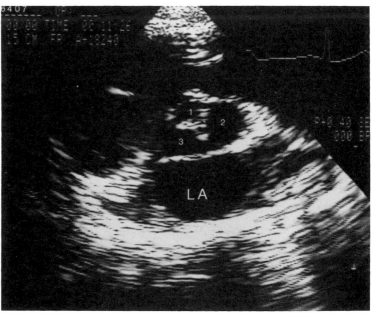

FIGURE 16–61
BICUSPID AORTIC VALVE
Short-axis left parasternal view in a patient with an ejection click, eccentric closure of the aortic valve on M-mode echocardiography, and what would appear to be a tricuspid aortic valve. On closer inspection the smaller leaflet (1) appears to be the result of a raphe in the anterior leaflet of a bicuspid valve. LA = left atrium.

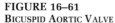

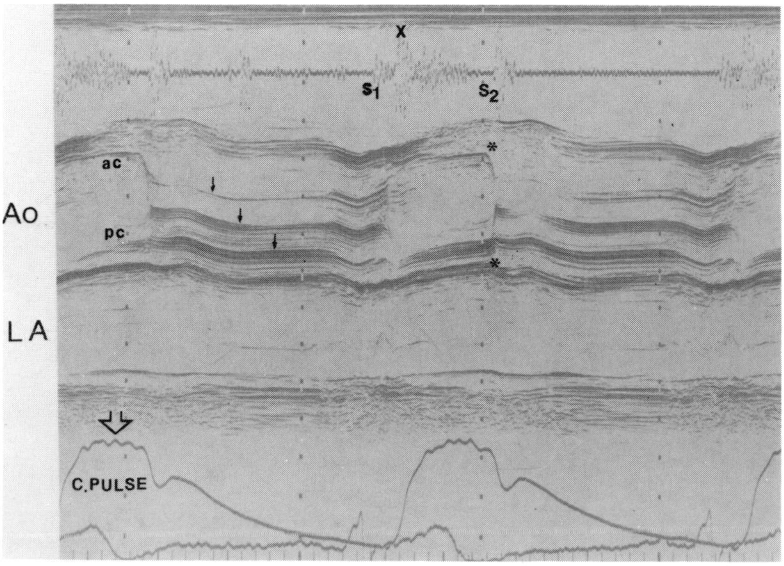

FIGURE 16–62
BICUSPID AORTIC VALVE, ECHO-PHONOCARDIOGRAM
Simultaneously recorded echocardiograms of the aortic valve and carotid pulse and a phonocardiogram recorded at the base in a 29-year-old man with bicuspid aortic valve and an aortic valve gradient of 50 mm Hg. The ejection click (x) coincides with the opening of the aortic valve. Multiple diastolic linear echoes are indicated (small arrows). The asterisks denote normal leaflet excursion. The large arrow points to carotid shudder. Ao = aorta; LA = left atrium.

DISCRETE SUBVALVULAR AORTIC STENOSIS

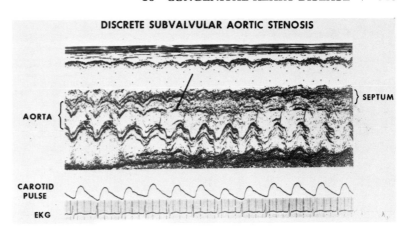

FIGURE 16–63
DISCRETE MEMBRANOUS SUBVAL-VULAR AORTIC STENOSIS
Echocardiographic scan in a patient with discrete subvalvular aortic stenosis. A band of echoes can be seen in the left ventricular outflow tract just below the aortic valve *(arrow)*.

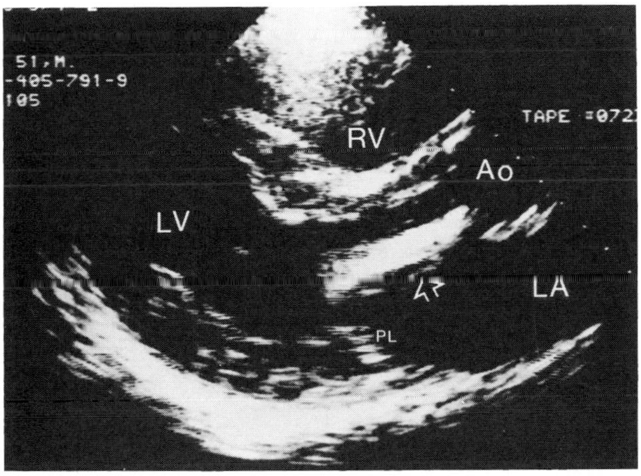

FIGURE 16–64
PSEUDO TUNNEL SUBAORTIC STENOSIS
Long-axis left parasternal view in a 51-year-old man with bicuspid aortic stenosis (gradient 50 mm Hg) and moderate aortic insufficiency with a band of calcium in the left ventricular outflow tract. No subvalvular gradient was present. LV = left ventricle; RV = right ventricle; Ao = aorta; LA = left atrium; PL = posterior leaflet.

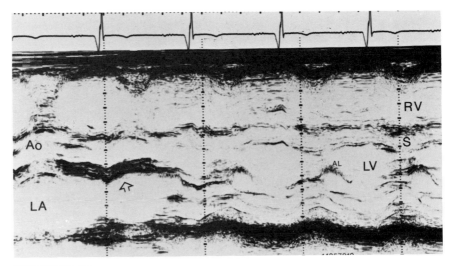

FIGURE 16–65
PSEUDO TUNNEL SUBAORTIC STENOSIS
An echocardiographic scan, from the aorta to the mitral valve in the same patient as in Figure 16–64 demonstrates the band of calcium *(arrow)* underneath the aortic valve in the left ventricular outflow tract. Ao = aorta; LA = left atrium; AL = anterior leaflet; RV = right ventricle; LV = left ventricle; S = septum.

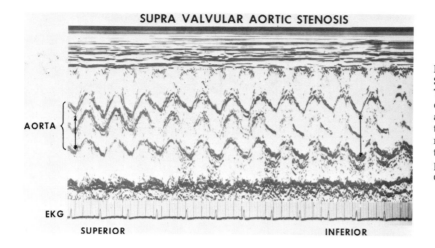

SUPRA VALVULAR AORTIC STENOSIS

AORTA

EKG

SUPERIOR   INFERIOR

FIGURE 16–66
SUPRAVALVULAR AORTIC STENOSIS
This echocardiogram of the aorta demonstrates a significant variation in the diameter of the aortic root when a superior-to-inferior angulation is made. Above the level of the aortic valve (superior) the diameter is significantly smaller.

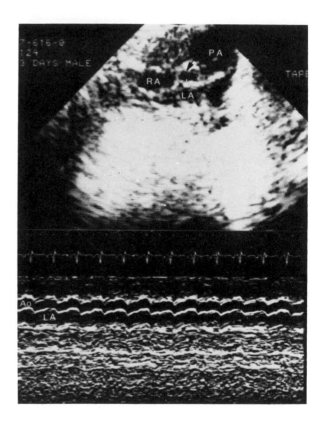

FIGURE 16–67
HYPOPLASTIC AORTA
Left parasternal short-axis view at the level of the great vessels in a newborn with hypoplastic aorta. The aorta (arrow) appears as a small circular structure in the center of the frame. It appears much smaller than the pulmonary artery (PA). RA = right atrium; LA = left atrium.

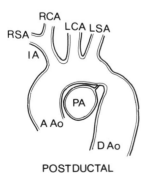

POSTDUCTAL

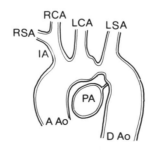

PREDUCTAL

FIGURE 16–68
COARCTATION OF THE AORTA
These diagrams demonstrate the usual location of a postductal coarctation as well as the more rare preductal location. RSA = right subclavian artery; RCA = right coronary artery; LCA = left coronary artery; LSA = left subclavian artery; PA = pulmonary artery; AAo = ascending aorta; DAo = descending aorta; IA = innominate artery.

FIGURE 16–69

PULMONIC STENOSIS, CLASSIFI-
CATION
Congenital obstruction in the
right ventricular outflow tract
can be classified as valvular,
infundibular, or supravalvular. TV = tricuspid valve; RA
= right atrium; Ao = aorta;
PV = pulmonic valve; PA =
pulmonary artery; RPA =
right pulmonary artery; LPA
= left pulmonary artery.

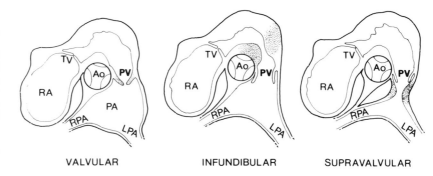

VALVULAR   INFUNDIBULAR   SUPRAVALVULAR

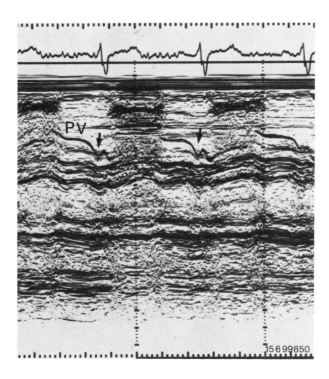

FIGURE 16–70

VALVULAR PULMONIC STENOSIS
Pulmonic valve (PV) recording in a 12-year-old
patient with valvular pulmonic stenosis (60 mm
Hg gradient). A large a wave *(arrow)*, a characteristic finding of this condition, can be seen.

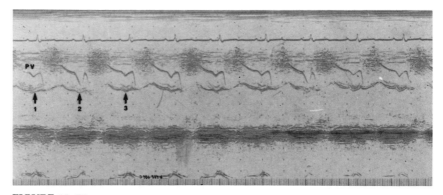

FIGURE 16–71

PSEUDO PULMONIC STENOSIS
Marked respiratory variation in the size of the pulmonic a wave is evident in this
recording from a patient with corrected transposition of the great vessels and no
pulmonic stenosis. In beat two the a wave measures more than 1 cm in depth. PV =
pulmonic valve.

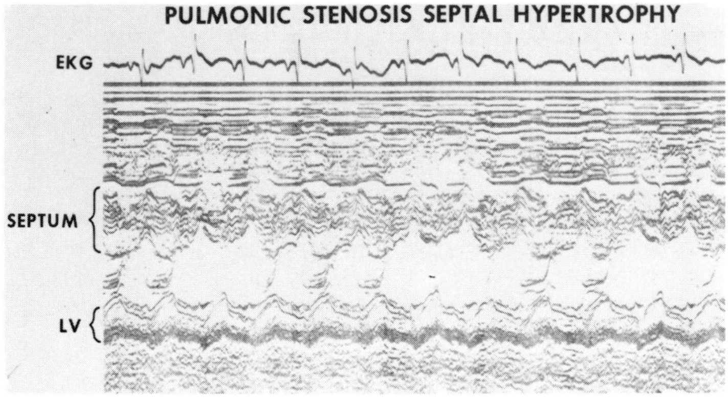

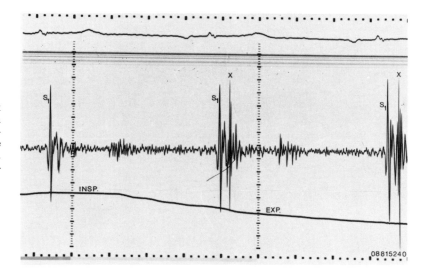

PULMONIC STENOSIS SEPTAL HYPERTROPHY

EKG

SEPTUM {

LV {

FIGURE 16–72
**PULMONIC STENOSIS, RIGHT VENTRICU-
LAR HYPERTROPHY**
Echocardiogram recorded at the ventricular level in a patient with severe
pulmonic stenosis. Increased free
right ventricular wall thickness as
well as septal hypertrophy can be
seen. The thickness of the posterior
left ventricular wall is normal. LV =
left ventricle.

FIGURE 16–73
PULMONIC STENOSIS
Phonocardiogram recorded at
the upper left sternal border in a
patient with mild pulmonic stenosis with a click that became
much louder with expiration (x).
INSP. = inspiration; EXP. = expiration.

S₁   X   S₁   X   S₁

INSP.

EXP.

08815240

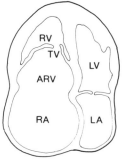

LONG-AXIS
PARASTERNAL VIEW

APICAL-FOUR
CHAMBER VIEW

FIGURE 16–74
EBSTEIN'S ANOMALY
These diagrams demonstrate the
characteristic downward displacement of the tricuspid valve (TV)
in a patient with Ebstein's anomaly. RV = right ventricle; LV =
left ventricle; Ao = aorta; LA =
left atrium; RA = right ventricle;
ARV = atrialized right ventricle.

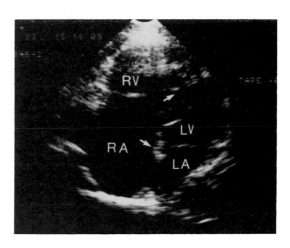

FIGURE 16–75
EBSTEIN'S ANOMALY
Apical four-chamber view in a patient with Ebstein's anomaly and significant downward displacement of the tricuspid valve. The arrows point to the tricuspid and mitral insertions in the septum. RV = right ventricle; RA = right atrium; LV = left ventricle; LA = left atrium.

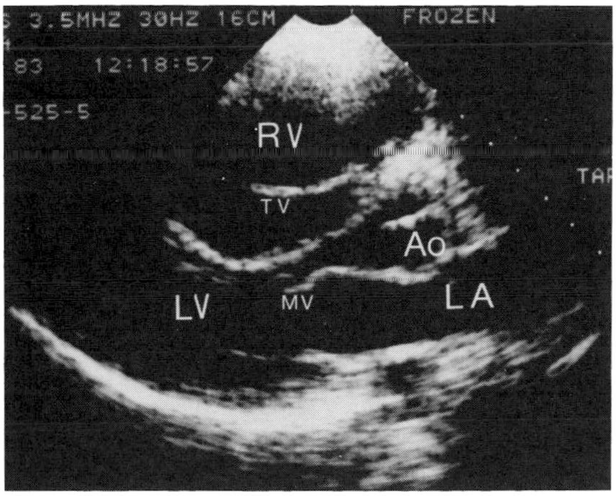

FIGURE 16–76
EBSTEIN'S ANOMALY
Long-axis left parasternal view in a patient with Ebstein's anomaly. A prominent tricuspid valve (TV) can be seen in a dilated right ventricular cavity. RV = right ventricle; LV = left ventricle; MV = mitral valve; Ao = aorta; LA = left atrium.

FIGURE 16–77
EBSTEIN'S ANOMALY
The tricuspid valve excursion is markedly increased in this view from a patient with Ebstein's anomaly. Delayed tricuspid valve closure produces a flail sound (F.S.).

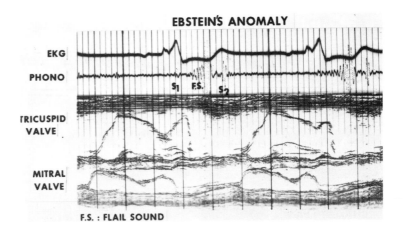

EBSTEIN'S ANOMALY

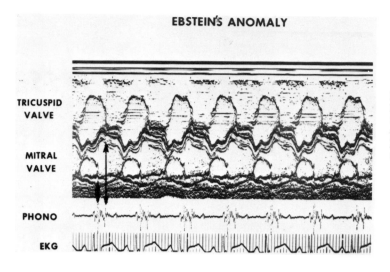

FIGURE 16–78
EBSTEIN'S ANOMALY
Simultaneous recording of the tricuspid and mitral valves in a patient with Ebstein's anomaly. Delayed tricuspid closure produces a flail sound after S_1.

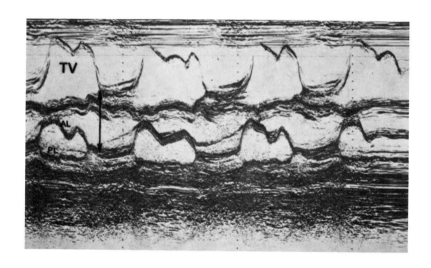

FIGURE 16–79
EBSTEIN'S ANOMALY
This echocardiogram recorded in a 14-year-old patient with Ebstein's anomaly and mild tricuspid regurgitation shows increased excursion and delayed closure of the tricuspid valve (TV). AL = anterior leaflet; PL = posterior leaflet.

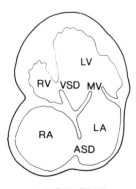

APICAL FOUR–
CHAMBER VIEW

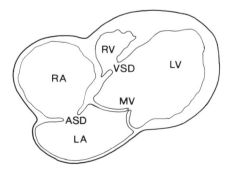

SUBCOSTAL FOUR–
CHAMBER VIEW

FIGURE 16–80
TRICUSPID ATRESIA
These diagrams demonstrate the characteristic findings of tricuspid atresia, which consist of a small right ventricle (RV), a large left ventricle (LV), and an atrial septal defect (ASD). A ventricular septal defect (VSD) is also frequently seen. MV = mitral valve; RA = right atrium; LA = left atrium.

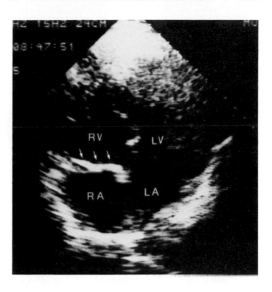

FIGURE 16–81
TRICUSPID ATRESIA
This apical four-chamber view shows a dense band of echoes at the level of the tricuspid ring. No tricuspid leaflets are seen. RV = right ventricle; LV = left ventricle; RA = right atrium; LA = left atrium.

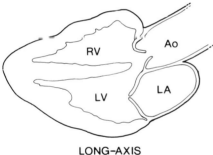

LONG-AXIS
PARASTERNAL VIEW

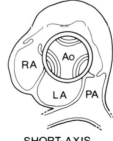

SHORT-AXIS
PARASTERNAL VIEW

FIGURE 16–82
FALLOT'S TETRALOGY
These diagrams demonstrate the characteristic abnormalities of patients with Fallot's tetralogy: aortic override, conotruncal ventricular septal defect, infundibular pulmonic stenosis, and right ventricular hypertrophy. RV = right ventricle; LV = left ventricle; Ao = aorta; LA = left atrium; PA = pulmonary artery.

FIGURE 16–83
FALLOT'S TETRALOGY
Left parasternal long-axis view in a 16-month-old boy with Fallot's tetralogy. This view demonstrates a conotruncal ventricular septal defect (arrow), aortic override, and a dilated aortic root. RV = right ventricle; LV = left ventricle; S = septum; Ao = aorta; LA = left atrium.

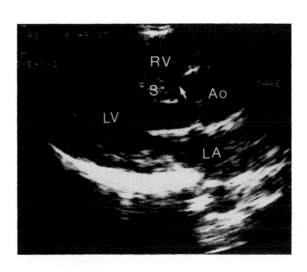

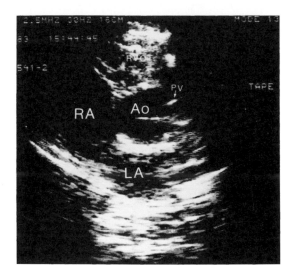

FIGURE 16–84
FALLOT'S TETRALOGY
Left parasternal short-axis view at the level of the aorta (Ao) in the same patient as in Figure 16–83. The dilated aorta, the narrowed right ventricular outflow tract (RVOT), and the presence of a pulmonic valve (PV) should be noted. RA = right atrium; LA = left atrium.

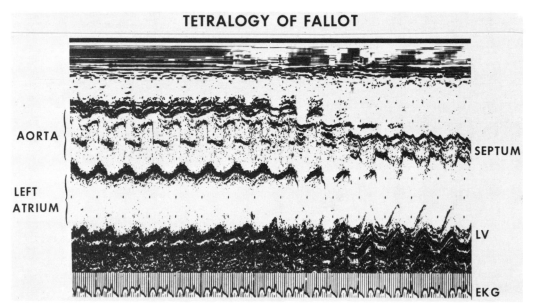

FIGURE 16–85
FALLOT'S TETRALOGY
This echocardiographic scan from the aorta to the left ventricle (LV) in a patient with Fallot's tetralogy demonstrates aortic override.

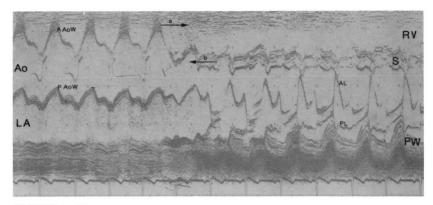

FIGURE 16–86
PSEUDO AORTIC OVERRIDE
Echocardiographic scan from the aorta to the left ventricle in a patient with acute pericarditis and no congenital heart disease. The transducer was placed high in the chest to produce a view of pseudo aortic override. Ao = aorta; LA = left atrium; AAoW = anterior aortic wall; PAoW = posterior aortic wall; AL = anterior leaflet; PL = posterior leaflet; RV = right ventricle; S = septum; PW = posterior wall.

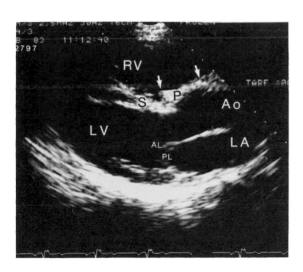

FIGURE 16–87
FALLOT'S TETRALOGY, AFTER REPAIR
Long-axis left parasternal view in a 19-year-old man with Fallot's tetralogy after corrective surgery. The arrows point to the patch (P) that was used to close the ventricular septal defect. RV = right ventricle; LV = left ventricle; S = septum; Ao = aorta; LA = left atrium; AL = anterior leaflet; PL = posterior leaflet.

FIGURE 16–88
FALLOT'S TETRALOGY, AFTER REPAIR
This short-axis left parasternal view in the same patient as in Figure 16–87 shows a right ventricular outflow tract of normal size, which is the result of infundibulectomy. RV = right ventricle; Ao = aorta; RA = right atrium; LA = left atrium.

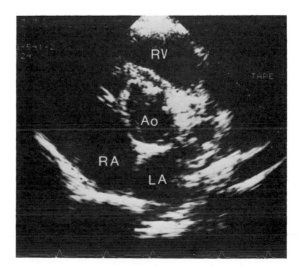

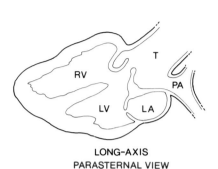

LONG-AXIS
PARASTERNAL VIEW

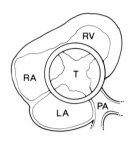

SHORT-AXIS
PARASTERNAL VIEW

FIGURE 16–89
TRUNCUS ARTERIOSUS
These diagrams of the long- and short-axis views in a patient with truncus arteriosus (T) demonstrate a large and single great vessel, a large septal defect, and absence of the pulmonic valve. RV = right ventricle; LV = left ventricle; LA = left atrium; PA = pulmonary artery; RA = right atrium.

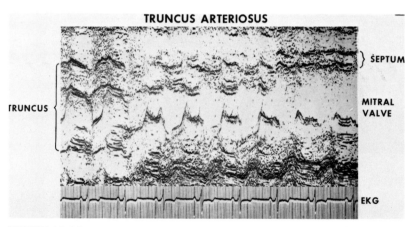

FIGURE 16–90
INCOMPETENT TRUNCUS ARTERIOSUS
Echocardiographic scan from the aorta to the mitral valve in a patient with an incompetent truncus arteriosus. The large great vessel and the flutter of the mitral valve and septum should be noted.

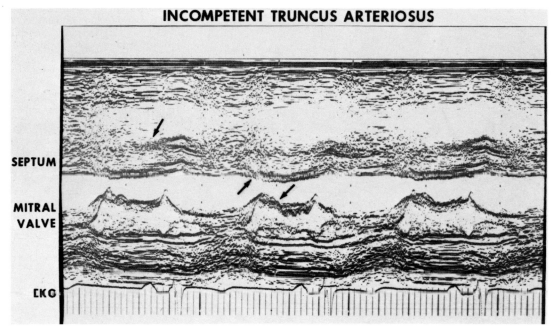

FIGURE 16–91
INCOMPETENT TRUNCUS ARTERIOSUS
Vibrations in both sides of the septum as well as in the mitral valve are seen in this recording from a patient with an incompetent truncus arteriosus.

FIGURE 16–92
TRANSPOSITION OF THE GREAT ARTERIES
These diagrams demonstrate the characteristic abnormalities of transposition of the great arteries. This includes anterior position of the aorta (Ao), which runs parallel to the posterior pulmonary artery (PA). A ventricular septal defect is also present. RV = right ventricle; LV = left ventricle; LA = left atrium; RA = right atrium.

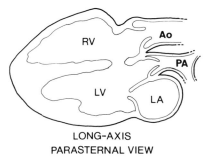
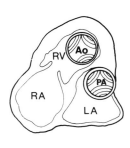

LONG-AXIS
PARASTERNAL VIEW

SHORT-AXIS
PARASTERNAL VIEW

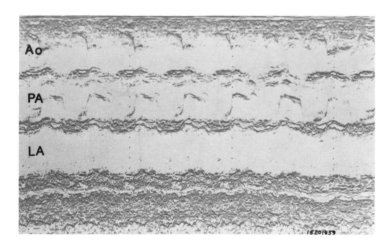

FIGURE 16–93
TRANSPOSITION OF THE GREAT ARTERIES
This echocardiogram of the great vessels shows that both semilunar valves can be recorded simultaneously. This finding is characteristic of transposition and is related to their parallel orientation. Ao = aorta; PA = pulmonary artery; LA = left atrium.

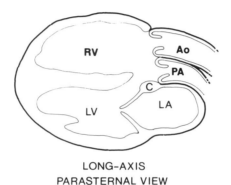

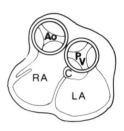

LONG-AXIS
PARASTERNAL VIEW

SHORT-AXIS
PARASTERNAL VIEW

FIGURE 16–94
DOUBLE OUTLET RIGHT VENTRICLE
Long-axis and short-axis views in a patient with double outlet right ventricle show the mitral great vessel discontinuity that is characteristic of this anomaly. A band of tissue (conus; C) separates these structures. RV = right ventricle; LV = left ventricle; Ao = aorta; PA = pulmonary artery; LA = left atrium; RA = right atrium; PV = pulmonary ventricle.

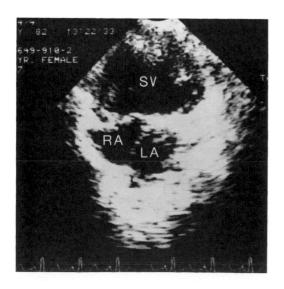

FIGURE 16–95
SINGLE VENTRICLE
This apical four-chamber view in a patient with single ventricle demonstates the absence of interventricular septum, a single ventricular chamber (SV), and two atria (right, RA, and left, LA).

REFERENCES

1 ECHOCARDIOGRAPHIC ANATOMY

1–1 THE HEART IN THE CHEST

1. Netter FH: Heart. Vol. 5. The Ciba collection of medical illustrations, 1969.

1–2 TOMOGRAPHIC ANATOMY OF THE HEART

2. McAlpine WA: Heart and Coronary Arteries: An Anatomic Atlas for Radiologic Diagnosis and Surgical Treatment. New York, Springer-Verlag, 1975.
3. Tajik AJ, Seward JB, Hagler DJ, Mair DD, Lie JT: Two-dimensional real-time ultrasonic imaging of the heart and great vessels. Technic, image orientation, structure identification, and validation. Mayo Clin Proc 53:271, 1978.
4. Edwards JE: Anatomic-pathologic foundations for echocardiography. Minn Med 63:838, 1980.
5. Edwards WD, Tajik AJ, Seward JB: Standardized nomenclature and anatomic basis for regional tomographic analysis of the heart. Mayo Clin Proc 56:479, 1981.

2 ECHOCARDIOGRAPHIC EXAMINATION AND MEASUREMENTS

2–1 TWO-DIMENSIONAL ECHOCARDIOGRAPHY

1. Tajik AJ, Seward JB, Hagler DJ, Mair DD, Lie JT: Two-dimensional real-time ultrasonic imaging of the heart and great vessels. Technique image orientation, structure identification, and validation. Mayo Clin Proc 53:271, 1978.
2. Bansal RC, Tajik AJ, Seward JB, Offord KP: Feasibility of detailed two-dimensional echocardiographic examination in adults. Prospective study of 200 patients. Mayo Clin Proc 55:291, 1980.
3. Henry WL, DeMaria A, Gramiak R, King DL, Kisslo JA, Popp RL, Sahn DJ, Schiller NB, Tajik A, Teichholz LE, Weyman AE: Report of the American Society of Echocardiography Committee on nomenclature and standards in two-dimensional echocardiography. Circulation 62:212, 1980.

2–2 COMBINED M-MODE AND TWO-DIMENSIONAL ECHOCARDIOGRAPHY

4. Chang S: M-mode echocardiographic techniques and pattern recognition. Philadelphia, Lea & Febiger, 1976.

2–3 M-MODE ECHOCARDIOGRAPHIC MEASUREMENTS

5. Sahn DJ, DeMaria A, Kisslo J, Weyman A: Recommendations regarding quantitation in M-mode echocardiography: Results of a survey of echocardiographic measurements. Circulation 58:1072, 1978.

2–4 TWO-DIMENSIONAL ECHOCARDIOGRAPHIC MEASUREMENTS

6. Schmittger I, Gordon EP, Fitzgerald PJ, Popp RL: Standardized intracardiac measurements of two-dimensional echocardiography. J Am Cardiol 2:934, 1983.

355

3 ECHOPHONOCARDI-OGRAPHY AND ECHOCARDIOGRAPHIC FINDINGS WITH ALTERED ELECTRICAL ACTIVATION

3–1 ECHOPHONOCARDIOGRAPHY

1. Burggraf GW, Craige E: The first heart sound in complete heart block. Phono-echocardiographic correlations. Circulation 50:17, 1974.
2. Laniaido S, Yellin E, Terdiman R, Meytes I, Stadler J: Hemodynamic correlates of the normal aortic valve echogram. A study of sound, flow, and motion. Circulation 54:729, 1976.
3. Mills PG, Brodie B, McLaurin L, Schall S, Craige E: Echocardiographic and hemodynamic relationships of ejection sounds. Circulation 56:430, 1977.
4. Mills P, Craige E: Echophonocardiography. Prog Cardiovasc Dis 20:337, 1978.

5. Burggraf GW: The first heart sound in the left bundle branch block: An echophonocardiographic study. Circulation 63:429, 1981.

3–2 SYSTOLIC TIME INTERVALS

6. Weissler AM, Garrard CL: Systolic time intervals in cardiac disease. Mod Concepts Cardiovasc Dis 40:1, 1971.

3–3 ALTERED ELECTRICAL ACTIVATION

7. Greenberg MA, Herman LS, Cohen MV: Mitral valve closure in atrial flutter. Circulation 59:902, 1979.

4 MITRAL VALVE DISEASE

4–1 MITRAL STENOSIS

1. Roberts WC: Clinical Cardiovascular Physiology. New York, Grune & Stratton, Inc., 1976.
2. Duchak JM, Chang S, Feigenbaum H: The posterior mitral valve echo and echocardiographic diagnosis of mitral stenosis. Am J Cardiol 29:628, 1972.
3. Weyman AE, Heger JJ, Kronik G, Wann LS, Dillon JC, Feigenbaum H: Mechanism of paradoxical early diastolic septal motion in patients with mitral stenosis: A cross-sectional echocardiographic study. Am J Cardiol 40:691, 1977.
4. Glover MU, Warren SE, Vieweg WVR, Ceretto WJ, Samtoy LM, Hagan AD: M-mode and two-dimensional echocardiographic correlation with findings at catheterization and surgery in patients with mitral stenosis. Am Heart J 105:98, 1983.
5. Cope GD, Kisslo JA, Johnson ML, Behar VS: A reassessment of the echocardiogram in mitral stenosis. Circulation 52:664, 1975.
6. Shiu MF: Mitral valve closure index: Echocardiographic index of severity of mitral stenosis. Br Heart J 39:839, 1977.
7. Shiu MF, Crowther A, Jenkins BS, Webb-Peploe MM: Echocardiographic and exercise evaluation of results of mitral valvotomy operations. Br Heart J 41:139, 1979.
8. Strunk BL, London EJ, Fitzgerald J, Popp RL, Barry WH: The assessment of mitral stenosis and prosthetic mitral valve obstruction using the posterior aortic wall echocardiogram. Circulation 55:885, 1977.
9. Wise JR: Echocardiographic evaluation of mitral stenosis using diastolic posterior left ventricular wall motion. Circulation 61:1037, 1980.
10. Henry WL, Griffith JM, Michaelis LL, McIntosh CL, Morrow AG, Epstein S: Measurement of mitral orifice area in patients with mitral valve disease by real-time two-dimensional echocardiography. Circulation 51:827, 1975.

11. Nichol PM, Gilbert BW, Kisslo JA: Two-dimensional echocardiography assessment of mitral stenosis. Circulation 55:120, 1977.
12. Wann LS, Weyman AE, Feigenbaum H, Dillon JC, Johnston KW, Eggleton RC: Determination of mitral valve area by cross-sectional echocardiography. Ann Intern Med 88:337, 1978.
13. Martin RP, Rakowski H, Kleiman JH, Beaver W, London E, Popp RL: Reliability and reproducibility of two-dimensional echocardiographic measurement of the stenotic mitral valve orifice area. Am J Cardiol 43:560, 1979.
14. Nanda NC, Gramiak R, Shah PM, DeWeese JA: Mitral commissurotomy versus replacement: Preoperative evaluation by echocardiography. Circulation 51:263, 1975.
15. Nicolosi GL, Atkins F, Dunn M: Echocardiographic evaluation of mitral stenosis in predicting mitral valve replacement vs. commissurotomy. Relation to hemodynamic measurements. Chest 77:147, 1980.
16. Heger JJ, Wann LS, Weyman AE, Dillon JC, Feigenbaum H: Long-term changes in mitral valve area after successful mitral commissurotomy. Circulation 59:443, 1979.
17. Nanda NC, Gramiak R, Shah PM, DeWeese JA, Mahoney EB: Echocardiographic assessment of left ventricular outflow width in the selection of mitral valve prosthesis. Circulation 48:1208, 1973.
18. Quinones MA, Gaash WH, Waisser E, Alexander JK: Reduction in the rate of diastolic descent of the mitral valve echogram in patients with altered left ventricular diastolic pressure-volume relations. Circulation 49:246, 1974.
19. Levisman JA, Abassi AS, Pearce ML: Posterior mitral leaflet motion in mitral stenosis. Circulation 51:511, 1975.
20. Glasser SP, Faris JV: Posterior leaflet motion in mitral stenosis. Chest 71:87, 1977.

4–2 MITRAL INSUFFICIENCY

21. Roberts WC, Perloff JK: Mitral valve disease: A clinicopathologic survey of the conditions causing the mitral valve to function abnormally. Ann Intern Med 77:939, 1972.
22. Selzer A, Katayama F: Mitral regurgitation: Clinical patterns, pathophysiology and natural history. Medicine 51:337, 1972.
23. Silverman ME, Hurst JW: The mitral complex. Am Heart J 76:399, 1968.
24. Patton R, Dragatakis L, Marpole D, Sniderman A: The posterior left atrial echocardiogram of mitral regurgitation. Circulation 57:1134, 1978.
25. Tei C, Tanaka H, Nakao S, Yoshimura H, Minagoe S, Kashima T, Kanehisa T: Motion of the interatrial septum in acute mitral regurgitation. Circulation 62:1080, 1980.
26. Gehl LG, Mintz GR, Kotler MN, Segal BL: Left atrial volume overload in mitral regurgitation: A two-dimensional echocardiographic study. Am J Cardiol 49:33, 1982.
27. Mintz GS, Kotler MN, Segal BL, Parry WR: Two dimensional echocardiographic evaluation of patients with mitral insufficiency. Am J Cardiol 44:670, 1979.

4–3 RHEUMATIC MITRAL INSUFFICIENCY

28. Wann LS, Feigenbaum H, Weyman AE, Dillon JC: Cross-sectional echocardiographic detection of rheumatic mitral regurgitation. Am J Cardiol 41:1258, 1978.

4–4 MITRAL VALVE PROLAPSE

29. Dillon JC, Haine CL, Chang S, Feigenbaum H: Use of echocardiography in patients with prolapsed mitral valve. Circulation 43:503, 1971.
30. Kerber RE, Isaeff DM, Hancock EW: Echocardiographic patterns in patients with the syndrome of systolic click and late systolic murmur. N Engl J Med 284:691, 1971.
31. Popp RL, Brown OR, Silverman IF, Harrison DC: Echocardiographic abnormalities in the mitral valve prolapse syndrome. Circulation 49:428, 1974.
32. DeMaria AN, King JF, Hugo GB, Lies JE, Mason DT: The variable spectrum of echocardiographic manifestations of the mitral valve prolapse syndrome. Circulation 50:33, 1974.
33. Markiewicz W, Stoner J, London E, Hunt SA, Popp RL: Mitral valve prolapse in 100 presumably healthy young females. Circulation 53:464, 1976.
34. Haikal M, Alpert MA, Whiting RB, Ahmad M, Kelly D: Sensitivity and specificity of M mode echocardiographic signs of mitral valve prolapse. Am J Cardiol 50:185, 1982.
35. Gilbert BW, Schatz RA, VonRamm OT, Behar VS, Kisslo JA: Mitral valve prolapse. Two-dimensional echocardiographic and angiographic correlation. Circulation 54:716, 1976.
36. Cohen MV: Real-time sector scan study of the mitral valve prolapse syndrome. Br Heart J 40:964, 1978.
37. Morganroth J, Mardelli TJ, Naito M, Chen CC: Apical cross-sectional echocardiography standard for the diagnosis of idiopathic mitral valve prolapse syndrome. Chest 79:23, 1981.
38. Chandraratna PAN, Langevin E: Limitations of the echocardiogram in diagnosing valvular vegetations in patients with mitral valve prolapse. Circulation 56:436, 1977.
39. Ormiston JA, Shah PM, Chuwa T, Wong M: Size and motion of mitral valve annulus in Man. II. Abnormalities in mitral valve prolapse. Circulation 65:713, 1982.
40. Winkle RA, Goodman DJ, Popp RL: Simultaneous echocardiographic phonocardiographic recordings at rest and during amyl nitrate administration in patients with mitral valve prolapse. Circulation 51:522, 1975.
41. Markiewicz W, London E, Popp RL: Effect of transducer placement on echocardiographic mitral valve motion. Am Heart J 96:555, 1978.
42. Yokota Y, Kawanishi H, Ohmori K, Oda A, Inoh T, Fukuzaki H: Studies on systolic anterior motion (SAM) pattern in idiopathic mitral valve prolapse by echocardiography. J Cardiogr 9:259, 1979.
43. Kerin NZ, Wajszczuk WJ, Cascade PN, Schairer J, Rubenfire M: Echocardiographic source of early anterior systolic motion in late systolic mitral valve prolapse. Chest 77:567, 1980.
44. Schreiber TL, Feigenbaum H, Weyman AE: Effect of atrial septal defect repair on left ventricular geometry and degree of mitral valve prolapse. Circulation 61:888, 1980.

4–5 RUPTURED CHORDAE TENDINEAE

45. Mintz GS, Kotler MN, Segal BL, Parry WR: Two-dimensional echocardiographic recognition of ruptured chordae tendineae. Circulation 57:244, 1978.
46. Mintz GS, Kotler MN, Parry WR, Segal BL: Statistical comparison of M-mode and two-dimensional echocardiographic diagnosis of flail mitral leaflets. Am J Cardiol 45:253, 1980.
47. Child JS, Skorton DJ, Taylor RD, Krivokapich J, Abbasi AS, Wong M, Shah PD: M-mode and cross-sectional echocardiographic features of flail posterior mitral leaflet. Am J Cardiol 44:1383, 1979.
48. Sweatman T, Selzer A, Kamagaki M, Cohn K: Echocardiographic diagnosis of mitral regurgitation due to ruptured chordae tendinae. Circulation 46:580, 1972.
49. Meyer JF, Frank MJ, Goldberg S, Cheng TO: Systolic mitral flutter, an echocardiographic clue to the diagnosis of ruptured chordae tendineae. Am Heart J 94:3, 1977.

4–6 PAPILLARY MUSCLE DYSFUNCTION

50. Ogawa S, Hubbard FE, Mardelli TJ, Dreifus LS: Cross-sectional echocardiographic spectrum of papillary muscle dysfunction. Am Heart J 97:312, 1979.
51. Godley RW, Wann LS, Rogers EW, Feigenbaum H, Weyman AE: Incomplete mitral leaflet closure in patients with papillary muscle dysfunction. Circulation 63:565, 1981.
52. Hayakawa M, Inoh T, Kawanishi H, Kaku K, Kumaki T, Toh S, Fukuzaki H: Two-dimensional echocardiographic findings of patients with papillary muscle dysfunction. J Cardiogr 12:137, 1982.

4–7 MITRAL ANNULUS CALCIFICATION

53. Fulkerson PK, Beaver BM, Auseon JC, Graber HL: Calcification of the mitral annulus: Etiology, clinical associations, complications and therapy. Am J Med 66:967, 1979.
54. D'Cruz IA, Cohen HC, Prabhu R, Bisla V, Glick G: Clinical manifestations of mitral annulus calcification with emphasis on its echocardiographic features. Am Heart J 94:367, 1977.
55. D'Cruz I, Panetta F, Cohen H, Glick G: Submitral

calcification or sclerosis in elderly patients: M-mode and two-dimensional echocardiography in "mitral annulus calcification." Am J Cardiol 44:31, 1979.

56. Mellino M, Salcedo EE, Lever HM, Vasudevan G, Kramer JR: Echographic-quantified severity of mitral annulus calcification. Prognostic correlation to related hemodynamic, valvular, rhythm, and conduction abnormalities. Am Heart J 103:222, 1982.

57. Mellino M, Salcedo EE: Fluoroscopy and echocardiography in patients with mitral annulus calcification. Non-invasive assessment of the cardiovascular system. Littleton, MA, John Wright/PSG, Inc, 1982, p. 159.

58. Nair CK, Aronow WS, Sketch MH, Mohiuddin SM,

Pagano T, Esterbrooks DJ, Hee TT: Clinical and echocardiographic characteristics of patients with mitral annular calcification. Comparison with age and sex-matched control subjects. Am J Cardiol 51:992, 1983.

59. Savage DD, Garrison RJ, Castelli WP, McNamara PM, Anderson SJ, Kammel WB, Feinleib M: Prevalence of submitral (annular) calcium and its correlates in a general population-based sample (The Framingham Study). Am J Cardiol 51:1375, 1983.

60. Takamoto T, Popp RL: Conduction disturbances related to the site and severity of mitral annular calcification: A two-dimensional echocardiographic and electrocardiographic correlative study. Am J Cardiol 51:1644, 1983.

5 AORTIC VALVE DISEASE

5-1 VALVULAR AORTIC STENOSIS

1. DeMaria AN, Bommer W, Joye J, Lee G, Bouteller J, Mason DT: Value and limitations of cross-sectional echocardiography of the aortic valve in the diagnosis and quantification of valvular aortic stenosis. Circulation 62:304, 1980.

2. Henry WL, Bonow RO, Borer JS, Kent KM, Ware JH, Redwood DR, Itscoitz SB, McIntosh CL, Morrow AG, Epstein SE: Evaluation of aortic valve replacement in patients with valvular aortic stenosis. Circulation 61:814, 1980.

3. Chang S, Clements S, Chang J: Aortic stenosis: Echocardiographic cusp separation and surgical description of aortic valve in 22 patients. Am J Cardiol 39:499, 1977.

4. Godley RW, Green D, Dillon JC, Rogers EW, Feigenbaum H, Weyman AE: Reliability of two-dimensional echocardiography in assessing the severity of valvular aortic stenosis. Chest 79:657, 1981.

5. Weyman AE, Feigenbaum H, Dillon JC, Chang S: Cross-sectional echocardiography in assessing the severity of valvular aortic stenosis. Circulation 52:828, 1975.

6. Bennett DH, Evans DW, Raj MVJ: Echocardiographic left ventricular dimensions in pressure and volume overload. Their use in assessing aortic stenosis. Br Heart J 37:971, 1975.

7. Johnson GL, Meyer RA, Schwartz DC, Korfhagen J, Kaplan S: Echocardiographic evaluation of fixed left ventricular outlet obstruction in children. Pre- and postoperative assessment of ventricular systolic pressures. Circulation 56:299, 1977.

8. Aziz KU, van Grondelle A, Paul MH, Muster AJ: Echocardiographic assessment of the relation between left ventricular wall and cavity dimensions and peak systolic pressure in children with aortic stenosis. Am J Cardiol 40:775, 1977.

9. Schwartz A, Vignola PA, Walker HJ, King ME, Goldblatt A: Echocardiographic estimation of aortic valve gradient in aortic stenosis. Ann Intern Med 89:329, 1978.

10. Blackwood RA, Bloom KR, Williams CM: Aortic stenosis in children; experience with echocardiographic prediction of severity. Circulation 57:263, 1978.

11. Gewitz MH, Werner JC, Kleinman CS, Hellenbrand WE, Talner NS: Role of echocardiography in aortic stenosis: Pre- and postoperative studies. Am J Cardiol 43:67, 1979.

12. DePace NL, Ren JF, Iskandrian AS, Kotler MN, Hakki AH, Segal BL: Correlation of echocardiographic wall stress and left ventricular pressure and function in aortic stenosis. Circulation 67:854, 1983.

13. Leo LR, Barrett MJ, Leddy CL, Wolf NM, Frankl WS: Determination of aortic valve area by cross-sectional echocardiography. Circulation 60:203, 1979.

14. Bonner AJ, Sacks HN, Tavel ME: Assessing the severity of aortic stenosis by phonocardiography and external carotid pulse recordings. Circulation 48:247, 1973.

15. Voelkel AG, Kendrick M, Pietro DA, Parisi AF, Voelkel V, Greenfield D, Askenazi J, Folland ED: Noninvasive tests to evaluate the severity of aortic stenosis. Limitations and reliability. Chest 77:155, 1980.

5-2 AORTIC INSUFFICIENCY

16. D'Cruz I, Cohen HC, Prabhu R, Ayabe T, Glick G: Flutter of left ventricular structures in patients with aortic regurgitation, with special reference to patients with associated mitral stenosis. Am Heart J 92:684, 1976.

17. Johnson AD, Gosink BB: Oscillation of left ventricular structures in aortic regurgitation. JCU 5:21, 1977.

18. Cope GD, Kisslo JA, Johnson ML, Myers S: Diastolic vibration of the interventricular septum in aortic insufficiency. Circulation 51:589, 1975.

19. Johnson AD, Alpert JS, Francis GS, Vieweg VR, Ockene I, Hagan AD: Assessment of left ventricular function in severe aortic regurgitation. Circulation 54:975, 1976.

20. Ambrose JA, Meller J, Teichholz LE, Herman MV: Premature closure of the mitral valve: Echocardiographic clue for the diagnosis of aortic dissection. Chest 73:121, 1978.

21. Mann T, McLaurin L, Grossman W, Craige E: Assessing the hemodynamic severity of acute aortic regurgitation due to infective endocarditis. N Engl J Med 293:108, 1975.

22. Weaver WF, Wilson CS, Rourke T, Caudill CC: Mid-diastolic aortic valve opening in severe acute aortic regurgitation. Circulation 55:145, 1977.

23. Pietro DA, Parisi AF, Harrington JJ, Askenazi J: Premature opening of the aortic valve: An index of

highly advanced aortic regurgitation. JCU 6:170, 1978.

24. Mardelli TJ, Morganroth J, Naito M, Chen CC: Cross-sectional echocardiographic detection of aortic valve prolapse. Am Heart J 101:295, 1980.

25. Krivokapich J, Child JS, Skorton DJ: Flail aortic valve leaflets: M-mode and two-dimensional echocardiographic manifestations. Am Heart J 99:425, 1980.

26. Henry WL, Bonow RO, Borer JS, Ware JH, Kent KM, Redwood DR, McIntosh CL, Morrow AG, Epstein SE: Observations on the optimum time for operative intervention for aortic regurgitation. I.

Evaluation of the results of aortic valve replacement in symptomatic patients. Circulation 61:471, 1980.

27. Henry WL, Bonow RO, Rosing DR, Epstein SE: Observations on the optimum time for operative intervention for aortic regurgitation. II. Serial echocardiographic evaluation of asymptomatic patients. Circulation 62:484, 1980.

28. Fioretti P, Roeland J, Bose R, Meltzer R, Hoogenhijze D, Serruys P, Nauta J, Hugenholtz P: Echocardiography in chronic aortic insufficiency. Is valve replacement too late when left ventricular end-systolic dimension reaches 55 mm? Circulation 67:216, 1983.

6 THE AORTA AND DISEASES OF THE AORTA

6–2 ECHOCARDIOGRAPHIC EXAMINATION OF THE AORTA

1. Gramiak R, Shah PM: Echocardiography of the aortic root. Invest Radiol 3:356, 1968.
2. Francis GS, Hagan AD, Oury J, O'Rourke RA: Accuracy of echocardiography for assessing aortic root diameter. Br Heart J 37:376, 1975.
3. Mintz GS, Kotler MN, Segal BL, Parry WR: Two-dimensional echocardiographic recognition of the descending thoracic aorta. Am J Cardiol 44:232, 1979.
4. Come PC: Improved cross-sectional echocardiographic technique for visualization of the retrocardiac descending aorta in its long axis. Normal findings and abnormalities in saccular and/or dissecting aneurysms. Am J Cardiol 51:1029, 1983.
5. Haaz WS, Mintz GS, Kotler MN, Parry W, Segal BL: Two-dimensional echocardiographic recognition of the descending thoracic aorta: Value in differentiating pericardial from pleural effusions. Am J Cardiol 46:739, 1980.
6. Leopold GR, Goldberger LE, Bernstein EF: Ultrasonic detection and evaluation of abdominal aortic aneurysms. Surgery 72:939, 1972.

6–4 ARTERIOSCLEROTIC AORTIC ANEURYSM

7. DeMaria AN, Bommer W, Neumann A, Weinert L, Bogren H, Mason DT: Identification and localization of aneurysms of the ascending aorta by cross-sectional echocardiography. Circulation 59:755, 1979.
8. D'Cruz IA, Jain DP, Hirsch L, Levinsky R, Cohen HC, Glick G: Echocardiographic diagnosis of dilatation of the ascending aorta using right parasternal scanning. Radiology 129:465, 1978.
9. Iliceto S, Antonelli G, Biasco G, Rizzo P: Two-dimensional echocardiographic evaluation of aneurysms of the descending thoracic aorta. Circulation 66:1045, 1982.

6–6 AORTIC DISSECTION

10. Roberts WC: Aortic dissection: Anatomy, consequences, and causes. Am Heart J 101:195, 1981.
11. Nanda NC, Gramiak R, Shah PM: Diagnosis of aortic root dissection by echocardiography. Circulation 48:506, 1973.
12. Yuste P, Aza V, Minguez I, Cerezo L, Martinez-

Bordiu C: Dissecting aortic aneurysm diagnosed by echocardiography. Br Heart J 36:111, 1974.
13. Brown OR, Popp RL, Kloster FE: Echocardiographic criteria for aortic root dissection. Am J Cardiol 36:17, 1975.
14. Moothart RW, Spangler RD, Blont SG Jr: Echocardiography in aortic root dissection and dilatation. Am J Cardiol 36:11, 1975.
15. Victor MF, Mintz GS, Kotler MN, Wilson AR, Segal BL: Two-dimensional echocardiographic diagnosis of aortic dissection. Am J Cardiol 48:1155, 1981.
16. Smuckler AL, Nomeir AM, Watts LE, Hackshaw BT: Echocardiographic diagnosis of aortic root dissection by M-mode and two-dimensional techniques. Am Heart J 103:897, 1982.
17. Nicholson WJ, Cobbs BW Jr: Echocardiographic oscillating flap in aortic root dissecting aneurysm. Chest 70:305, 1976.
18. Krueger SK, Starke H, Forker AD, Eliot RS: Echocardiographic mimics of aortic root dissection. Chest 67:441, 1975.
19. Matsumoto M, Matsuo H, Ohara T, Yoshioka Y, Abe H: A two-dimensional echoaortocardiographic approach to dissecting aneurysms of the aorta to prevent false-positive diagnoses. Radiology 127:491, 1978.
20. Kasper W, Meinertz T, Kersting F, Lang K, Just H: Diagnosis of dissecting aortic aneurysm with suprasternal echocardiography. Am J Cardiol 42:291, 1978.

6–7 ANEURYSM OF THE SINUS OF VALSALVA

21. Sakakibara S, Konno S: Congenital aneurysm of the sinus of Valsalva associated with ventricular septal defect: Anatomy and classification. Am Heart J 75:595, 1968.
22. Rothbaum DA, Dillon JC, Chang S, Feigenbaum H: Echocardiographic manifestation of right sinus of Valsalva aneurysm. Circulation 49:768, 1974.
23. Wong BYS, Bogart DB, Dunn MI: Echocardiographic features of an aneurysm of the left sinus of Valsalva. Chest 73:105, 1978.
24. Cooperberg P, Mercer EN, Mulder DS, Winsberg F: Rupture of a sinus Valsalva aneurysm: Report of a case diagnosed preoperatively by echocardiography. Radiology 113:171, 1974.
25. Matsumoto M, Matsuo H, Beppu S, Yoshioka Y,

servations during and after healing of active bacterial endocarditis limited to the mitral valve. Am Heart J 101:37, 1981.

16. Pasternak RC, Cannom DS, Cohen LS: Echocardiographic diagnosis of large fungal verruca attached to the mitral valve. Br Heart J 38:1209, 1976.

17. Martinez EC, Burch GE, Giles TD: Echocardiographic diagnosis of vegetative aortic bacterial endocarditis. Am J Cardiol 34:845, 1974.

18. Gottlieb S, Khuddus SA, Balooki H, Dominguez AE, Myerburg RJ: Echocardiographic diagnosis of aortic valve vegetations in candida endocarditis. Circulation 50:826, 1974.

19. DeMaria AN, King JF, Salel AF, Caudill CC, Miller RR, Mason DT: Echography and phonography of acute aortic regurgitation in bacterial endocarditis. Ann Intern Med 82:329, 1975.

20. Hirschfeld DS, Schiller N: Localization of aortic valve vegetations by echocardiography. Circulation 53:280, 1976.

21. Busch UW, Garcia E, Pechacek LW, DeCastro CM Jr, Hall RJ: Cross-sectional echocardiographic findings in vegetative aortic valve endocarditis. Cardiovasc Dis 5:328, 1978.

22. Wray TM: The variable echocardiographic features in aortic valve endocarditis. Circulation 52:658, 1975.

23. Wray TM: Echocardiographic manifestations of flail aortic valve leaflets in bacterial endocarditis. Circulation 51:832, 1975.

24. Kleiner JP, Brundage BH, Ports TA, Thomas HM: Echocardiographic manifestation of flail right and noncoronary aortic valve leaflets: Studies in patients with bacterial endocarditis. Chest 74:301, 1978.

25. Kisslo J, Von Ramm OT, Haney R, Jones R, Juk SS, Behar VS: Echocardiographic evaluation of tricuspid valve endocarditis: An M-mode and two-dimensional study. Am J Cardiol 38:502, 1976.

26. Berger M, Delfin LA, Jelveh M, Goldberg E: Two-dimensional echocardiographic findings in right-sided infective endocarditis. Circulation 61:855, 1980.

27. Ginzton LE, Siegel RJ, Criley JM: Natural history of tricuspid valve endocarditis: A two-dimensional echocardiographic study. Am J Cardiol 49:1853, 1982.

28. Chandraratna PAN, Aronow WS: Spectrum of echocardiographic findings in tricuspid valve endocarditis. Br Heart J 42:528, 1979.

29. Andy JJ, Sheikh MU, Ali N, Barnes BO, Fox LM, Curry CL, Roberts WC: Echocardiographic observations in opiate addicts with active infective endocarditis. Am J Cardiol 40:17, 1977.

30. Kramer NE, Gill SS, Patel R, Towne WD: Pulmonary valve vegetations detected with echocardiography. Am J Cardiol 39:1064, 1977.

31. Sheikh MU, Ali N, Covarrubias E, Fox LM, Morjaria M, Dejo J: Right-sided infective endocarditis: An echocardiographic study. Am J Med 66:283, 1979.

32. Chiang CW, Lee YS, Chang CH, Hung JS, Chen L: Preoperative and postoperative echocardiographic studies of pulmonic valvular endocarditis. Chest 80:232, 1981.

33. Weiss RJ, LeMire MS, Bajor M, Buda AJ: Two-dimensional echocardiographic detection of pulmonic valve endocarditis. JCU 10:452, 1982.

34. Nakamura K, Satomi G, Sakai T, Ando M, Hashimoto A, Koyanagi H, Hirosawa K, Takao A: Clinical and echocardiographic features of pulmonary valve endocarditis. Circulation 67:198, 1983.

9–3 NONVALVULAR ENDOCARDITIS

35. Eichhorn EJ, Winters WL, Crawford ES, Musher DM, Middleton JW, Hettig RA: Bacterial endocarditis and right atrial vegetation. Detection by two-dimensional echocardiography. JAMA 246:2724, 1981.

9–4 VALVE RING ABSCESS

36. Arnett EN, Roberts WC: Valve ring abscess in active infective endocarditis. Frequency, location, and clues to clinical diagnosis from the study of 95 necropsy patients. Circulation 54:140, 1976.

37. Arnett EN, Roberts WC: Prosthetic valve endocarditis. Clinicopathologic analysis of 22 necropsy patients with comparison of observations in 74 patients with active infective endocarditis involving natural left-sided cardiac valves. Am J Cardiol 38:281, 1976.

38. Mardelli TJ, Ogawa S, Hubbard FE, Dreifus LS, Meixell LL: Cross-sectional echocardiographic detection of aortic ring abscess in bacterial endocarditis. Chest 74:576, 1978.

39. Scanlan JG, Seward JB, Tajik AJ: Valve ring abscess in infective endocarditis: Visualization with wide angle two-dimensional echocardiography. Am J Cardiol 49:1794, 1982.

40. Nakamura K, Suzuki S, Satomi G, Hayashi H, Hirosawa K: Detection of mitral ring abscess by two-dimensional echocardiography. Circulation 65:816, 1982.

10 PROSTHETIC VALVES

10–2 GENERAL ECHOCARDIOGRAPHIC FINDINGS

1. Mintz GS, Carlson ED, Kotler MN: Comparison of noninvasive techniques in evaluation of the nontissue cardiac valve prostheses. Am J Cardiol 49:39, 1982.

2. Kotler MN, Mintz GS, Panidis I, Morganroth J, Segal BL, Ross J: Noninvasive evaluation of normal and abnormal prosthetic valve function. J Am Coll Cardiol 2:151, 1983.

10–3 CAGED-BALL VALVES

3. Pfeifer J, Goldschlager N, Sweatman T, Gerbode F, Selzer A: Malfunction of mitral ball valve prosthesis due to thrombus. Am J Cardiol 29:95, 1972.

4. Wann LS, Pyhel HJ, Judson WE, Tavel ME, Feigenbaum H: Ball variance in a Harken mitral prosthesis: Echocardiographic and phonocardiographic features. Chest 72:785, 1977.

5. Belenkie I, Carr M, Schlant RC, Nutter DO, Sybmas PN: Malfunction of a Cutter-Smeloff mitral ball valve prosthesis: Diagnosis by phonocardiography and echocardiography. Am Heart J 86:399, 1973.

6. Brodie BR, Grossman W, McLaurin L, Starek PJK, Craige E: Diagnosis of prosthetic mitral valve malfunction with combined echophonocardiography. Circulation 53:93, 1976.

10–4 CAGED-DISC VALVES

7. Johnson ML, Holmes JH, Paton BC: Echocardiographic determination of mitral disc valve excursion. Circulation 47:1274, 1973.
8. Oliva PB, Johnson ML, Pomerantz M, Levene A: Dysfunction of the Beall mitral prosthesis and its detection by cinefluoroscopy and echocardiography. Am J Cardiol 31:393, 1973.
9. Kawai N, Segal BL, Linhart JW: Delayed opening of Beall mitral prosthetic valve detected by echocardiography. Chest 67:239, 1975.

10–5 TILTING-DISC VALVES

10. Douglas JE, Williams GD: Echocardiographic evaluation of Björk-Shiley prosthetic valve. Circulation 50:52, 1974.
11. Ben-Zvi J, Hildner FJ, Chandraratna PA, Samet P: Thrombosis on Björk-Shiley aortic valve prosthesis: Clinical, arteriographic, echocardiographic, and therapeutic observations in seven cases. Am J Cardiol 4:538, 1974.
12. Chandraratna PAN, Lopez JM, Hildner FJ, Samet P, Ben-Zvi J, Gindlesperger D: Diagnosis of Björk-Shiley aortic valve dysfunction by echocardiography. Am Heart J 91:318, 1976.
13. Yoganathan AP, Corcoran WH, Harrison EC, Carl JR: The Björk-Shiley aortic prosthesis: Flow characteristics, thrombus formation, and tissue overgrowth. Circulation 58:70, 1978.
14. Bernal-Ramirez JA, Phillips JH: Echocardiographic study of malfunction of the Björk-Shiley prosthetic heart valve in the mitral position. Am J Cardiol 40:449, 1977.
15. Copans H, Lakier JB, Kinsley RH, Colsen PR, Fritz VU, Barlow JB: Thrombosed Björk-Shiley mitral prostheses. Circulation 61:169, 1980.
16. Mintz GS, Carlson EB, Kotler MN: Comparison of noninvasive techniques in evaluation of the nontissue cardiac valve prosthesis. Am J Cardiol 49:39, 1982.
17. Gibson TC, Starek JK, Moos S, Craige E: Echocardiographic and phonocardiographic characteristics of the Lillehei-Kaster mitral valve prosthesis. Circulation 49:434, 1974.
18. Estevez R, Mookherjee S, Potts J, Fulton M, Obeid AI: Phonocardiographic and echocardiographic features of Lillehei-Kaster mitral prosthesis. JCU 5:153, 1977.

10–6 BILEAFLET VALVES

19. Amann FW, Burckhardt D, Hasse J, Gradel E: Echocardiographic features of the correctly functioning St. Jude medical valve prosthesis. Am Heart J 101:45, 1981.
20. DePace NL, Kotler MN, Mintz GB, Lichtenberg R, Goel IP, Segal BL: Echocardiographic and phonocardiographic assessment of the St. Jude cardiac valve prosthesis. Chest 80:272, 1981.
21. Feldman HJ, Gray RJ, Chaux A, Halpern SW, Kraus R, Allen HN, Matloff JM: Noninvasive in vivo and in vitro study of the St. Jude mitral valve prosthesis. Evaluation using two-dimensional and M-mode echocardiography, phonocardiography and cinefluoroscopy. Am J Cardiol 49:1101, 1982.

10–8 HETEROGRAFTS

22. Horowitz MS, Tecklenberg PL, Goodman DJ, Harrison DC, Popp RL: Echocardiographic evaluation of the stented mounted aortic bioprosthetic valve in the mitral position, in vitro and in vivo studies. Circulation 54:91, 1976.
23. Bloch WN, Felner JM, Wickliffe C, Symbas PN, Schlant RC: Echocardiogram of the porcine aortic bioprosthesis in the mitral position. Am J Cardiol 38:293, 1976.
24. Bloch WN Jr, Felner JM, Schlant RC, Symbas PN, Jones EL: The echocardiogram of the porcine aortic bioprosthesis in the aortic position. Chest 72:640, 1977.
25. Harston WE Jr, Robertson RM, Friesinger GC: Echocardiographic evaluation of porcine heterograft valves in the mitral and aortic positions. Am Heart J 96:448, 1978.
26. Horowitz MS, Goodman DJ, Hancock EW, Popp RL: Noninvasive diagnosis of complications of the mitral bioprosthesis. J Thorac Cardiovasc Surg 71:450, 1976.
27. Alam M, Madrazo AC, Magilligan DJ, Goldstein S: M-mode and two-dimensional echocardiographic features of porcine valve dysfunction. Am J Cardiol 43:502, 1979.
28. Schapira JN, Martin RP, Fowles RE, Rakowski H, Stinson EB, French JW, Shumway NE, Popp RL: Two-dimensional echocardiographic assessment of patients with bioprosthetic valves. Am J Cardiol 43:510, 1979.
29. Alam M, Lakier JB, Pickard SD, Goldstein S: Echocardiographic evaluation of porcine bioprosthetic valves: Experience with 309 normal and 59 dysfunctioning valves. Am J Cardiol 52:309, 1983.
30. Alam M, Garcia R, Goldstein S: Echo-phonocardiographic features of regurgitant porcine mitral and tricuspid valves presenting with musical murmurs. Am Heart J 105:456, 1983.
31. Bloch WN Jr, Felner JM, Wickliffe C, Symbas PN: Echocardiographic diagnosis of thrombus on a heterograft aortic valve in the mitral position. Chest 70:399, 1976.
32. Mikell FL, Asingh RW, Rourke T, Hodges M, Sharma B, Francis G: Two-dimensional echocardiographic demonstration of left atrial thrombi in patients with prosthetic mitral valves. Circulation 60:1183, 1979.
33. Szkopiec RL, Torstveit J, Desser KB, Savajiyani RD, Benchimol A, Solomon DK: M-mode and 2-dimensional echocardiographic characteristics of the Ionescu-Shiley valve in the mitral and aortic positions. Am J Cardiol 51:973, 1983.

10–9 AUTOGRAFT VALVES

34. Mary DAS, Pakrashi BC, Catchpole RW, Ionescu MI: Echocardiographic studies of stented fascia lata grafts in the mitral position. Circulation 49:237, 1974.

10–10 PROSTHETIC VALVE ENDOCARDITIS

35. Wilson WOR: In Duma RS (ed.): Infections of Prosthetic Heart Valves and Vascular Grafts. Baltimore, University Park Press, 1977, pp. 3–13.

10–12 CARPENTIER RING

36. Kronzon I, Mercurio P, Winer HE, Colvin S: Echocardiographic evaluation of Carpentier mitral valvuloplasty. Am Heart J 106:362, 1983.

11 LEFT VENTRICLE

11–1 LEFT VENTRICULAR SIZE AND FUNCTION

1. Pombo JF, Troy BL, Russell RO: Left ventricular volumes and ejection fraction by echocardiography. Circulation 43:480, 1971.
2. Fortuin NJ, Hood WP, Craige E: Evaluation of left ventricular function by echocardiography. Circulation 46:26, 1972.
3. Gibson DG: Estimation of left ventricular size by echocardiography. Br Heart J 35:128, 1973.
4. Quinones MA, Gaasch WH, Alexander JK: Echocardiographic assessment of left ventricular function, with special reference to normalized velocities. Circulation 50:42, 1974.
5. Teichholz LE, Kreulen T, Herman MV, Gorlin R: Problems in echocardiographic volume determinations: Echocardiographic-angiographic correlations in the presence or absence of asynergy. Am J Cardiol 37:7, 1976.
6. Sahn DJ, DeMaria A, Kisslo J, Weyman AE: Recommendations regarding quantitation in M-mode echocardiography: Results of a survey of echocardiographic measurements. Circulation 58:1072, 1978.
7. Schiller NB, Acquatella H, Ports TA, Drew D, Goerke J, Ringertz H, Silverman NH, Brundage B, Botvinick EH, Boswell R, Carlsson E, Parmley WW: Left ventricular volume from paired biplane two-dimensional echocardiography. Circulation 60:547, 1979.
8. Bommer W, Chun T, Kwan OL, Neumann A, Mason DT, DeMaria AN: Biplane apex echocardiography versus biplane cineangiography in the assessment of left ventricular volume and function: Validation by direct measurements. Am J Cardiol 45:471, 1980.
9. Wyatt HL, Heng MK, Meerbaum S, Gueret P, Hestenes J, Dula E, Corday E: Cross-sectional echocardiography: II. Analysis of mathematic models for quantifying volume of formalin fixed left ventricle. Circulation 61:1119, 1980.
10. Gueret P, Wyatt J, Meerbaum S, Corday E: A practical two-dimensional echocardiographic model to assess volume in the ischemic left ventricle. Am J Cardiol 45:471, 1980.
11. Wahr DW, Wang YS, Schiller NB: Left ventricular volumes determined by two-dimensional echocardiography in a normal adult population. J Am Coll Cardiol 1:863, 1983.
12. Tortoledo FA, Quinones MA, Fernandez GC, Waggoner AD, Winters WL Jr: Quantification of left ventricular volumes by two-dimensional echocardiography: A simplified and accurate approach. Circulation 67:579, 1983.
13. Feigenbaum H, Popp RL, Wolfe SB, Pombo JF, Troy BL, Haine CL, Dodge HT: Ultrasound measurements of left ventricle correlative study with angiocardiography. Arch Intern Med 129:461, 1972.
14. Troy BL, Pombo J, Rackley CE: Measurements of left ventricular wall thickness and mass by echocardiography. Circulation 45:602, 1972.
15. Wyatt H, Heng MK, Meerbaum S, Hestenes JD, Cobo JM, Davidson RM, Corday E: Cross-sectional echocardiography. I. Analysis of mathematic models for quantifying mass of the left ventricle in dogs. Circulation 60:1104, 1979.
16. Helak J, Reichek N, Pearlman E, Weber K, Pietra G, Kastor JA: Quantitation of human left ventricular (LV) mass and volume by cross-sectional echocardiography: In vitro anatomic validation. Am J Cardiol 45:470, 1980.
17. Reichek N, Helak J, Plappert T, Sutton MS, Weber K: Anatomic validation of left ventricular mass estimates from clinical two-dimensional echocardiography: Initial results. Circulation 67:348, 1983.
18. McFarland TM, Alam M, Goldstein S, Pickard SD, Stein PD: Echocardiographic diagnosis of left ventricular hypertrophy. Circulation 57:140, 1978.
19. Devereux R, Reichek N: Echocardiographic determination of left ventricular mass in man. Circulation 55:613, 1977.
20. Kronic G, Slany J, Mosslacher H: Comparative value of eight M-mode echocardiographic formulas for determining left ventricular stroke volume. Circulation 60:1308, 1979.
21. Rasmussen S, Corya BC, Feigenbaum H, Black MJ, Lovelace DE, Phillips J, Noble RJ, Knoebel SB: Stroke volume calculated from the mitral valve echogram in patients with and without ventricular dyssynergy. Circulation 58:125, 1978.
22. Lalani AV, Lee SJK: Echocardiographic measurement of cardiac output using the mitral valve and aortic root echo. Circulation 54:738, 1976.
23. Massie BM, Schiller NB, Ratshin RA, Parmley WW: Mitral-septal separation: New echocardiographic index of left ventricular function. Am J Cardiol 39:1008, 1977.
24. D'Cruz IA, Lalmalani GG, Sambasivan V, Cohen HC, Glick G: The superiority of mitral E-point ventricular septum separation to other echocardiographic indicators of left ventricular performance. Clin Cardiol 2:140, 1979.
25. Carr K, Engler RL, Forsythe JR, Johnson AD, Gosink B: Measurement of left ventricular ejection fraction by mechanical cross-sectional echocardiography. Circulation 59:1196, 1979.
26. Folland ED, Parisi AF, Moynihan PF, Jones DR, Feldman CL, Tow DE: Assessment of left ventricular ejection fraction and volumes by real-time two-dimensional echocardiography. Circulation 60:760, 1979.
27. Quinones MA, Waggoner AD, Reduto LA, Nelson JG, Young JB, Winters WL, Ribeiro LG, Miller RR: A new simplified and accurate method for determining ejection fraction with two-dimensional echocardiography. Circulation 64:744, 1981.
28. Cooper RH, O'Rourke RA, Karliner JS, Peterson KL, Leopold GR: Comparison of ultrasound and cineangiographic measurements of the mean rate of circumferential fiber shortening in man. Circulation 46:914, 1972.

11–2 LEFT VENTRICULAR HYPERTROPHY

29. Devereux RB, Reichek N: Left ventricular hypertrophy. Cardiovasc Rev Rep 1:55, 1980.
30. Abbasi AS, MacAlpin RN, Eber LM, Pearce ML: Left ventricular hypertrophy diagnosed by echocardiography. N Engl J Med 289:118, 1973.
31. Reichek N, Devereux RB: Left ventricular hypertrophy: Relationship of anatomic, echocardiographic, and electrocardiographic findings. Circulation 63:1391, 1981.
32. Kansal S, Roitman D, Sheffield LT: Interventricu-

lar septal thickness and left ventricular hypertrophy. An echocardiographic study. Circulation 60:1058, 1979.

33. Hanrath P, Mathey DG, Seigert R, Bleifeld W: Left ventricular relaxation and filling pattern in different forms of left ventricular hypertrophy: An echocardiographic study. Am J Cardiol 45:15, 1980.

11–3 LEFT VENTRICULAR SIZE AND FUNCTION IN SYSTEMIC HYPERTENSION

34. Savage DD, Drayer JIM, Henry WL, Mathews EC, Ware JH, Gardin JM, Cohen ER, Epstein SE, Laragh JH: Echocardiographic assessment of cardiac anatomy and function in hypertensive subjects. Circulation 59:623, 1979.

35. Kotler MN, Mintz GS, Segal BL: The use of echocardiography in the assessment of the patient with essential hypertension. Practical Cardiol 7:85, 1981.

36. Cohen A, Hagan AD, Watkins J, Mitas J, Schvartzman M, Mazzoleni A, Cohen IM, Warren SE, Vieweg WVR, Elias W, Samtoy L: Clinical correlates in hypertensive patients with left ventricular hypertrophy diagnosed with echocardiography. Am J Cardiol 47:335, 1981.

37. Drayer JIM, Weber MA, DeYoung JL: BP as determinant of cardiac left ventricular muscle mass. Arch Intern Med 143:90, 1981.

38. Culpepper WS, Sodt PC, Messerli FH, Ruschhaupt DG, Arcilla RA: Cardiac status in juvenile borderline hypertension. Ann Intern Med 90.1, 1983.

39. Dreslinski GR, Frohlich ED, Dunn FG, Messerli FH, Suarez DH, Reisin E: Echocardiographic diastolic ventricular abnormality in hypertensive heart disease: Atrial emptying index. Am J Cardiol 47:1087, 1981.

11–4 LEFT VENTRICULAR SIZE AND FUNCTION IN ATHLETES

40. Allen HD, Goldberg SJ, Sahn DJ, Schy N, Wojcik R: A quantitative echocardiographic study of champion childhood swimmers. Circulation 55:142, 1977.

41. Cohen JL, Gupta PK, Lichstein E, Chadda KD: The heart of a dancer: Noninvasive cardiac evaluation of professional ballet dancers. Am J Cardiol 45:959, 1980.

42. Nishimura T, Yamada Y, Kawai C: Echocardiographic evaluation of long-term effects of exercise on left ventricular hypertrophy and function in professional bicyclists. Circulation 61:832, 1980.

43. Stein RA, Michielli D, Diamond J, Horwitz B, Krasnow N: The cardiac response to exercise training. Echocardiographic analysis at rest and during exercise. Am J Cardiol 46:219, 1980.

11–5 CONGESTIVE CARDIOMYOPATHY

44. Corya BC, Feigenbaum H, Rasmussen S, Black MJ: Echocardiographic features of congestive cardiomyopathy compared with normal subjects and patients with coronary artery disease. Circulation 49:1153, 1974.

45. Epstein SE, Henry WL, Clark CE, Roberts WC, Maron BJ, Ferrans VJ, Redwood DR, Morrow AG: Asymmetric septal hypertrophy. Ann Intern Med 81:650, 1974.

46. Shah PM: Hypertrophic cardiomyopathy. Annu Rev Med 28:235, 1977.

47. Henry WL, Clark CE, Roberts WC, Morrow AG, Epstein SE: Differences in distribution of myocardial abnormalities in patients with obstructive and nonobstructive asymmetrical septal hypertrophy: Echocardiographic and gross anatomic findings. Circulation 50:447, 1974.

48. Tajik AJ, Giuliani ER: Echocardiographic observations in idiopathic hypertrophic subaortic stenosis. Mayo Clin Proc 49:89, 1974.

49. Martin RP, Rakowski H, French J, Popp RL: Idiopathic hypertrophic subaortic stenosis viewed by wide-angle, phased-array echocardiography. Circulation 59:1206, 1979.

50. Shapiro LM, McKenna WJ: Distribution of left ventricular hypertrophy in hypertrophic cardiomyopathy: A two-dimensional echocardiographic study. J Am Coll Cardiol 2:437, 1983.

51. Henry WL, Clark CE, Epstein SE: Asymmetric septal hypertrophy: Echocardiographic identification of the pathognomonic anatomic abnormality of IHSS. Circulation 47:225, 1973.

52. Yamaguchi H, Ishimura T, Nishiyama S, Nagasaki F, Nakanishi S, Takatsu F, Nishijo T, Umeda T, Machii K: Hypertrophic nonobstructive cardiomyopathy with giant negative T-waves (apical hypertrophy): Ventriculographic and echocardiographic features in 30 patients. Am J Cardiol 44:401, 1979.

53. Maron BJ, Bonow RO, Seshagiri TNR, Roberts WC, Epstein SE: Hypertrophic cardiomyopathy with ventricular septal hypertrophy localized to the apical region of the left ventricle (apical hypertrophic cardiomyopathy). Am J Cardiol 49:1838, 1982.

54. Maron BJ, Gottdiener JS, Bonow RO, Epstein S: Hypertrophic cardiomyopathy with unusual locations of left ventricular hypertrophy undetectable by M-mode echocardiography. Identification by wide-angle two-dimensional echocardiography. Circulation 63:409, 1981.

55. Gehrke J: New observations on systolic anterior motion of mitral valve leaflets in hypertrophic cardiomyopathy. Br Heart J 38:314, 1976.

56. Gilbert BW, Pollick C, Adelman AG, Wigle ED: Hypertrophic cardiomyopathy: Subclassification by M-mode echocardiography. Am J Cardiol 45:861, 1980.

57. Gramiak R, Shah PM: Cardiac ultrasonography. A review of current applications. Radiol Clin North Am 9:469, 1971.

58. St. John Sutton MG, Tajik AJ, Gibson DG, Brown DJ, Seward JB, Giuliani ER: Echocardiographic assessment of left ventricular filling and septal and posterior wall dynamics in idiopathic hypertrophic subaortic stenosis. Circulation 57:512, 1978.

59. Feigenbaum H: Echocardiography. 2nd ed. Philadelphia, Lea & Febiger, 1976, p. 137.

60. Greenwald J, Yap JF, Franklin M, Lichtman AM: Echocardiographic mitral systolic motion in left ventricular aneurysm. Br Heart J 37:684, 1975.

61. Maron BJ, Gottdiener JS, Roberts WC, Henry WL, Savage DD, Epstein SE: Left ventricular outflow tract obstruction due to systolic anterior motion of the anterior mitral leaflet in patients with concentric left ventricular hypertrophy. Circulation 57:527, 1978.

62. Maron BJ, Edwards JE, Moller JH, Epstein SE: Prevalence and characteristics of disproportionate ventricular septal thickening in infants with congenital heart disease. Circulation 59:126, 1979.

63. Maron BJ, Edwards JE, Epstein SE: Prevalence and characteristics of disproportionate ventricular septal hypertrophy in patients with systemic hypertension. Chest 73:466, 1978.

64. Maron BJ, Savage DD, Clark CE, Henry WL, Vlodaver Z, Edwards JE, Epstein S: Prevalence and characteristics of disproportionate ventricular septal thickening in patients with coronary artery disease. Circulation 57:250, 1978.

65. Fowles RE, Martin RP, Popp RL: Apparent asymmetric septal hypertrophy due to angled interventricular septum. Am J Cardiol 46:386, 1980.

66. Chew CYC, Ziady GM, Raphael MJ, Nellen M, Oakley CM: Primary restrictive cardiomyopathy. Nontropical endomyocardial fibrosis and hypereosinophilic heart disease. Br Heart J 39:399, 1977.

67. Benotti JR, Grossman W, Cohn PF: Clinical profile of restrictive cardiomyopathy. Circulation 61:1206, 1980.

68. Roberts WC, Waller BF: Cardiac amyloidosis causing cardiac dysfunction: Analysis of 54 necropsy patients. Am J Cardiol 52:137, 1983.

69. Child JS, Krivokapich J, Abbasi AS: Increased right ventricular wall thickness on echocardiography in amyloid infiltrative cardiomyopathy. Am J Cardiol 44:1391, 1979.

70. Siqueira-Filho AG, Cunha CLP, Tajik AJ, Seward JB, Schattenberg TT, Giuliani ER: M-mode and two-dimensional echocardiographic features in cardiac amyloidosis. Circulation 63:188, 1981.

71. Sutton MG, Reichek N, Kastor JA, Giuliani ER: Computerized M-mode echocardiographic analysis of left ventricular dysfunction in cardiac amyloid. Circulation 66:790, 1982.

72. Henry WL, Neinhuis AW, Wiener M, Miller DR, Canale VC, Piomelli S: Echocardiographic abnormalities in patients with transfusion-dependent anemia and secondary myocardial iron deposition. Am J Med 64:547, 1978.

73. Silverman KJ, Hutchins GM, Bulkley BH: Cardiac sarcoid: A clinicopathologic study of 84 unselected patients with systemic sarcoidosis. Circulation 58:1204, 1978.

74. Rizzato G, Pezzano A, Sala G, Merlini R, Ladelli L, Tausini G, Montarani G, Bertoli L: Right heart impairment in sarcoidosis: Haemodynamic and echocardiographic study. Eur J Respir Dis 64:121, 1983.

75. Acquatella H: Two-dimensional echocardiography in endomyocardial disease. Postgrad Med J 59:157, 1983.

76. Puigbo JJ, Combellas I, Acquatella H, Marsiglia I, Tortoledo F, Casal H, Suarez JA: Endomyocardial disease in South America—report on 23 cases in Venezuela. Postgrad Med J 59:162, 1983.

77. Acquatella H, Schiller NB, Puigbo JJ, Gomez-Mancebo JR, Suarez C, Acquatella G: Value of two-dimensional echocardiography in endomyocardial disease with and without eosinophilia. A clinical and pathologic study. Circulation 67:1219, 1983.

11–6 CARDIAC INVOLVEMENT IN SYSTEMIC DISEASES

78. Borer JS, Henry WL, Epstein SE: Echocardiographic observation in patients with systemic infiltrative disease involving the heart. Am J Cardiol 39:184, 1977.

79. Howard RJ, Drobac M, Rider WD, Keane TJ, Finlayson J, Silver MD, Wigle ED, Rakowski H: Carcinoid heart disease: Diagnosis by two-dimensional echocardiography. Circulation 66:1059, 1982.

80. Callahan JA, Wroblewski EM, Reeder GS, Edwards WD, Seward JB, Tajik AJ: Echocardiographic features of carcinoid heart disease. Am J Cardiol 50:762, 1982.

81. Schieken RM, Kerber RE, Ionasescu VV, Zellweger H: Cardiac manifestations of the mucopolysaccharidoses. Circulation 52:700, 1975.

82. Goldberg SJ, Feldman L, Reinecke C, Stern LZ, Sahn DJ, Allen HD: Echocardiographic determination of contraction and relaxation measurements of the left ventricular wall in normal subjects and patients with muscular dystrophy. Circulation 62:1061, 1980.

83. Goldberg SJ, Stern LZ, Feldman L, Allen HD, Sahn DJ, Baldez-Cruz LM: Serial two-dimensional echocardiography in Duchenne muscular dystrophy. Neurology 32:1101, 1982.

84. Hunsaker RH, Fulkerson PK, Barry FJ, Lewis RP, Leier CV, Unverferth DV: Cardiac function in Duchenne's muscular dystrophy. Results of 10-year follow-up study and non-invasive tests. Am J Med 73:235, 1982.

85. Weiss E, Kronzon I, Winder HE, Berger AR: Case report: Echocardiographic observations in patients with Friedreich's ataxia. Am J Med Sci 282:136, 1981.

86. Gaffney FA, Anderson RJ, Nixon JV, Blomqvist CG: Cardiovascular function in patients with progressive systemic sclerosis (scleroderma). Clin Cardiol 5:569, 1982.

87. Gottdiener JS, Katin MJ, Borer JS, Bacharach SL, Green MV: Late cardiac effects of therapeutic mediastinal irradiation: Assessment by echocardiography and radionuclide angiography. N Engl J Med 308:569, 1983.

88. Kupari M: Acute cardiovascular effects of ethanol: A controlled noninvasive study. Br Heart J 49:174, 1983.

89. Legha SS, Benjamin RS, Mackay B, Ewer M, Wallace S, Valdivieso M, Rasmussen SL, Blumenschein GR, Freireich EJ: Reduction of doxorubicin cardiotoxicity by prolonged continuous intravenous infusion. Ann Intern Med 96:133, 1982.

90. Moodie DS, Salcedo EE: Cardiac function in adolescents and young adults with anorexia nervosa. J Adolesc Health Care 4:9, 1983.

11–7 LEFT VENTRICULAR MASSES

91. Ports TA, Cogan J, Schiller NB, Rapaport E: Echocardiography of left ventricular masses. Circulation 58:528, 1978.

92. DeJoseph RL, Shiroff RA, Levenson LW, Martin CE, Zelis RF: Echocardiographic diagnosis of intraventricular clots. Chest 71:417, 1977.

93. Van den Bos AA, Vletter WB, Hagemeijer F: Progressive development of a left ventricular thrombus. Detection and evolution studied with echocardiographic techniques. Chest 74:307, 1978.

94. DeMaria AN, Bommer W, Neumann A, Grehl T, Weinart L, DeNardo S, Amsterdam EA, Mason DT: Left ventricular thrombi identified by cross-sectional echocardiography. Ann Intern Med 90:14, 1979.

95. Meltzer RS, Guthaner D, Rakowski H, Popp RL, Martin RP: Diagnosis of left ventricular thrombi by two-dimensional echocardiography. Br Heart J 42:261, 1979.

96. Stratton JR, Lightly GW, Pearlman AS, Ritchie JL: Detection of left ventricular thrombus by two-dimensional echocardiography: Sensitivity, specificity and causes of uncertainty. Circulation 66:156, 1982.

97. Visser CA, Kan G, David GK, Lie KI, Durrer D: Two-dimensional echocardiography in the diagnosis of left ventricular thrombus. A prospective study of 67 patients with anatomic validation. Chest 83:228, 1983.

98. Levisman JA, MacAlpin RN, Abbasi AS, Ellis N, Eber LM: Echocardiographic diagnosis of a mobile, pedunculated tumor in the left ventricular cavity. Am J Cardiol 36:957, 1975.

99. Meller J, Teichholz LE, Pichard AD, Matta R, Litwak R, Herman MV, Massie KF: Left ventricular myxoma. Echocardiographic diagnosis and review of the literature. Am J Med 63:816, 1977.

100. Morgan DL, Palazola J, Reed W, Bell HH, Kindred LH, Beauchamp GD: Left heart myxomas. Am J Cardiol 40:611, 1977.

101. Chandraratna PAN, Littman BB, Serafini A, Whayne T, Robinson H: Echocardiographic evaluation of extracardiac masses. Br Heart J 40:741, 1978.

102. Koch PC, Kronzon I, Winer HE, Adams P, Trubek M: Displacement of the heart by a giant mediastinal cyst. Am J Cardiol 40:445, 1977.

103. Roberts WC: Anomalous left ventricular band. An unemphasized cause of a precordial murmur. Am J Cardiol 23:735, 1969.

104. Nishimura T, Kondo M, Umadome H, Shimono Y: Echocardiographic features of false tendons in the left ventricle. Am J Cardiol 48:177, 1981.

105. Perry LW, Ruckman RN, Chapiro SR, Kuehl KS, Galioto FM, Scott LD: Left ventricular false tendons in children: Prevalence as detected by 2-dimensional echocardiography and clinical significance. Am J Cardiol 52:1264, 1983.

12 CORONARY ARTERY DISEASE

12–1 CORONARY ARTERY VISUALIZATION

1. Weyman AE, Feigenbaum H, Dillon JC, Johnston KW, Eggleton RC: Noninvasive visualization of left main coronary artery by cross-sectional echocardiography. Circulation 54:169, 1976.

2. Ogawa S, Chen CC, Hubbard FE, Pauletto FJ, Mardelli TJ, Morganroth J, Dreifus LS, Akaishi M, Nakamura Y: A new approach to visualize the left main coronary artery using apical cross-sectional echocardiography. Am J Cardiol 45:301, 1980.

3. Chen CC, Morganroth J, Ogawa S, Mardelli TJ: Detecting left main coronary artery disease by apical cross-sectional echocardiography. Circulation 62:288, 1980.

4. Chandraratna PAN, Aronow WS, Murdock K, Milholland H: Left main coronary arterial patency assessed with cross-sectional echocardiography. Am J Cardiol 46:91, 1980.

5. Morganroth J, Chen CC, David D, Naito M, Mardelli TJ: Echocardiographic detection of coronary artery disease. Detection of effects of ischemia on regional myocardial wall motion and visualization of left main coronary artery disease. Am J Cardiol 46:1178, 1980.

6. Rink LD, Feigenbaum H, Godley RW, Weyman AE, Dillon JC, Phillips JF, Marshall JE: Echocardiographic detection of left main coronary artery obstruction. Circulation 65:719, 1982.

7. Reeder GS, Seward JB, Tajik AJ: The role of two-dimensional echocardiography in coronary artery disease. A critical appraisal. Mayo Clin Proc 57:247, 1982.

8. Fisher EA, Sepehri B, Lendrum B, Luken J, Levitsky S: Two-dimensional echocardiographic visualization of the left coronary artery in anomalous origin of the left coronary artery from the pulmonary artery. Pre- and postoperative studies. Circulation 63:698, 1981.

9. Yoshikawa J, Kataa H, Yamagihara K, Takagi Y, Okumachi F, Yoshida K, Tomita Y, Fukaya T, Baba K: Noninvasive visualization of the dilated main coronary arteries in coronary artery fistulas by cross sectional echocardiography. Circulation 65:600, 1982.

10. Chen W, Woo KS, Kong SM, Mok CK: Coronary artery to left ventricle fistulas: Echocardiographic features. Cardiovasc Interven Radiol 5:241, 1982.

11. Yoshikawa J, Yanagihara K, Owaki T, Kato H, Takagi Y, Okumachi F, Fukaya T, Tomita Y, Baba K: Cross-sectional echocardiographic diagnosis of coronary artery aneurysms in patients with the mucocutaneous lymph node syndrome. Circulation 59:133, 1979.

12. Chung KJ, Brandt L, Fulton DR, Kreidberg MB: Cardiac and coronary arterial involvement in infants and children from New England with mucocutaneous lymph node syndrome (Kawasaki disease). Angiographic-echocardiographic correlations. Am J Cardiol 50:136, 1982.

12–2 LEFT VENTRICULAR FUNCTION IN CORONARY ARTERY DISEASE

13. Kisslo JA, Robertson D, Gilbert BW, von Ramm O, Behar VS: A comparison of real-time, two-dimensional echocardiography and cineangiography in detecting left ventricular asynergy. Circulation 55:134, 1977.

14. Chandraratna PAN, Rashid A, Tolentino A, Hilder FJ, Fester A, Samet P, Littman BB, Sabharwal S, Gindlesperger D: Echocardiographic assessment of left ventricular function in coronary artery disease. Br Heart J 39:139, 1977.

15. Folland ED, Parisi AF, Moynihan PF, Jones DR, Feldman CL, Tow DE: Assessment of left ventricular ejection fraction and volumes by real-time, two-dimensional echocardiography: A comparison of cineangiographic and radionuclide techniques. Circulation 60:760, 1979.

16. Carr KW, Engler RL, Forsythe JR, Johnson AD, Gosink B: Measurement of left ventricular ejection fraction by mechanical cross-sectional echocardiography. Circulation 59:1196, 1979.

17. Stefadouros MA, Grossman W, Shahawy ME, Stefadouros F, Witham AC: Non-invasive study of effect of isometric exercise on left ventricular performance in normal man. Br Heart J 36:988, 1974.

18. Mason SJ, Weiss JL, Weisfeldt ML, Garrison JB, Fortuin NJ: Exercise echocardiography: Detection of wall motion abnormalities during ischemia. Circulation 59:50, 1979.

19. Sugishita Y, Koseki S: Dynamic exercise echocardiography. Circulation 60:743, 1979.

20. Wann LS, Faris JV, Childress RH, Dillon JC, Weyman AE, Feigenbaum H: Exercise cross-sectional echocardiography in ischemic heart disease. Circulation 60:1300, 1979.

21. Crawford MH, White DH, Amon KW: Echocardiographic evaluation of left ventricular size and performance during handgrip and supine and upright bicycle exercise. Circulation 59:1188, 1979.

22. Morganroth J, Chen CC, David D, Sawin HS, Naito M, Parrotto C, Meixell L: Exercise cross-sectional echocardiographic diagnosis of coronary artery disease. Am J Cardiol 47:20, 1981.

23. Zwehl W, Gueret P, Meerbaum S, Holt D, Corday E: Quantitative two-dimensional echocardiography during bicycle exercise in normal subjects. Am J Cardiol 47:866, 1981.

24. Crawford MH, Amon KW, Vance WS: Exercise 2-dimensional echocardiography. Quantitation of left ventricular performance in patients with severe angina pectoris. Am J Cardiol 51:1, 1983.

25. Limacher MC, Quinones MA, Poliner LR, Nelson JG, Winters WL Jr, Waggoner AD: Detection of coronary artery disease with exercise two-dimensional echocardiography. Description of a clinically applicable method and comparison with radionuclide ventriculography. Circulation 67:1211, 1983.

12–3 ACUTE MYOCARDIAL INFARCTION

26. Corya BC, Rasmussen S, Knoebel SB, Feigenbaum H: Echocardiography in acute myocardial infarction. Am J Cardiol 36:1, 1975.

27. Heikkila J, Nieminen M: Echoventriculographic detection, localization, and quantification of left ventricular asynergy in acute myocardial infarction: A correlative echo and electrocardiographic study. Br Heart J 37:46, 1975.

28. Horowitz RS, Morganroth J, Parrotto C, Chen CC, Soffer J, Pauletto FJ: Immediate diagnosis of acute myocardial infarction by two-dimensional echocardiography. Circulation 65:323, 1982.

29. Heger JJ, Weyman AE, Wann LS, Dillon JC, Feigenbaum H: Cross-sectional echocardiography in acute myocardial infarction: Detection and localization of regional left ventricular asynergy. Circulation 60:531, 1979.

30. Heger JJ, Weyman AE, Wann LS, Rogers EW, Dillon JC, Feigenbaum H: Cross-sectional echocardiographic analysis of the extent of left ventricular asynergy in acute myocardial infarction. Circulation 61:113, 1980.

31. Nixon JV, Narahara KA, Smitherman TC: Estimation of myocardial involvement in patients with acute myocardial infarction by two-dimensional echocardiography. Circulation 62:1248, 1980.

32. Visser CA, Inglie K, Kan G, Meltzer R, Durrer D: Detection and quantification of acute, isolated myocardial infarction by two-dimensional echocardiography. Am J Cardiol 47:1020, 1981.

33. Gibson RS, Bishop HL, Stamm RB, Crampton RS, Beller GA, Martin RP: Value of early two-dimensional echocardiography in patients with acute myocardial infarction. Am J Cardiol 49:1110, 1982.

34. Asinger RW, Mikell FL, Elsperger J, Hodges M: Incidence of left ventricular thrombosis after acute transmural myocardial infarction. N Engl J Med 305:297, 1981.

12–4 MYOCARDIAL SCAR

35. Corya BC, Feigenbaum H, Rasmussen S, Black MJ: Anterior left ventricular wall echoes in coronary artery disease. Linear scanning with a single element transducer. Am J Cardiol 34:652, 1974.

36. Feigenbaum H, Corya BC, Dillon JC, Weyman AE, Rasmussen S, Black MJ, Chang S: Role of echocardiography in patients with coronary artery disease. Am J Cardiol 37:775, 1976.

37. Corya BC, Rasmussen S, Feigenbaum H, Knoebel SB, Black MJ: Systolic thickening and thinning of the septum and posterior wall in patients with coronary artery disease, congestive cardiomyopathy and atrial septal defect. Circulation 55:109, 1977.

38. Cody RJ, Salcedo EE, Phillips DF, Tarazi R: M-mode echocardiography in anteroseptal myocardial infarction: Lack of sensitivity. Chest 77:781, 1980.

39. Jacobs JJ, Feigenbaum H, Corya BC, Phillips JF: Detection of left ventricular asynergy by echocardiography. Circulation 48:263, 1973.

12–5 LEFT VENTRICULAR ANEURYSM

40. Dillon JC, Feigenbaum H, Weyman AE, Corya BC, Peskoe S, Chang S: M-mode echocardiography in the evaluation of patients for aneurysmectomy. Circulation 53:657, 1976.

41. Weyman AE, Peskoe SM, Williams ES, Dillon JC, Feigenbaum H: Detection of left ventricular aneurysms by cross-sectional echocardiography. Circulation 54:936, 1976.

42. Barrett MJ, Charuzi Y, Corday E, Sullivan P: Ventricular aneurysm: Cross-sectional echocardiographic approach. Am J Cardiol 46:1133, 1980.

43. Visser CA, Kan G, David GK, Lie KI, Durrer D: Echocardiographic-cineangiographic correlation in detecting left ventricular aneurysm: A prospective study of 422 patients. Am J Cardiol 50:337, 1982.

44. El Togby S, Salcedo EE, Loop FD: Value and limitations of cross-sectional echocardiography in the diagnosis of myocardial aneurysm. Cleve Clin Q 50:231, 1983.

12–6 LEFT VENTRICULAR PSEUDOANEURYSM

45. Katz RJ, Simpson A, Dibianco R, Fletcher RD, Bates HR, Sauerbrunn BJL: Non-invasive diagnosis of left ventricular pseudoaneurysm. Role of two-dimensional echocardiography and radionuclide gated pool imaging. Am J Cardiol 44:372, 1979.

46. Catherwood E, Mintz GS, Kotler MN, Parry WR, Segal BL: Two-dimensional echocardiographic recognition of left ventricular pseudoaneurysm. Circulation 62:294, 1980.

47. Gatewood RP, Nanda NC: Differentiation of left ventricular pseudoaneurysm from true aneurysm with two-dimensional echocardiography. Am J Cardiol 46:869, 1980.

48. Roelandt J, Van Den Brand M, Vletter WB, Nauta J, Hugenholtz PG: Echocardiographic diagnosis of

pseudoaneurysm of the left ventricle. Circulation 52:466, 1975.
49. Morcerf FP, Duarte EP, Salcedo EE, Siegel W: Echocardiographic findings in false aneurysm of the left ventricle. Cleve Clin Q 43:71, 1976.
50. Mills PG, Rose JD, Brodie BR, Delaney DJ, Craige E: Echophonocardiographic diagnosis of left ventricular pseudoaneurysm. Chest 72:365, 1977.

12–7 VENTRICULAR SEPTAL RUPTURE
51. Hutchins GM: Rupture of interventricular septum complicating myocardial infarction: Pathological analysis of ten patients with clinically diagnosed perforations. Am Heart J 97:165, 1979.
52. Chandraratna PAN, Balachandran PK, Shah PM, Hodges M: Echocardiographic observations on ventricular septal rupture complicating acute myocardial infarction. Circulation 51:506, 1975.
53. DeJoseph RL, Seides SF, Lindner A, Damato AN: Echocardiographic findings of ventricular septal rupture in acute myocardial infarction. Am J Cardiol 36:346, 1975.
54. Scanlan JG, Seward JB, Tajik AJ: Visualization of ventricular septal rupture utilizing wide-angle two-dimensional echocardiography. Mayo Clin Proc 54:381, 1979.
55. Bishop HL, Gibson RS, Stamm RB, Beller GA, Martin RP: Role of two-dimensional echocardiography in the evaluation of patients with ventricular septal rupture post myocardial infarction. Am Heart J 102:965, 1981.
56. Drobac M, Gilbert B, Howard R, Baigrie R, Rakowski H: Ventricular septal defect after myocardial infarction: Diagnosis by two-dimensional contrast echocardiography. Circulation 67:335, 1983.

12–8 PAPILLARY MUSCLE DYSFUNCTION
57. Tallury VK, DePasquale NP, Burch GE: The echocardiogram in papillary muscle dysfunction. Am Heart J 83:12, 1972.
58. Ogawa S, Hubbard FE, Mardelli TJ, Dreifus LS: Cross-sectional echocardiographic spectrum of papillary muscle dysfunction. Am Heart J 97:312, 1979.

12–9 MURAL THROMBUS
59. Meltzer RS, Guthaner D, Rakowski H, Popp RL, Martin RP: Diagnosis of left ventricular thrombi by two-dimensional echocardiography. Br Heart J 42:261, 1979.
60. DeMaria AN, Bommer W, Neumann A, Grehl T, Weinart L, DeNardo S, Amsterdam EA, Mason DT: Left ventricular thrombi identified by cross-sectional echocardiography. Ann Intern Med 90:14, 1979.
61. Reeder GS, Tajik AJ, Seward JB: Left ventricular mural thrombus. Two-dimensional echocardiographic diagnosis. Mayo Clin Proc 56:82, 1981.
62. Keating EC, Gross SA, Schlamowitz RA, Glassman J, Mazur JH, Pitt WA, Miller D: Mural thrombi in myocardial infarctions. Prospective evaluation by two-dimensional echocardiography. Am J Med 74:989, 1983.

12–10 RIGHT VENTRICULAR INFARCTION
63. Sharpe DN, Botvinick EH, Shames DM, Schiller NB, Massie BM, Chatterjee K, Parmley WW: The noninvasive diagnosis of right ventricular infarction. Circulation 57:483, 1978.
64. Lorell B, Leinbach RC, Pohost GM, Gold HK, Dinsmore RE, Hutter AM, Pastore JO, Desanctis RW: Right ventricular infarction. Clinical diagnosis and differentiation from cardiac tamponade and pericardial constriction. Am J Cardiol 43:465, 1979.
65. D'Arcy B, Nanda NC: Two-dimensional echocardiographic features of right ventricular infarction. Circulation 65:167, 1982.
66. Lopez-Sendon J, Garcia-Fernandez MA, Coma-Canella I, Yanguela MM, Banuelos F: Segmental right ventricular function after acute myocardial infarction: Two-dimensional echocardiographic study in 63 patients. Am J Cardiol 51:390, 1983.

13 THE LEFT ATRIUM

13–1 LEFT ATRIAL ENLARGEMENT
1. Brown OR, Harrison DC, Popp RL: An improved method for echographic detection of left atrial enlargement. Circulation 50:58, 1974.

13–2 LEFT ATRIAL MYXOMA
2. Nasser WK, Davis RH, Dillon JC, Tavel ME, Helmen CH, Feigenbaum H, Fisch C: Atrial myxoma. I. Clinical and pathologic features in nine cases. Am Heart J 83:694, 1972.
3. Nasser WK, Davis RH, Dillon JC, Tavel ME, Helmen CH, Feigenbaum H, Fisch C: Atrial myxoma. II. Phonocardiographic, echocardiographic, hemodynamic, and angiographic features in nine cases. Am Heart J 83:810, 1972.
4. Bass NM, Sharratt GP: Left atrial myxoma diagnosed by echocardiography with observations on tumour movement. Br Heart J 35:1332, 1973.
5. Abdulla AM, Stefadouros MA, Mucha E, Moore HV, O'Malley GA: Left atrial myxoma: Echocardiographic diagnosis and determination of size. JAMA 238:510, 1977.
6. Lappe DL, Bulkley BH, Weiss JL: Two-dimensional echocardiographic diagnosis of left atrial myxoma. Chest 74:55, 1978.
7. Salcedo EE, Adams KV, Lever HM, Gill CC, Lombardo H: Echocardiographic findings in 25 patients with left atrial myxoma. J Am Coll Cardiol 1:1162, 1983.
8. Giuliani ER, Lemire F, Schattenberg TT: Unusual echocardiographic findings in a patient with left atrial myxoma. Mayo Clin Proc 53:469, 1978.
9. Chadda KD, Pochaczevsky R, Gupta PK, Lichstein E, Schwartz IS: Nonprolapsing atrial myxoma: Clinical echocardiographic and angiographic correlations. Angiology 29:179, 1978.
10. Tway KP, Shah AA, Rahimtoola SH: Multiple bilateral myxomas demonstrated by two-dimensional echocardiography. Am J Med 71:896, 1981.

13–3 LEFT ATRIAL THROMBUS
11. Poehlmann HW, Basta LL, Brown RE: Left atrial thrombus detected by ultrasound: A case report. JCU 3:65, 1975.

12. Graboys TB, Sloss LJ, Ockene IA: Echocardiographic diagnosis of left atrial thrombus—a case report. JCU 5:284, 1977.
13. DePace NL, Soulen RL, Kotler MN, Nintz GS: Two-dimensional echocardiographic detection of intra-atrial masses. Am J Cardiol 48:954, 1981.
14. Shrestha NK, Moreno FL, Narciso FV, Torres L, Calleja HB: Two-dimensional echocardiographic diagnosis of left atrial thrombus in rheumatic heart disease. A clinicopathologic study. Circulation 67:341, 1983.

13–4 CORONARY SINUS

15. Snider AR, Ports TA, Silverman NH: Venous anomalies of the coronary sinus: Detection of M-mode, two-dimensional and contrast echocardiography. Circulation 60:721, 1979.
16. Cohen BE, Winer HE, Kronzon I: Echocardiographic findings in patients with left superior vena cava and dilated coronary sinus. Am J Cardiol 44:158, 1979.

13–5 CONGENITAL ANEURYSM OF THE LEFT ATRIUM

17. Foale RA, Gibson TC, Guyer DE, Gillam L, King ME, Weyman AE: Congenital aneurysms of the left atrium: Recognition by cross-sectional echocardiography. Circulation 66:1065, 1982.

14 RIGHT ATRIUM AND RIGHT VENTRICLE

14–2 RIGHT ATRIAL MASSES

1. Farooki ZQ, Henry JG, Green EW: Echocardiographic diagnosis of right atrial extension of Wilms' tumor. Am J Cardiol 36:363, 1975.
2. Farooki ZQ, Green EW, Arciniegas E: Echocardiographic pattern of right atrial tumour motion. Br Heart J 38:580, 1976.
3. Broadbent JC, Tajik AJ, Wallace RB: Thrombus of inferior vena cava presenting as right atrial tumor: Roentgenographic phonoechocardiographic, angiographic, and surgical findings. J Thorac Cardiovasc Surg 72:422, 1976.
4. Come PC, Kurland GS, Vine HS: Two-dimensional echocardiography in differentiating right atrial and tricuspid valve mass lesions. Am J Cardiol 44:1207, 1979.
5. Riggs T, Paul MH, DeLeon S, Ilbawi M, Pajcic S: Two-dimensional echocardiography in the evaluation of right atrial masses: Five cases in pediatric patients. Am J Cardiol 48:961, 1981.
6. Manno BV, Panidis IP, Kotler MN, Mintz GS, Ross J: Two-dimensional echocardiographic detection of right atrial thrombi. Am J Cardiol 51:615, 1983.
7. Charuzi Y, Kraus R, Swan HJC: Echocardiographic interpretation in the presence of Swan-Ganz intracardiac catheters. Am J Cardiol 40:989, 1977.

14–3 VENOUS CATHETERS

8. Reeves WC, Nanda NC, Barold SS: Echocardiographic evaluation of intracardiac pacing catheters: M-mode and two-dimensional studies. Circulation 58:1049, 1978.
9. Gondi B, Nanda NC: Real-time two-dimensional echocardiographic features of pacemaker perforation. Circulation 64:97, 1981.
10. Meier B, Felner JM: Two dimensional echocardiographic evaluation of intracardiac transvenous pacemaker leads. JCU 10:421, 1982.
11. Nanda NC, Barold SS: Usefulness of echocardiography in cardiac pacing. Pace 5:222, 1982.
12. Iliceto S, Di-Biase M, Antonelli G, Favale S, Rizzon P: Two-dimensional echocardiographic recognition of a pacing catheter perforation of the interventricular septum. Pace 5:934, 1982.

14–4 THE EUSTACHIAN VALVE AND THE CHIARI NETWORK

13. Werner JA, Cheitlin MD, Gross BW, Speck SM, Ivey TD: Echocardiographic appearance of the Chiari network: Differentiation from right heart pathology. Circulation 63:1104, 1981.

14–5 RIGHT VENTRICULAR VOLUME OVERLOAD

14. Weyman AE, Wann S, Feigenbaum H, Dillon JC: Mechanism of abnormal septal motion in patients with right ventricular volume overload. Circulation 54:179, 1976.

14–7 RIGHT VENTRICULAR HYPERTROPHY

15. Prakash R, Matsukubo H: Usefulness of echocardiographic right ventricular measurements in estimating right ventricular hypertrophy and right ventricular systolic pressure. Am J Cardiol 51:1036, 1983.
16. Child JS, Krivokapich J, Abbasi AS: Increased right ventricular wall thickness on echocardiography in amyloid infiltrative cardiomyopathy. Am J Cardiol 44:1391, 1979.

14–8 RIGHT VENTRICULAR TUMORS

17. Asayama J, Kunishige H, Katsume H, Watanabe T, Matsukubo H, Endo N, Matsuura T, Ijichi H, Onouchi Z, Tomizawa M, Goto M, Nakata K: The ultrasound cardiographic findings of myxoma in the right ventricular wall. Cardiovasc Sound Bull 5:129, 1975.
18. Ports TA, Schiller NB, Strunk BL: Echocardiography of right ventricular tumors. Circulation 56:439, 1977.
19. Nanda NC, Barold SS, Gramiak R, Ong LS, Heinle RA: Echocardiographic features of right ventricular outflow tumor prolapsing into the pulmonary artery. Am J Cardiol 40:272, 1977.
20. Chandraratna PAN, San Pedro S, Elkins RC, Grantham N: Echocardiographic, angiocardiographic, and surgical correlations in right ventricular myxoma simulating valvar pulmonic stenosis. Circulation 55:619, 1977.

15 PERICARDIAL DISEASES

15–1 PERICARDIAL EFFUSION

1. Feigenbaum H: Echocardiographic diagnosis of pericardial effusion. Am J Cardiol 26:475, 1970.
2. Horowitz MS, Schultz CS, Stinson EB, Harrison DC, Popp RL: Sensitivity and specificity of echocardiographic diagnosis of pericardial effusion. Circulation 50:239, 1974.
3. Tajik AJ: Echocardiography in pericardial effusion. Am J Med 63:29, 1977.
4. Martin RP, Rakowski H, French J, Popp RL: Localization of pericardial effusion with wide angle phased array echocardiography. Am J Cardiol 42:904, 1978.
5. Krueger SK, Zucker RP, Dzindzio BS, Forker AD: Swinging heart syndrome with predominant anterior pericardial effusion. JCU 4:113, 1976.
6. Levisman JA, Abbasi AS: Abnormal motion of the mitral valve with pericardial effusion: Pseudo-prolapse of the mitral valve. Am Heart J 91:18, 1976.
7. Nanda NC, Gramiak R, Gross CM: Echocardiography of cardiac valves in pericardial effusion. Circulation 54:500, 1976.
8. Haaz WS, Mintz GS, Kotler MN, Parry W, Segal BL: Two-dimensional echocardiographic recognition of the descending thoracic aorta: Value in differentiating pericardial from pleural effusions. Am J Cardiol 46:739, 1980.
9. Ratshin RA, Smith M, Hood WP Jr: Possible false-positive diagnosis of pericardial effusion by echocardiography in presence of large left atrium. Chest 65:112, 1974.
10. Reeves WC, Ciotola T, Babb JD, Buonocore E, Leaman D, Beers E, Papich L: Prolapsed left atrium behind the left ventricular posterior wall: Two-dimensional echocardiographic and angiographic features. Am J Cardiol 47:708, 1981.

15–2 CARDIAC TAMPONADE

11. Settle HP, Adolph RJ, Fowler NO, Engel P, Agruss NS, Levenson NI: Echocardiographic study of cardiac tamponade. Circulation 56:951, 1977.
12. Schiller NB, Botvinick EH: Right ventricular compression as a sign of cardiac tamponade: An analysis of echocardiographic ventricular dimensions and their clinical implications. Circulation 56:774, 1977.
13. D'Cruz IA, Cohen HC, Prabhu R, Glick G: Diagnosis of cardiac tamponade by echocardiography: Changes in mitral valve motion and ventricular dimensions with special reference to paradoxical pulse. Circulation 52:460, 1975.
14. Engel PJ, Hon H, Fowler NO, Plummer S: Echocardiographic study of right ventricular wall motion in cardiac tamponade. Am J Cardiol 50:1018, 1982.
15. Armstrong WF, Schilt BF, Helper DJ, Dillon JC, Feigenbaum H: Diastolic collapse of the right ventricle with cardiac tamponade. An echocardiographic study. Circulation 65:1491, 1982.
16. Vignola PA, Pohost GM, Curfman GD, Myers GS: Correlation of echocardiographic and clinical findings in patients with pericardial effusion. Am J Cardiol 37:701, 1976.

15–3 CONSTRICTIVE PERICARDITIS

17. Pool PE, Seagren SC, Abbasi AS, Charuzi Y, Kraus R: Echocardiographic manifestations of constrictive pericarditis: Abnormal septal motion. Chest 68:684, 1975.
18. Schnittger I, Bowden RE, Abrams J, Popp RL: Echocardiography: Pericardial thickening and constrictive pericarditis. Am J Cardiol 42:388, 1978.
19. Candell-Riera J, Del Castillo G, Permanyer-Miralda G, Soler-Soler J: Echocardiographic features of the interventricular septum in chronic constrictive pericarditis. Circulation 57:1154, 1978.
20. Voelkel AG, Pietro DA, Folland ED, Fisher ML, Parisi AF: Echocardiographic features of constrictive pericarditis. Circulation 58:871, 1978.
21. Wann LS, Weyman AE, Dillon JC, Feigenbaum H: Premature pulmonary valve opening. Circulation 55:128, 1977.
22. Lewis BS: Real-time two-dimensional echocardiography in constrictive pericarditis. Am J Cardiol 49:1789, 1982.

16 CONGENITAL HEART DISEASE

16–1 DEDUCTIVE ECHOCARDIOGRAPHY

1. Henry WL: Evaluation of older children and adults with congenital heart disease by M-mode and cross-sectional echocardiography. Cardiovasc Clin 10:139, 1979.
2. Huhta JC, Smallhorn JF, Macartney FJ: Two-dimensional echocardiographic diagnosis of situs. Br Heart J 48:97, 1982.
3. Foale R, Stefanini L, Rickards A, Somerville J: Left and right ventricular morphology in complex congenital heart disease defined by two-dimensional echocardiography. Am J Cardiol 49:93, 1982.

16–2 CARDIAC MALPOSITIONS

4. Huhta JC, Hagler DJ, Seward JB, Tajik AJ, Julsrud PR, Ritter DG: Two-dimensional echocardiographic assessment of dextrocardia: A segmental approach. Am J Cardiol 50:1351, 1982.
5. Hagler DJ, Tajik AJ, Seward JB, Edwards WD, Mair DD, Ritter DG: Atrioventricular and ventriculoarterial discordance (corrected transposition of the great arteries). Wide-angle two-dimensional echocardiographic assessment of ventricular morphology. Mayo Clin Proc 56:591, 1981.

16–3 ABNORMALITIES OF THE INTERATRIAL SEPTUM

6. Diamond MA, Dillon JC, Haine CL, Chang S, Feigenbaum H: Echocardiographic features of atrial septal defect. Circulation 32:129, 1971.
7. Tajik AJ, Gau GT, Ritter DG, Schattenberg TT: Echocardiographic pattern of right ventricular dia-

hemodynamic correlation in transposition of the great arteries. Circulation 57:291, 1978.

70. Bierman FZ, Williams RG: Prospective diagnosis of d-transposition of the great arteries in neonates by subxiphoid two-dimensional echocardiography. Circulation 60:1496, 1979.

16–19 DOUBLE OUTLET RIGHT VENTRICLE

71. DiSessa TG, Hagan AD, Pope C, Samtoy L, Friedman WF: Two-dimensional echocardiographic characteristics of double outlet right ventricle. Am J Cardiol 44:1146, 1979.

16–20 SINGLE VENTRICLE

72. Felner JM, Brewer DB, Franch RH: Echocardiographic manifestations of single ventricle. Am J Cardiol 38:80, 1976.

73. Seward JB, Tajik AJ, Hagler DJ, Giuliani ER, Gau GT, Ritter DG: Echocardiogram in common (single) ventricle: Angiographic-anatomic correlation. Am J Cardiol 39:217, 1977.

74. Mortera C, Hunter S, Terry G, Tynan M: Echocardiography of primitive ventricle. Br Heart J 39:847, 1977.

75. Rigby ML, Anderson RH, Gibson D, Jones OD, Joseph MC, Shinebourne EA: Two-dimensional echocardiographic categorization of the univentricular heart. Ventricular morphology, type, and mode of atrioventricular connection. Br Heart J 46:603, 1981.

76. Sahn DJ, Harder JR, Freedom RM, Duncan WJ, Rowe RD, Allen HD, Baldes-Cruz, Goldberg SJ: Cross-sectional diagnosis and subclassification of univentricular hearts: Imaging studies of atrioventricular valves, septal structures and rudimentary outflow chambers. Circulation 66:1070, 1982.

INDEX

Page numbers in *italics* refer to figures; page numbers followed by t refer to tables.

A₂, 52

A_2, 52
a wave, *45, 84,* 100
  absent, *59, 290*
    in pulmonary hypertension, 151–152, *153, 154*
  accentuated, with low E point, 201
  decreased, *82*
  in mitral stenosis, 63
  in mitral valve, as reference for fourth heart sound, 57
  in sinus arrhythmia, *58*
  large, *345*
  of apexcardiogram, *52, 57*
  of mitral valve, *52, 61*
  of pulmonic valve, 317
  prominent, *237*
a wave amplitude, *47*
  definition of, 14
  in pulmonary hypertension, 14
  in pulmonic stenosis, 14
  normal, 14
Abdomen, *321*
Abdominal aorta, echocardiographic examination of, 128
Abdominal viscera, position of, *321*
Abnormal septal motion. See *Septal motion, abnormal.*
Abscess, myocardial, 161
  ring, 161, 179
    valve, 163
      M-mode echocardiography for, 163
      two-dimensional echocardiography for, 163
Adenocarcinoma, metastatic, *304*
Adriamycin, left ventricular dysfunction in patients receiving, 208
Alcoholic cardiomyopathy, 208
Allograft, 178
  classification of, 175t
Amplitude of opening, *47*
  definition of, 14
  in pulmonary hypertension, 14
  normal, 14
Amyl nitrate administration, disappearance of diastolic flutter after, *117.* See also under *Amyl nitrate inhalation.*
  SAM after, 206
Amyl nitrate inhalation, absent SAM after, *235*
  in mitral valve prolapse, 67
  mitral valve prolapse before and after, *92*

Amyl nitrate inhalation (*Continued*)
  nonobstructive hypertrophic cardiomyopathy after, *232*
  phonocardiography in hypertrophic cardiomyopathy before and after, *238*
  SAM after, *229*
Amyloidosis, cardiac, 207, *239*
Anatomy, cardiac, 307
Aneurysm, aortic, aortic root dimension in, 14
  arteriosclerotic, 128, *135*
    classification of, 128
    syphilitic, 128
  congenital, of left atrium, 265
  dissecting, of aorta, 107
  fusiform, of ascending aorta, 129
  mycotic, 161
  of pulmonary artery, 159
  septal, atrial. See *Atrial septal aneurysm.*
  septal, ventricular, 311, *330*
  sinus of Valsalva, 128, 129, *138, 139*
  ventricular, *258*
    left, *251–252, 259, 260*
      in inferior wall, *260*
      two-dimensional echocardiography for, 251
    with thrombus, *259*
Aneurysmal dilatation, 294
  of aorta, *140, 142*
  of left atrium, *75*
Angell-Shiley xenograft, *181*
Ankylosing spondylitis, 107, 130, 208
Annular hypoplasia, 314
Annuloplasty, Carpentier ring for, 179
Annulus, mitral. See *Mitral annulus.*
  tricuspid, 317
Anomalous pulmonary venous drainage, 313
  atrial septal defect with, 313
Anomalous pulmonary venous return, 313
  classification of, 313
  echocardiographic abnormalities in, 313
Anomalous venous connection, direct visualization of pulmonary vein to exclude, 313
  partial, 313
  total, 313, *336*
Anorexia nervosa, decreased left ventricular mass in, 208
Anterior leaflet, *36, 37*
  arcing of, *88*
  diastolic flutter of, *158*
  doming of, *70, 72*
  E to F slope of, *72, 79, 81*

375

Anterior leaflet excursion, in mitral stenosis, 71
Anterior leaflet flutter, 97
Anterior leaflet thickening, 90
Anterior mitral annulus calcification, 103
Anterior mitral leaflet, diastolic flutter of, 116, 124
Anterior mitral leaflet vibration, septal and, 118
Anterior motion, diastolic, of posterior leaflet, 84
    pseudosystolic, 230, 231
    systolic, 86, 93, 226–229
Anterior motion, systolic, of mitral valve. See SAM.
Anterior view, of heart, 3
Anterior wall, 213
    two-dimensional echocardiography of, 202
Anterolateral papillary muscle, 69
Anteroposterior diameter, of left ventricle, formula for, 198
Anteroposterior left ventricular dimension, 198
Aorta, 22, 44, 46, 48
    abdominal, echocardiographic examination of, 128
    anatomic considerations of, 127
    and diseases of aorta, 127–142
    and left atrium, sector plane to view, 22
    aneurysm of, aortic root dimension in, 14
        classification of, 128
    aneurysmal dilatation of, 140, 142
    anteroposterior dimension of, 49
    ascending, echocardiographic examination of, 127
        fusiform aneurysm of, 129
        location of, 127
        long-axis parasternal view of, 131
        M-mode echocardiogram of, 131
        short-axis parasternal view of, 132
    coarctation of, 129, 163, 316–317, 344
    descending, 132–134
        echocardiographic examination of, 128
        location of, 127
        short-axis left parasternal view of, 134
        short-axis view of, 134
    dextroposition of, 318
    dilatation of, 129, 135, 255, 350
    diseases of, and aorta, 127–142
    dissecting aneurysm of, 107
    echocardiographic examination of, 12, 39, 127–128
    hypoplasia of, 316, 344
    in long-axis section, 2
    in parasternal long-axis view, 15
    in parasternal short-axis view, 15
    in short-axis left parasternal view, 10
    in short-axis section, 2
    long axis of, 34
    M-mode echocardiographic measurement of, 13
    normal, 39
    postductal coarctation of, 344
    preductal coarctation of, 316, 344
    short axis of, 34
    short-axis view of, 6
    shunt from, to pulmonary artery, 313
Aortic and mitral caged-ball prosthesis, 182

Aortic aneurysm, arteriosclerotic, 128, 135
    syphilitic, 128
Aortic arch, echocardiographic examination of, 127
    location of, 127
    long axis of, 34
    long-axis view of, 11
    right, 318
    short-axis view of, 12
Aortic Björk-Shiley prosthesis, 186, 187
Aortic closure, mid-systolic, 233, 234
Aortic conduit, 196
Aortic disease, aortic insufficiency secondary to, 107
Aortic dissection, 128, 129, 136–138
    DeBakey Type I, 129, 135
    DeBakey Type II, 129, 136
    DeBakey Type III, 129
Aortic gradient, 106
Aortic Hancock valve, mitral and, 192
Aortic insufficiency, 80, 81, 88, 107–109, 112, 115–124, 129, 135, 136, 139, 339, 343
    abnormal septal motion in, 108
    absent diastolic flutter in, 109
    acute, 109, 122
    aortic root dimension in, 14
    aortic valve prolapse in, 108
    aortic valve replacement in, 108
    conditions complicating diagnosis of, 109
    congenital deformities as cause of, 107
    depressed left ventricular function in, 108
    dilated aortic root in, 108
    diastolic flutter around mitral valve in, 109
    diastolic flutter of mitral valve without, 125
    early closure of mitral valve in, 109
    echocardiographic diagnosis of, 107
    echocardiographic examination of, 130
    end-systolic diameter of left ventricle in, 108
    flail aortic leaflet in, 108
    infective endocarditis as cause of, 107
    left ventricular volume overload in, 108
    lack of leaflet coaptation in, 108
    leaflet thickening in, 108
    left ventricular volume overload in, 108
    mitral valve vibration in, 116
    percentage of fractional shortening in, 108
    premature aortic valve opening in, 108
    premature mitral valve closure in, 108
    rheumatic, 107
    secondary effects of, 163
    secondary to aortic disease, 107
    secondary to bacterial endocarditis, 167, 171
    septal vibration in diagnosis of, with mitral stenosis, 81
    severe, 123
        with short diastole, 109
    severity of, 108
    systolic anterior motion of mitral valve in, 109
    valve prolapse as cause of, 107
    valvular, causes of, 107
    with mitral stenosis, 66, 109
    with systolic anterior movement of mitral valve, 126
Aortic leaflet, fibrosis of, 105
    flail, 162

Aortic leaflet (*Continued*)
  flail, in aortic insufficiency, 108
  thickening of, 105, *110, 112, 120*
    irregular, 162
Aortic leaflet motion, restricted, 105
Aortic lumen, 316
Aortic orifice, narrow, 106
Aortic override, *349, 350*
  pseudo, *351*
Aortic position, caged-ball prosthesis in, *183*
  porcine valve in, *187*
Aortic prosthesis, of caged-ball valve, 176
Aortic regurgitation, 129
Aortic ring, 127
Aortic root, 48
  dilated, *112, 120, 135, 140, 141, 349*
    diagnosis of, 128
    echocardiographic examination of, 130
    in aortic insufficiency, 108
    in aortic stenosis, 106
  location of, 127
Aortic root calcification, *113*
Aortic root diameter, *46*, 127, *344*
Aortic root dimension, 46
  at end-diastole, definition of, 14
  in aneurysm of the aorta, 14
  in aortic insufficiency, 14
  normal, 14
  ratio of left atrium to, 14
Aortic root fibrosis, and calcification, with
  aortic stenosis, 106
Aortic root movement, 12
Aortic sclerosis, *113*
  with aortic stenosis, 106
Aortic sinus, 316
Aortic stenosis, *79, 81, 110–112, 114, 115,*
  124, 143, 214, 339
  aortic root fibrosis and calcification with,
    106
  aortic sclerosis with, 106
  bicuspid, 316, *343*
  calcific, echocardiographic findings in, 105
  classification of, *337*
  conditions complicating diagnosis of, 106
  congenital, 105, 106, 314–316, 338, 339
    after valvulotomy, *338*
  decreased cardiac output with, 106
  decreased left ventricular compliance in,
    106
  dilated aortic root in, 106
  echophonocardiography in, 107
  fibrocalcific, senile, *110*
  hypertrophic cardiomyopathy with, *236,*
    237
  leaflet motion restriction in, 106
  leaflet motion to estimate severity of, 106
  left atrial enlargement in, 106
  left ventricular dilatation and dysfunction
    in, 106
  left ventricular hypertrophy in, 106
  membranous, 314
  murmur of, 107
  senile, fibrocalcific, 105
  rheumatic, 105
  severity of, 106
  subvalvular, 314, 316, *337*
    fibromuscular, 314–316
    membranous, discrete, 315–316, *343*

Aortic stenosis (*Continued*)
  supravalvular, 314, 316, *337, 344*
    membranous type, 316
  tunnel, 315, 316
  valvular, 105–107, 314, *337*
Aortic valve, *39, 46,* 127, *327*
  as reference for ejection click, 51
  bicuspid, 114, 115, 119, 129, 314–316,
    339–342
    eccentric closure of, *342*
    echophonocardiogram of, *342*
    formula for eccentricity index with, 315
    pseudo, *342*
  calcification of, 105
  coaptation of pulmonic and, 52
  cusps of, 315
  diastolic flutter of, 108, *120*
  doming of, 314, 315, *338*
  eccentric closure of, 315, *341*
    and transducer position, *342*
  echocardiographic examination of, 12
  endocarditis involving, *171*
  flutter of, 316
  in end-systole, *40*
  in short axis, *22*
  in systole, *40*
  long-axis view of, *41*
  M-mode echocardiographic measurement of,
    13
  mid-closure of, *224*
  mid-systolic closure of, 129, *140*
  mid-systolic notching of, *200, 222*
  mid-systolic semiclosure of, 206
  mitral valve vegetation from, *167*
  motion of, *9, 59*
  narrow, *111*
  noncoronary cusps of, *59*
  normal, *39*
    in short-axis view, *22*
  position of, 1
  presystolic closure of, 201
  semiclosure of, *83*
  short-axis view of, *41*
  systolic mid-closure of, 316
  thickened, *124*
Aortic valve area, 106
Aortic valve closure, *138*
  early, *83*
    in mitral insufficiency, 66
  in relation to second heart sound, 55
Aortic valve disease, 105–126
Aortic valve excursion, decreased, *124*
Aortic valve gradient, *112*
Aortic valve leaflet separation, 13, *46*
Aortic valve opening, in mitral insufficiency,
  83
  premature, *123*
    in aortic insufficiency, 108
Aortic valve orifice, narrowing of, 105, 314
Aortic valve prolapse, as cause of aortic insuf-
  ficiency, 107
  in aortic insufficiency, 108
Aortic valve replacement, *88*
  in aortic insufficiency, 108
Aortic valve vegetation, 162, *170, 171*
  two-dimensional echocardiography for, 162
Aortic wall, *39*
Aortic wall thickness, 129

Aortitis, syphilitic, 107
Aperture motion, 65
Apex, foreshortened, 18
  in long-axis section, 2
  in long-axis view of left ventricle, 9
  short-axis view of, 7
  true, 18, 30
  two-dimensional echocardiography of, 202
  ventricular, 213
Apexcardiogram, a wave of, 52, 57
  in diagnosis of hypertrophic cardiomyopa-
    thy, 206
  in mitral stenosis, 82
  of left atrial myxoma, 277
Apexcardiogram phonocardiogram, 51
Apexphonocardiogram, in hypertrophic cardiomyopathy, 237
Apical area, 1
Apical five-chamber view, 11, 28
  transducer position in, 28
Apical four-chamber view. See Four-chamber
  view, apical.
Apical hypertrophy, 205
  electrocardiogram of, of heart, 225
Apical level, left ventricle at, 26
  short-axis left parasternal view at, 10
  short-axis parasternal view at, 212
Apical long-axis view, 11, 30
  for segmental wall motion, 201
  transducer position in, 30
Apical transducer position, 10, 27
Apical two-chamber view, 11, 29
  for segmental wall motion, 201
  transducer position in, 29
Apical view, 212
  of mitral valve prolapse, 89
Arch, aortic. See Aortic arch.
Arcing, of anterior leaflet, 88
  of mitral valve leaflet, 88
  of tricuspid valve, 150
Area-length method, for calculation of left
  ventricular volume, 199, 210
Arrhythmia, 52
  sinus, 52, 58, 59
    a wave in, 58
    effects of, in normal mitral valve, 58
Arteriosclerotic aortic aneurysm, 128, 135
Artery(ies), bronchial, large, 319
  carotid, common, left, origin of, 128
  coronary. See Coronary artery.
  great. See Great artery(ies).
  innominate, origin of, 128
  pulmonary. See Pulmonary artery.
  subclavian, left, 316
    origin of, 128
Artery anomalies, coronary, congenital, 250
Artery bifurcation, pulmonary, 160, 337
Artery dilatation, pulmonary, 160
  in increased pulmonary blood flow, 152
  in pulmonary hypertension, 152
  pulmonic valve in, 160
Artery disease, coronary, 249–261
  confused with myocardial disease, 204
  left ventricular function, 250–251
Artery fistula, coronary, 250
Artery pressure, pulmonary, diastolic, increased, 151
Artery stenosis, coronary, echocardiography
  of, 249

Artery visualization, coronary, 249–250
  transducer position in, 249
Arthritis, rheumatoid. See Rheumatoid arthritis.
Ascending aorta. See Aorta, ascending.
ASH, 205. See also under Asymmetric septal
  hypertrophy.
Asymmetric septal hypertrophy, 205, 224, 231
  in hypertrophic cardiomyopathy, 206
  septal thickness in, 14
Ataxia, Friedreich's, 207
    congestive cardiomyopathy in, 207
    idiopathic hypertrophic subaortic stenosis
     in, 207
Athletes, enlargement of left ventricular end-
    diastolic dimension in, 203
  increased left ventricular wall thickness in,
    203
  increased stroke volume in, 203
  left ventricular hypertrophy in, 218
Atresia, mitral, 314
  pulmonary, with ventricular septal defect,
    318, 319
  tricuspid, 318, 348, 349
Atrial contraction, 59
Atrial diameter, left, definition of, 14
    normal, 14
    with ventricular septal defects, 311
Atrial emptying index, left, definition of, 64
Atrial endocarditis, 163, 174
Atrial enlargement, left, 233, 266, 313, 336
    in aortic stenosis, 106
    in hypertrophic obstructive cardiomyopa-
     thy, 206
    in mitral insufficiency, 66
    M-mode echocardiography for, 263
    two-dimensional echocardiography for, 263
  right, 281, 284
Atrial fibrillation, 52, 60
  caged-ball prosthesis in, 183
  diastolic flutter with, 109
  normal sinus rhythm after, 60
  wave pattern in, 60
Atrial flutter, 61
Atrial function, left, in atrioventricular sequential pacing, 282
Atrial kick, 59
Atrial level, right-to-left shunt at, 309, 324
  contrast study of, 324
Atrial mass, left, pseudo, 303
  right, 281, 284
    two-dimensional echocardiography for,
    281
Atrial myxoma, calcified, 273
  left. See Left atrial myxoma.
  right. See Right atrial myxoma.
Atrial rhabdomyosarcoma, left, 276
Atrial septal aneurysm, 310, 326, 327
  after injection of contrast material, 327
Atrial septal defect, 308–309, 318, 319, 321,
  322, 348
  classification of, 323
  echocardiographic findings in, 309
  ostium primum, 308, 323
    echocardiographic views of, 326
    echocardiography in, 309
    with cleft mitral valve, 311
  ostium secundum, 68, 308, 323
    echocardiographic views of, 324

Atrial septal defect (Continued)
ostium secundum, echocardiography in, 309
sinus venosus, 323
with anomalous pulmonary venous drainage, 313
with cor triatriatum, 314
with negative contrast effect, 325
Atrial septum, 311
absent, 309, 326
Atrial sound, 51
Atrial systole, 17
caged-ball prosthesis in, 182
mitral valve in, 37
Atrial thrombus, left, 64, 277
in mitral stenosis, 66
M-mode echocardiography for, 264
two-dimensional echocardiography for, 264
Atrial tumor, left, confused with left atrial myxoma, 264
right, 163
Atrial volume overload, left, in mitral insufficiency, 66
right, in tricuspid insufficiency, 144
Atrial wall, left, pulsation of, in mitral insufficiency, 66
Atriopulmonary sulcus, 163
Atrioventricular block, first-degree, 52, 61, 123
and premature mitral closure, 108
Atrioventricular canal, common, tricuspid insufficiency in, 143
incomplete, 309
partial, 309
Atrioventricular canal defect, 332, 333
Atrioventricular canal ventricular septal defect, 311, 335
Atrioventricular groove, hyperactive, 91
in mitral valve prolapse, 67
Atrioventricular sequential pacemaker, DDD, 290
Atrioventricular sequential pacing, 290
left atrial function in, 282
Atrioventricular valve, common, 320
echocardiographic examination of, 307
straddling, 312
ventricular septal defect in, 312
Atrioventricular valve motion, 52
Atrium, common, 309, 326
echocardiographic examination of, 307
left. See Left atrium.
right. See Right atrium.
Autograft, classification of, 175t
Autograft valve, 178

B notch, 200, 221
prominent, 227
in tricuspid valve, 290, 291
Bacterial endocarditis, 120, 121, 173, 192
aortic insufficiency secondary to, 167, 171
organic tricuspid insufficiency in, 143
subacute, 123
Ball variance, in caged-ball valve, 176
Bicuspid aortic stenosis, 316, 343
Bicuspid aortic valve. See Aortic valve, bicuspid.
Bidirectional shunt, 329

Bifurcation, artery, pulmonary, 160
Bigeminy, ventricular, 59
Bileaflet valve, 177–178
classification of, 175t
echocardiographic appearance of, 177–178
Bispherins carotid pulse, 234, 238
in hypertrophic cardiomyopathy, 206
Bisection, of heart, 2
Björk-Shiley prosthesis, 177
aortic, 186, 187
opening click of, 187
Björk-Shiley valve, 180. See also under Björk-Shiley prosthesis.
Blood flow, pulmonary, increased, pulmonary artery dilatation in, 152
Bovine valve, 178
Breast carcinoma, 242, 295
Bronchial arteries, large, 319
"Bullet" method, for calculation of left ventricular volume, 199, 211
Bundle branch block, left, 52, 62
right, 52

Caged-ball prosthesis. See also under Caged-ball valve.
aortic and mitral, 182
in aortic position, 183
in atrial fibrillation, 183
in atrial systole, 182
in mitral position, 182, 183
transducer position to evaluate poppet motion in, 182
Caged-ball valve. See also under Caged-ball prosthesis.
aortic prosthesis of, 176
ball variance in, 176
classification of, 175t
closing click of, 176
echocardiographic appearance of, 176
echophonocardiography for poppet motion in, 176
mitral and tricuspid, echophonocardiography to identify, 186
mitral prosthesis of, 176
opening click of, 176
Starr-Edwards, 180
thrombosis, of, 184
Caged-disc valve, 177
echocardiographic appearance of, 177
motion of strut in, 176
poppet motion in, 176
suture ring of, 176
Calcific aortic stenosis, echocardiographic findings in, 105
Calcification, aortic root fibrosis and, with aortic stenosis, 106
mitral annulus. See Mitral annulus calcification.
of aortic valve, 105
of medial commissure, 64
of papillary muscle, 69
root, aortic, 113
Calcified leaflet, 78
Calcified mitral annulus, in mitral stenosis, 66
Calcified mitral ring, 81
Calcium, absence of, in mitral stenosis, 65
in left ventricular outflow tract, 343

Carcinoid, malignant, as cause of tricuspid stenosis, 143
  pulmonic stenosis with, 152
Carcinoid heart disease, 146, 148, 149, 207
  involving tricuspid valve, 144
Carcinoid syndrome, bacterial endocarditis in, 143
Carcinoma, breast, 242, 295
  lung, 295
Cardiac amyloidosis, 207, 239
Cardiac anatomy, 307
Cardiac apex, echocardiographic view from, 27
Cardiac catheterization, 76, 87, 148
Cardiac contusion. See Contusion, cardiac.
Cardiac cycle, 17
  echocardiographic view of, 18
  frame-by-frame analysis of, 9
  mitral valve motion during, 46
Cardiac enlargement, in congestive cardiomyopathy, 204
Cardiac involvement, in systemic disease, 207–208
  physical and toxic causes of, 208
Cardiac malposition, 308
Cardiac motion, alteration in, 52
Cardiac output, decreased, 219–221
  in aortic stenosis, 106
  in mitral stenosis, 66
Cardiac pacemaker, 281
Cardiac tamponade, 294–295, 304, 305
  pericardial effusion in, 294
  right ventricular compression in, 295
Cardiac valve, 1
  anterior view of, 4
  lateral view of, 4
Cardiomyopathy, 203–207
  alcoholic, 208
  classification of, 203
  congestive, 203, 218–221, 244, 277
    cardiac enlargement in, 204
    decreased stroke volume in, 204
    differential diagnosis in, 204
    global left ventricular dysfunction in, 204
    in Friedreich's ataxia, 207
  hypertrophic, 204, 226, 227, 230, 233, 234, 238
    apexcardiogram in diagnosis of, 206
    apexphonocardiogram in, 237
    bispherins carotid pulse in, 206
    carotid pulse in, 238
    carotid pulse in diagnosis of, 206
    differential diagnosis of, 206
    echocardiographic findings in, 205
    echophonocardiography in diagnosis of, 206
    nonobstructive, 206, 231–233
      after amyl nitrate inhalation, 232
    obstructive. See Cardiomyopathy, obstructive, hypertrophic.
    phonocardiography in, before and after amyl nitrate inhalation, 238
    septal hypertrophy in conditions other than, 204
    with aortic stenosis, 236, 237
  increased diastolic pressure in, 204
    pericardial effusion in, 204
    right ventricular thrombus with, 283
  obstructive, hypertrophic, 222–225, 229, 315
    left atrial enlargement in, 206

Cardiomyopathy (Continued)
  restrictive, 206
    abnormal diastolic function in, 206
    causes of, 206
    echocardiographic findings in, 206
Cardiovascular abnormalities, of Marfan's syndrome, 129
Cardiovascular disease, 235
  hypertensive, 217
Carditis, radiation, 242
  rheumatic, as cause of mitral stenosis, 63
    as cause of ruptured chordae tendineae, 68
Carotid pulse, 52, 56, 114, 342
  bispherins, 234, 238
    in hypertrophic cardiomyopathy, 206
  in diagnosis of hypertrophic cardiomyopathy, 206
  in hypertrophic cardiomyopathy, 238
Carotid pulse tracing, 51
  in patient with complete heart block, 54
Carotid upstroke, delayed, 107, 110
Carpentier ring, echocardiographic appearance of, 179
  for annuloplasty, 179
  in mitral position, 196
Carpentier-Edwards bioprosthesis, 181. See also under Carpentier-Edwards prosthesis and Carpentier-Edwards valve.
Carpentier-Edwards prosthesis. 189. See also under Carpentier-Edwards bioprosthesis and Carpentier-Edwards valve.
  mitral, 188
Carpentier-Edwards valve, 178
Catheter, echocardiographic appearance of, 281
  Swan-Ganz, 281, 288
  venous, 281–282
Catheter displacement, 281
Catheter tip, intracardiac localization of, 281
Catheterization, cardiac. See Cardiac catheterization.
Central venous pressure, elevated, 294
Chemotherapy, extracardiac tumor after, 245
Chest, heart in, 1, 3
  trauma to, cardiac contusion from, 208
Chiari network, eustachian valve and, 282
Chordae, flail, 94
Chordae level, left ventricular minor axis dimension at, 15
Chordae tendineae, 44
  excessive motion of, 93
  fibrosis of, 64, 110
  in left ventricular outflow tract, 230, 231
  ruptured. See Ruptured chordae tendineae.
  severed, 195
  shortening of, 64
  thickening of, 74
Chronic renal failure, 103
Circulation, venous, 323
Circumferential fiber shortening, formula for, 200
Cleft mitral valve. See Mitral valve, cleft.
Closing click, of caged-ball valve, 176
  of Smeloff-Cutter valve, 185
Closure, delayed, of tricuspid valve, 318
  early, of mitral valve, 137
    in aortic insufficiency, 109
  eccentric, of aortic valve, 315, 341

Closure (*Continued*)
  eccentric, of aortic valve, and transducer position, *342*
    of bicuspid aortic valve, *342*
    pseudo, 315
  mid-systolic, in pulmonary hypertension, 151
    of aortic valve, 129, *140*, *233*, *234*
    of pulmonic valve, *153*, *154*
  of tricuspid valve, delayed, *347*, *348*
  premature, of mitral valve, 122, *123*, *171*
  presystolic, of mitral valve, 201
Coaptation, of aortic and pulmonic valves, 52
Coarctation, of aorta, 129, 163, 316–317, 344
  postductal, of aorta, *344*
  preductal, of aorta, 316, *344*
Collagen disease, 207
Combined M-mode and two-dimensional echocardiography, 12–13
Commissure, 315
  medial, calcification of, 64
  raphe confused with, 315
  single, *340*
Commissure fusion, 63, *71*, 105
Commissurotomy, *78*
  E to F slope after, *79*
  for mitral stenosis, 65
  mitral stenosis after, *79*, *80*
  mitral stenosis before, *79*
Common atrioventricular valve, 320
Common atrium, 309, *326*
Common carotid artery, left, origin of, 128
Common pulmonary venous chamber, 313
Complete endocardial cushion defect, 311, *331*, *332*
  and cleft mitral valve, echocardiographic findings in, 311–312
  classification of, 311
  cleft mitral valve in, 311, 312
  direct visualization of, 311, 312
  mitral insufficiency secondary to cleft mitral valve in, 312
  narrowed left ventricular outflow tract with, 311, 312
  Rastelli Type A, 311, *330*
    Type B, 311, *330*
    Type C, 311, *330*
  right ventricular volume overload with, 311, 312
  tricuspid-mitral alignment with, 311, 312
Complete heart block, 52, 54, 55
  carotid pulse tracing in patient with, 54
  pulmonic valve in, *153*
  relationship of mitral valve closure and first heart sound in, 51
Concentric left ventricular hypertrophy, *214*
Conduit, 179
  aortic, *196*
  echocardiographic appearance of, 179
  Lillehie-Kaster, 179
Congenital aneurysm, of left atrium, 265
Congenital aortic stenosis, 105, 106, 314–316, *338*, *339*
  after valvulotomy, *338*
Congenital deformities, as cause of aortic insufficiency, 107
Congenital disease, as cause of tricuspid stenosis, 143
Congenital heart disease, 307–354
  deductive echocardiography in, 307–308

Congenital mitral stenosis, 314
Congenital valvular pulmonic stenosis, 152
Congestive cardiomyopathy. See *Cardiomyopathy, congestive.*
Congestive heart failure, 99, *103*, 221, 239, *276*, 301
Connective tissue disorders, as cause of ruptured chordae tendineae, 68
Conotruncal abnormalities, classification of, 318
Conotruncal ventricular septal defect, 311, 318, *349*
Constrictive pericarditis, 295, *306*
  abnormal septal motion in, 295
  heart size in, 295
  idiopathic, *305*
  premature opening of pulmonic valve in, 295
  slope of diastolic posterior wall motion in, 295
  thickened pericardium in, 295
  two-dimensional echocardiographic findings in, 295
Contraction, ventricular, premature, *115*
Contrast echocardiography. See also under *Contrast study* and *Contrast two-dimensional echocardiography.*
  for left-to-right shunt in patent ductus arteriosus, 314
  for shunt at ventricular level, 311
  for transposition, 308
Contrast material, inferior vena cava before and after injection of, *149*
  regurgitant, in tricuspid insufficiency, 144
Contrast study, of corrected transposition of great vessels, *323*
  of right-to-left shunt, at atrial level, *324*
  of tricuspid insufficiency, *146*, *147*
  of ventricular septal defect, *328*, *329*, *330*
Contrast two-dimensional echocardiography, for left superior vena cava draining into coronary sinus, 265
Contusion, cardiac, from trauma to chest, 208
  right ventricular thrombus after, 283, *292*
Conus, subpulmonary, 320
Cor triatriatum, 314, *337*
  atrial septal defect with, 314
Coronary artery, left, 254
  anomalous origin of, from pulmonary artery, 250
  echocardiography of, 249
  right, *254*, *255*
  echocardiography of, 249
Coronary artery anomalies, congenital, 250
Coronary artery disease, 60, 250–261
  confused with myocardial disease, 204
  left ventricular function in, 250–251
Coronary artery fistula, 250
Coronary artery stenosis, echocardiography of, 249
Coronary artery visualization, 249–250
  transducer position in, 249
Coronary cusp, left. See *Left coronary cusp.*
  right. See *Right coronary cusp.*
Coronary sinus, 264–265, 313
  dilated, 264
  left superior vena cava draining into, *278*, *279*
  movement of, *133*

Coronary sinus (*Continued*)
    two-dimensional echocardiography for left
        superior vena cava draining into, 265
Crista ventricularis, 310
Cross-sectional transducer, multi-element, 12
Cusp, coronary, left, 10
    right. See *Right coronary cusp*.
    noncoronary. See *Noncoronary cusp*.
    of aortic valve, 315
Cusp separation, maximal, *112*

D³ method, for calculation of left ventricular
    volume, 198, *210*
DDD atrioventricular sequential pacemaker,
    290
DE excursion, 65
DeBakey Type I aortic dissection, 129, *135*
    Type II aortic dissection, 129, *136*
    Type III aortic dissection, 129
Delrin stent, *181*
Delta wave, *62*
Dermatomyositis, 208
Descending aorta. See *Aorta, descending*.
Dextrocardia, *150*, 308, *321*
Dextroposition, of aorta, 318
    of great arteries, 319
Dextroversion, 308
Diagnosis, differential, in congestive cardio-
        myopathy, 204
    of mitral stenosis, 65
    echocardiographic, of papillary muscle dys-
        function, 69
    of aortic insufficiency, conditions compli-
        cating, 109
    of aortic root dilatation, 128
    of aortic stenosis, conditions complicating,
        106
    of mitral valve prolapse, conditions obscur-
        ing, 68
Diagnostic accuracy, in mitral valve prolapse,
    67
Diastole, *17*
    early, mitral valve in, *37*
    left ventricle at mitral valve level during, *24*
    left ventricle in, *43*
    mitral valve during, *23*
    posterior motion of right ventricular wall
        during, 295
    short, severe aortic insufficiency with, 109
Diastolic abnormalities, of mitral valve mo-
        tion, *97*
Diastolic anterior motion, of posterior leaflet,
    63, *84*, *314*
Diastolic dip, early, of interventricular sep-
        tum, in mitral stenosis, 74
Diastolic doming, absence of, *84*
    in tricuspid stenosis, 143
    of mitral leaflet, 63
Diastolic filling, ventricular, left, impaired,
    294
Diastolic filling rate, ventricular, 295
Diastolic flutter, *81*, *314*, *335*
    absent, in aortic insufficiency, 109
    after mitral valve replacement, 109
    around mitral valve, in aortic insufficiency,
        109
    disappearance of, after amyl nitrate admin-
        istration, *117*

Diastolic flutter (*Continued*)
    in normal individuals, 109
    of anterior leaflet, *158*
    of anterior mitral leaflet, *116*, *124*
    of anterior mitral valve leaflet, *116*
    of aortic valve, 108, *120*
        in infective endocarditis, 162
    of interventricular septum, 107
        in rheumatic mitral valve disease, 107
    of mitral valve, *81*, 107, *117*, *120*, *126*, 130,
        139, 163
        without aortic insufficiency, *125*
    of posterior mitral leaflet, *80*
    of tricuspid leaflet, *159*
    of tricuspid valve, in pulmonic insuffi-
        ciency, 152
    with atrial fibrillation, 109
    with hand grip, *117*
    with ruptured chordae tendineae, 109
Diastolic function, abnormal, in restrictive
        cardiomyopathy, 206
Diastolic motion, of mitral valve, *61*
Diastolic murmur, 115
Diastolic posterior wall motion, early, *305*
    slope of, in constrictive pericarditis, 295
Diastolic posterior wall velocity, decreased,
    217
Diastolic pressure, increased, in congestive
        cardiomyopathy, 204
    ventricular, left. See *Left ventricular dia-
        stolic pressure*.
Diastolic pulmonary artery pressure, in-
        creased, 151
Diastolic slope, decreased, in tricuspid steno-
        sis, 143
Diastolic vibration, of interventricular septum,
    118, *119*
    of mitral valve, 117
Differential diagnosis. See *Diagnosis, differen-
        tial*.
Dilatation, aneurysmal, 294
    of aorta, *140*, *142*
    of left atrium, *75*
    artery, pulmonary, *160*
        in increased pulmonary blood flow, 152
        in pulmonary hypertension, 152
        pulmonic valve in, *160*
    artrial, left, with ventricular septal defects,
        311
    globular, of left ventricle, *219*
    of aorta, 129, *135*
    of aortic root, *112*, *135*, *138*, *140*, *141*
        diagnosis of, 128
        echocardiographic examination of, 130
    of left atrium, 110, 111, *217*, *266*
    of left ventricle, *136*, *137*, 204, *218*
        and dysfunction, in aortic stenosis, 106
        with ventricular septal defects, 311
    of noncoronary sinus of Valsalva, *141*
    of pulmonary artery, 152
    of right atrium, 281
    of right ventricle, 64, 111, 143, 146, 155,
        157, *258*, *282*, 309, *321*, *322*, *331*, *336*
        in pulmonary hypertension, 154
    of valve ring, as cause of pulmonic insuffi-
        ciency, 152
    poststenotic, 317
        in pulmonic stenosis, 152
    ventricular. See *Dilatation, of left ventricle*
        and *Dilatation, of right ventricle*.

Dilated and pulsatile inferior vena cava, in intricuspid insufficiency, 144
Dilated aortic root, 120
  in aortic insufficiency, 108
  in aortic stenosis, 106
Dilated mitral ring, 130
Disc excursion, in prosthetic valve, 177
Dissecting aneurysm, of aorta, 107
Dissection, aortic, 128, 129, 136–138
    DeBakey Type I, 129, 135
    DeBakey Type II, 129, 136
    DeBakey Type III, 129
  of heart, 2
Domed tricuspid valve, 148
Doming, diastolic, absence of, 84
    in tricuspid stenosis, 143
    of mitral leaflet, 63
  of anterior leaflet, 70, 72
  of aortic valve, 314, 315, 338
  of leaflets, 339
  of mitral valve, 73
  of posterior leaflet, 72
  of pulmonic valve, 317
Double outlet right ventricle, 318, 320
  echocardiographic views of, 354
  ventricular septal defect with, 320
Down's syndrome, 331, 332, 335
Duchenne's muscular dystrophy, 207
Ductus arteriosus, direct visualization of, 313
  patent, 163, 313–314, 316, 319, 336, 337
    contrast echocardiography for left-to-right shunt in, 314
    echocardiographic findings in, 313–314
Dura mater prosthesis, 178
Dynamic ergometry, regional wall motion abnormalities during, 250
Dyskinesia, 259

E point, absent, with decreased mitral valve opening, 107
    low, with accentuated a wave, 201
E to F slope, 46, 47, 59, 61, 82
  absent, in mitral stenosis, 71
  after commissurotomy, 79
  decreased, 80, 84, 314
    in mitral stenosis, 63, 70, 71
    in pulmonary hypertension, 151, 153
  definition of, 13, 14
  in mitral stenosis, 64
  in rheumatic mitral insufficiency, 65
  increased, in mitral insufficiency, 66
  mitral, decreased, with inspiration, 295
  normal, 14
  of anterior leaflet, 72, 79, 81
  of anterior tricuspid valve, 318
  of mitral echocardiogram, 56
  of mitral valve, 52, 57, 83
    in aortic insufficiency, 109
Ebstein's anomaly, 317–318, 346–348
  echocardiographic views of, 346
  interatrial septal defect in, 317
  tricuspid insufficiency in, 143
Eccentric closure, of aortic valve, 315, 341
    and transducer position, 342
  of bicuspid aortic valve, 342
  pseudo, 315
Eccentric left ventricular hypertrophy, 216

Eccentricity index, formula for, with bicuspid aortic valve, 315
Echo dropout, 329, 332
  with membranous ventricular septal defect, 310
Echocardiogram, for evaluation of heart sounds and murmurs, 51
  M-mode, of ascending aorta, 131
  of mitral valve, 53
Echocardiographic, phonocardiographic, and graphic recording, correlation of, 53
Echocardiographic abnormalities, in anomalous pulmonary venous return, 313
  in mitral valve prolapse, 67
  in systemic hypertension, 203
  in tricuspid stenosis, 143
  secondary, with mitral regurgitation, 66
  with ruptured chordae tendineae, 68
Echocardiographic anatomy, 1–7
Echocardiographic appearance, M-mode, of rheumatic mitral insufficiency, 67
  of bioleflet valve, 177–178
  of caged-ball valve, 176
  of caged-disc valve, 177
  of Carpentier ring, 179
  of catheter, 281
  of conduit, 179
  of mitral annulus calcification, 69
  of mitral valve, with alteration in heart rate, 59
  of porcine valve, 178
  of tilting-disc valve, 177
Echocardiographic calculation, of left ventricular volume, 198
Echocardiographic diagnosis, of aortic insufficiency, 107
  of papillary muscle dysfunction, 69
Echocardiographic differentiation, between pleural and pericardial effusion, 294
Echocardiographic examination, and measurements, 9–50
  in Fallot's tetralogy, 318
  of abdominal aorta, 128
  of aorta, 12, 39, 127–128
  of aortic arch, 127
  of aortic insufficiency, 130
  of aortic root dilatation, 130
  of aortic valve, 12
  of ascending aorta, 127
  of atrium, 307
  of cleft mitral valve, 312
  of descending aorta, 128
  of great vessels, 308
  of inferior vena cava, 307
  of left ventricle, 13, 42
  of mitral valve, 12, 35
  of mitral valve prolapse, 130
  of pulmonic valve, 13
  of semilunar valve, 308
  of transposition of great arteries, 319
  of tricuspid valve, 13
  of ventricle, 307
Echocardiographic findings, for prosthetic valve, 175
  in atrial septal defect, 309
  in calcific aortic stenosis, 105
  in complete endocardial cushion defect and cleft mitral valve, 311–312
  in hypertrophic cardiomyopathy, 205

Echocardiographic findings (*Continued*)
  in infective endocarditis, 161
  in Marfan's syndrome, 130
  in mitral stenosis, 63
  in patent ductus arteriosus, 313–314
  in restrictive cardiomyopathy, 206
  with altered electrical activation, echo-
    phonocardiography and, 51–62
Echocardiographic measurement, M-mode.
    See *M-mode echocardiographic measure-
    ment.*
  two-dimensional, 15
Echocardiographic scan, 13
Echocardiographic view(s), from cardiac apex,
    27
  long-axis, of left ventricle, *17, 18*
  M-mode, of left ventricle, *209*
  of cardiac cycle, *18*
  of double outlet right ventricle, *354*
  of Fallot's tetralogy, *349*
  of membranous ventricular septal defect,
    327
  of ostium primum atrial septal defect, *326*
  of transposition of great arteries, *353*
  short-axis, of left ventricle, at mitral valve
    level, *23*
  two-dimensional, of left ventricle, *209*
    of mitral stenosis, *70*
Echocardiographic windows, *4*
  definition of, *1*
Echocardiography, contrast, for left-to-right
    shunt in patent ductus arteriosus, 314
    for shunt at ventricular level, 311
  deductive, in congenital heart disease,
    307–308
  for analysis of segmental wall motion, 201
  for pericardial effusion, 293
  for tricuspid insufficiency, 143
  in ostium primum atrial septal defect, 309
  in ostium secundum atrial septal defect, 309
  in sinus venosus, 309
  M-mode. See *M-mode echocardiography.*
  of coronary artery stenosis, 249
  of right coronary artery, 249
  two-dimensional. See *Two-dimensional
    echocardiography.*
Echophonocardiogram, of bicuspid aortic
    valve, *342*
Echophonocardiography, 51–52
  and echocardiographic findings with altered
    electrical activation, 51–62
  for mitral and tricuspid caged-ball valve,
    186
  for poppet motion in caged valve, 176
  for ruptured chordae tendineae, 69
  in aortic stenosis, 107
  in diagnosis of hypertrophic cardiomyopa-
    thy, 206
  in diagnosis of myxoma, 264
EDD, 14, 199. See also under *End-diastolic
    diameter.*
Effusion, loculated, 294
Effusion, pericardial. See *Pericardial effusion.*
  pleural, *299, 200, 301*
  pleuropericardial, *301, 302*
Ejection, *39, 45*
Ejection click, 315, 317, *342*
  aortic valve as reference for, 51
  pulmonic valve as reference for, 51
  systolic, *115*

Ejection fraction, formula for, 200
Ejection murmur, systolic, *110, 113, 114*
Ejection phase indices, 200
Ejection time, 51
  ventricular, *46, 62*
    left, *13, 52, 53, 58*
    right, *53*
Electrical activation, altered, 52
  echophonocardiography and echocardi-
    ographic findings with, 51–62
Electric alternans, 294–295, *304*
Electrocardiogram, of apical hypertrophy of
    heart, *225*
Electromechanical systole, right, total, *58*
Electromechanical time, total, 52
Elgiloy frame, *181*
Embolism, pulmonary, 157
End-diastole, aortic root dimension, definition
    of, 14
End-diastolic diameter, *47*
  of left ventricle, 121, 198
    definition of, 14
    dilated, *124*
    normal, 14
  of right ventricle, 14
    in right ventricular volume overload, 14
    increased, 282
    normal, 14
End-diastolic dimension, of left ventricle,
    enlargement of, in athletes, 203
  of right ventricle, *47*
End-diastolic posterior wall thickness, *47*
End-diastolic pressure, of left ventricle, in-
    creased, 221
  of right ventricle, increased, 151, *290, 291*
End-diastolic septal thickness, *47*
Endocardial cushion defect, 311–312, *331–334*
  classification of, 311, *330*
  complete. See *Complete endocardial cush-
    ion defect.*
  incomplete, 311
  long-axis parasternal view of, *332*
  partial, 311
Endocardial cushion defect malformation, 309
Endocardial fibroelastosis, 207, 239, 240
  as cause of tricuspid stenosis, 143
  from radiation therapy, 208
Endocarditis, 67, 99
  atrial, 163, 174
  bacterial. See *Bacterial endocarditis.*
  fungal, *193*
  infective. See *Infective endocarditis.*
  involving aortic valve, 171
  Löffler's, 206
  nonvalvular, 163
  pacemaker, 163, *173*
  prosthetic valve, 179
    Klebsiella in, 179
    Pseudomonas in, 179
    Staphylococcus in, 179
    Streptococcus in, 179
    valve dehiscence in, 179
  valve, mitral, ruptured chordae tendineae
    in, 162
Endocardium, posterior wall, mitral annulus
    calcification in front of, *102*
End-systole, aortic valve in, *40*
  mitral valve at, *36*
End-systolic diameter, *47*
  definition of, 14

End-systolic diameter (*Continued*)
  left ventricular, 106
  normal, 14
  of left ventricle, *121, 198*
    dilated, *124*
    in aortic insufficiency, 108
Epicardium, 293, 296
Ergometry, dynamic regional wall motion abnormalities during, 250
ESD, 14. See also under *End-systolic diameter.*
Ethyl alcohol, in cardiomyopathy, 208
Eustachian valve, *290*
  and Chiari network, 282
Exercise, isometric, regional wall motion abnormalities during, 250
Exercise-induced wall motion abnormalities, ischemia with, 250
Extracardiac tumor, 208, *244–246*
  after chemotherapy, *245*

F point, *56, 61*
F wave, 52
Fallot's tetralogy, 311, 317–319, *349–351*
  after repair, *351*
  echocardiographic examination in, 318
  echocardiographic views of, *349*
False lumen, 128
False tendon, *246, 247*
  of left ventricle, 208
Fascia lata graft, 178
Fenestration, of leaflet, 161
Fetal state, septal hypertrophy in, 204
Fiber hypertrophy, myocardial, 205
Fiber shortening, circumferential, formula for, 200
Fibrillation, atrial. See *Atrial fibrillation.*
Fibrocalcific aortic stenosis, senile, *110*
Fibrocalcific senile aortic stenosis, 105
Fibroelastosis, endocardial. See *Endocardial fibroelastosis.*
Fibromuscular subvalvular aortic stenosis, 314–316
Fibromuscular subvalvular stenosis, 316
Fibrosis, of aortic leaflet, 105
  endocardial, from radiation therapy, 208
  myocardial, from radiation therapy, 208
  of chordae tendineae, 64
  of papillary muscle, 69
  pericardial, from radiation therapy, 208
Fibrotic chordae tendineae, *110*
First heart sound, 51, *53–55, 82, 87, 115*
  loud, 51, *267*
  mitral valve closure in relation to, 53
  relationship of mitral valve closure and, in complete heart block, 51
  tricuspid valve closure in relation to, 53
First-degree atrioventricular block, 52, *61, 123*
  and premature mitral closure, 108
Fistula, artery, coronary, 250
Five-chamber view, apical, 11, *28*
  transducer position in, *28*
Flail aortic leaflet, 162
  in aortic insufficiency, 108
Flail chordae, *94*
  visualization of, 68
Flail leaflet, *171*
  with ruptured chorade tendineae, 68

Flutter, diastolic. See *Diastolic flutter.*
  of anterior leaflet, *97*
  of aortic valve, 316
  of left ventricular thrombus, *125*
  of mitral prosthesis, *190*
  of mitral valve, *352*
  of posterior leaflet, *80*
  of pulmonic valve, 317
  of septum, *352, 353*
  septal, in persistent truncus arteriosus, 319
  systolic, *99*
    of mitral valve, *99*
    of prosthetic leaflet, *191*
    of right coronary cusp, *233*
    of tricuspid valve, 282
Foramen ovale, patent, 309–310
Fossa ovalis, 314, *329*
Four-chamber section, mitral valve in, 2
  of heart, 2, *7*
  septum in, 2
  tricuspid valve in, 2
Four-chamber view, apical, 10, *15, 27, 50*
  for segmental wall motion, 201
  left ventricular minor axis dimension in, 15
  normal left ventricular minor axis dimension in, 15
  normal right ventricular minor axis dimension in, 15
  right ventricular minor axis dimension in, 15
  subcostal, 11, *32*
  transducer position in, *32*
Fourth heart sound, 52, 57, *100*
  a wave in mitral valve as reference for, 57
  loud, 57
Fractional shortening, *124, 198*
  percentage of, in aortic insufficiency, 108
Friedreich's ataxia, 207
  congestive cardiomyopathy in, 207
  idiopathic hypertrophic subaortic stenosis in, 207
Fungal endocarditis, *193*
Fusiform aneurysm, of ascending aorta, 129
Fusion, commissure, 63, *71*

Graft, fascia lata, 178
Graphic recording, echocardiographic, phonocardiographic, and, correlations of, *53*
Great artery(ies), dextroposition of, 319
  transposition of, 319–320, *354*
    echocardiographic examination of, 319
    echocardiographic views of, *353*
Great vessels, echocardiographic examination of, 308
  transposition of, 318, 320
    corrected, *322, 323*
    contrast study of, *323*

Hand grip, diastolic flutter with, *117*
Hancock bioprosthesis, *181.* See also under *Hancock prosthesis* and *Hancock valve.*
Hancock prosthesis, *187, 189.* See also under *Hancock bioprosthesis* and *Hancock valve.*
  mitral, *188*

Hancock valve, 178. See also under *Hancock bioprosthesis* and *Hancock prosthesis.*
　mitral, *193*
　　and aortic, *192*
Heart, anterior view of, *3*
　bisection of, *2*
　electrocardiogram of, apical hypertrophy of, *225*
　four-chamber section of, 2, *7*
　in chest, 1, *3*
　lateral view of, *3*
　long-axis section of, 2, *5*
　orthogonal section of, *5*
　pericardial effusion surrounding, *297, 304*
　position of, *1*
　　normal, 308
　short-axis section of, 2, *5*
　short-axis view of, *20*
　　transducer position in, *20*
　swinging of, *298, 299, 304*
　tomographic anatomy of, 1–2
Heart block, complete. See *Complete heart block.*
Heart disease, carcinoid, *146, 148, 149,* 207
　involving tricuspid valve, 144
Heart disease, congenital, 307–354
　deductive echocardiography in, 307–308
　rheumatic, as cause of tricuspid stenosis, 143
　　organic tricuspid insufficiency in, 143
　　tricuspid insufficiency secondary to, *147*
　　with mitral and tricuspid stenosis, *145*
　valvular, vegetation with, 161
Heart failure, congestive. See *Congestive heart failure.*
Heart motion, with pericardial effusion, 293
Heart murmur, *85*
Heart rate, alteration in, *59*
　echocardiographic appearance of mitral valve with alteration in, *59*
Heart size, in constrictive pericarditis, 295
Heart sound, and murmurs, echocardiogram for evaluation of, 51
　first. See *First heart sound.*
　fourth. See *Fourth heart sound.*
　second. See *Second heart sound.*
　third. See *Third heart sound.*
Heart syndrome, hypoplastic, 314
Hemochromatosis, 207
Hemorrhagic pericardial effusion, *306*
Hepatic vein, *31, 306*
　dilated, 295
　with subcostal transducer position, 11
Heterograft, 178
　classification of, 175t
　thrombus with, 178
High-frequency murmur, holosystolic, *100*
Hodgkin's lymphoma, *242*
Holosystolic high-frequency murmur, *100*
Holosytolic mitral valve prolapse, *86, 92*
Holosystolic murmur, *89*
Holosystolic prolapse, 68
Homograft, 178
　classification of, 175t
Hourglass deformity, 316
Hunter's syndrome, *341*
Hyperactive atrioventricular groove, *91*
　in mitral valve prolapse, 67
Hypercalcemia, infantile, 316

Hyperkinetic left ventricular contractility, 311
　with ventricular septal defect, 311
Hypernephroma, 281, *284*
Hypertension, chronic, *216*
　pulmonary. See *Pulmonary hypertension.*
　systemic, *215*
　　echocardiographic abnormalities in, 203
　　ventricular size and function in, 203
Hypertensive cardiovascular disease, *217*
Hypertrophic cardiomyopathy. See *Cardiomyopathy, hypertrophic.*
Hypertrophic obstructive cardiomyopathy, 222–225, 229, 315
　left atrial enlargement in, 206
Hypertrophic subaortic stenosis, idiopathic. See *Idiopathic hypertrophic subaortic stenosis.*
Hypertrophy, apical, 205
　of heart, electrocardiogram of, *225*
　fiber, myocardial, 205
　in unusual locations, 205, *226*
　ᵐyocardial, 202
　septal, *291, 317, 346*
　　asymmetric, 205, 222, 224, 231
　　　in hypertrophic cardiomyopathy, 206
　　　thickness in, 14
　　disproportionate, 205
　　in conditions other than hypertrophic cardiomyopathy, 204
　　in fetal state, 204
　　in left ventricular hypertrophy, 204, *235*
　　in neonates and infants, 204
　　in right ventricular hypertrophy, 204, *235*
　ventricular, left. See *Left ventricular hypertrophy.*
　ventricular, right. See *Right ventricular hypertrophy.*
　wall, posterior, *234*
　　septal, *234*
Hyperventilation, *125*
Hypoplasia, annular, 314
　of aorta, 316, *344*
　of left ventricular outflow tract, 316
Hypoplastic heart syndrome, 314
Hypotension, 294

Idiopathic causes, of ruptured chordae tendineae, 68
Idiopathic constrictive pericarditis, *305*
Idiopathic hypertrophic subaortic stenosis, 68, 69
　in Friedreich's ataxia, 207
　septal thickness in, 14
Idiopathic left ventricular hypertrophy, 204
Impaired left ventricular function, *124*
Incomplete atrioventricular canal, 308
Incomplete endocardial cushion defect, 311
Infantile hypercalcemia, 316
Infants, neonates and, septal hypertrophy in, 204
Infarction, 143
　myocardial, *261*
　　acute, 251
　　　M-mode echocardiography in, 251
　　　two-dimensional echocardiography in, 251
　　anteroapical, *243, 257*
　　lateral wall, *101*

Infarction (Continued)
  ventricular, right, echocardiograpic findings
    in, 253
Infection, of tricuspid valve, in intravenous
    drug user, 163
Infective endocarditis, 161–174, 164, 165, 167,
    172, 173
  as cause of aortic insufficiency, 107
  as cause of pulmonic insufficiency, 152
  as cause of ruptured chordae tendineae, 68
  diastolic flutter of aortic valve in, 162
  echocardiographic finding in, 161
  general considerations in, 161
  myxomatous valvular degeneration with,
    162
  valvular necrosis in, 162
  vegetation in, 161
Inferior vena cappa, with subcostal transducer
    position, 11
Inferior vena cava, 31
  before and after injection of contrast mate-
    rial, 149
  before and after injection of normal saline
    solution, 146
  dilated, 146, 295, 306
    and pulsatile, in tricuspid insufficiency,
      144
  echocardiographic examination of, 307
  in tricuspid insufficiency, 147
Inferior wall, 214
  left ventricular aneurysm in, 260
  two-dimensional echocardiography of, 202
Inflow obstruction, ventricular, left, 314
Inflow tract, ventricular, left, 2
    long-axis view of, 10, 19
    right, 148
Infundibular pulmonic stenosis, 152, 291, 345,
    349
Infundibular stenosis, 318
Infundibular subvalvular pulmonic stenosis,
    317
Infundibulectomy, 351
Inlet ventricular septal defect, 311
Innominate artery, origin of, 128
Innominate vein, left, 313
Inspiration, decreased left ventricular size
    during, 295
  decreased mitral E to F slope with, 295
Insufficiency, mitral, secondary findings of, 69
Interatrial septal defect, 318
  in Ebstein's anomaly, 317
Interatrial septal motion, abnormal, in mitral
    insufficiency, 66
Interatrial septum, 324, 325–327, 329
  abnormalities of, 308–310
  absent, 326
  bulging of, 295
Internal diameter, percentage of shortening of,
    formula for, 14
Interventricular septum, 213, 311, 316, 317,
    328, 331
  abnormalties of, 310–311
  absent, 320, 354
  angled, 235, 236
  bulging of, 295
  diastolic flutter of, 107
    in rheumatic mitral valve disease, 107
  diastolic vibration in, 118, 119
  early diastolic dip of, in mitral stenosis, 74

Interventricular septum (Continued)
  flattening of, 64
  movement of, 42
  thickening of, 240
  two-dimensional echocardiography of, 202
Intima, tear of, 128
Intimal flap, 129, 135–138
Intracardiac shunt, as cause of pulmonary hy-
    pertension, 152
Intravenous drug user, infection of tricuspid
    valve in, 163
Ionescu-Shiley prosthesis, 178
Ischemia, with exercise-induced wall motion
    abnormalities, 250
Isolated mitral cleft, 311
Isolated tricuspid cleft, 311
Isometric exercise, regional wall motion ab-
    normalities during, 250
IVC. See Inferior vena cava.
IVS, 199

Klebsiella, in prosthetic valve endocarditis,
    179

Laplace's law, 202
Late systolic mitral valve prolapse, 92, 93
Late systolic murmur, 86, 87
Lateral view, of heart, 3
Lateral wall, 214
  two-dimensional echocardiography of, 202
Lateral wall myocardial infarction, 101
Leaflet, anterior. See Anterior leaflet.
  aortic, flail, 162
    thickening of, 110, 112
  calcified, 78
  fenestration of, 161
  flail, 171
    with ruptured chordae tendineae, 68
Leaflet, mitral. See Mitral leaflet.
Leaflet, mitral valve. See Mitral leaflet.
  perforation of, 161
  posterior. See Posterior leaflet.
  prosthetic, systolic flutter of, 191
  redundant, 93, 340
    in mitral valve prolapse, 67
  thickened, in tricuspid insufficiency, 144
  tricuspid, diastolic flutter of, 159
Leaflet abnormalities, in complete endocardial
    cushion defect, 311
Leaflet aperture, 84
Leaflet coaptation, absent, 122, 130, 141
  in aortic insufficiency, 108
Leaflet degeneration, 190
Leaflet excursion, 119, 338, 342
  anterior, in mitral stenosis, 71
  restricted, 143
Leaflet motion, 112
  aortic, restricted, 105
  exaggerated, with ruptured chordae tendi-
    neae, 68
  mitral, posterior, 79
  posterior, 84
    abnormal, in mitral stenosis, 70
    normal, 80
      in mitral stenosis, 65

Leaflet motion (Continued)
  restricted, 111
    in aortic stenosis, 106
    to estimate severity of aortic stenosis, 106
Leaflet separation, aortic valve, 13, 46
  decreased, 314, 338
  restricted, 112
  with cleft mitral valve, 312
Leaflet thickening, 70, 73, 80, 84, 111, 117, 143, 145
  anterior, 90
  aortic, 120
    irregular, 162
  in aortic insufficiency, 108
  mitral, 168
  in mitral valve prolapse, 67
    M-mode echocardiography for, 63
    two-dimensional echocardiography for, 63
  posterior, 87, 91, 94
Leaflet vibration, mitral, septal and anterior, 118
Left atrial diameter, definition of, 14
  normal, 14
Left atrial dilatation, with ventricular septal defects, 311
Left atrial enlargement. See Atrial enlargement, left.
Left atrial emptying index, definition of, 64
Left atrial function, in atrioventricular sequential pacing, 282
Left atrial mass, pseudo, 303
Left atrial myxoma, 263–264, 266–277
  apexcardiogram of, 277
  cleft mitral valve confused with, 264
  conditions complicating diagnosis of, 264
  in mitral stenosis, 66
  left atrial tumor confused with, 264
  mitral stenosis confused with, 264
  mitral valve prolapse confused with, 264
  mitral valve vegetation confused with, 166, 264
  M-mode echocardiography for, 263
  nonprolapsing, 274, 275
  pathologic specimen of, 268
  transducer position in M-mode echocardiography of, 275
  two-dimensional echocardiogrpahy for, 263
Left atrial rhabdomyosarcoma, 276
Left atrial thrombus. See Atrial thrombus, left.
Left atrial volume overload, in mitral insufficiency, 66
Left atrial wall, pulsation of, in mitral insufficiency, 66
Left atrium, 22, 48
  aneurysmal dilatation of, 75
  anteroposterior dimension of, 49
  aorta and, sector plane to view, 22
  compression of, 135
  congenital aneurysm of, 265
  dilatation of, 83, 110, 111, 217, 266
  enlarged, 277
  in long-axis section, 2
  in parasternal long-axis view, 15
  in short-axis left parasternal view, 10
  in short-axis parasternal view, 15
Left atrium, large, 222, 223
  major axis of, 15, 50
  minor axis of, 15, 50
  mitral valve prolapse into, 96

Left atrium (Continued)
  mitral valve vegetation prolapsing into, 166
  M-mode echocardiographic measurement of, 14
  normal, 46
  positive of, 1
  prolapse of, 294
  ratio of, to aortic root dimension, 14
  ruptured chordae tendineae in, 95
  short-axis view of, 6
  systolic bowing of mitral valve toward, 67
  vegetation prolapsing into, 162, 168, 169
Left bundle branch block, 52, 62
Left common carotid artery, origin of, 128
Left coronary artery, 254
  anomalous origin of from pulmonary artery, 250
  echocardiography of, 249
Left coronary cusp, 10
Left innominate vein, 313
Left main trunk, 254
Left main trunk lesion, false-positive, 256
  nonvisualization of, 256
Left main trunk stenosis, 255, 256
Left parasternal transducer position, 9, 16, 17
Left parasternal view, long-axis. See Long-axis view, parasternal, left.
Left parasternal view, short-axis. See Short-axis view, parasternal, left.
Left subclavian artery, 316
  origin of, 128
Left superior vena cava, draining into coronary sinus, 278, 279
  two-dimensional echocardiography for, 265
Left ventricle, 47, 197–247, 321
  anteroposterior diameter of, formula for, 198
  apex in long-axis view of, 9
  at apical level, 26
  at mitral valve level, 23
    during diastole, 24
    during systole, 24
    short-axis echocardiographic view of, 23
  at papillary muscle level, 25
  compressed, 155, 157
Left ventricle, dilatation of, 83, 84, 111, 258, 336
  distortion of, 156
  in pulmonary hypertension, 151, 155
Left ventricle, echocardiographic examination of, 13, 42
  end-systolic diameter of, in aortic insufficiency, 108
  false tendons of, 208
  globular dilatation of, 219
  in diastole, 43
  in short-axis section, 2
  in systole, 43
  inflow tract of, 2
  large, 348
  long axis of, 50
  long-axis dimension of, 198, 209
  long-axis echocardiographic view of, 17, 18
  long-axis view of, 9, 16, 17
  M-mode echocardiograhic measurement of, 14
  M-mode echocardiographic view of, 209
  M-mode long-axis view of, 44
  M-mode short-axis view, 44

Leaf ventricle (*Continued*)
  movement of posterior wall of, 42
  normal, 42
  outflow tract of, 2
  posterior wall of, 43
  prolapse of myxoma into, 272
  pseudoaneurysm of, 260, 294
  right atrial myxoma prolapsing into, 287
  short axis of, 50
  short-axis left parasternal view of, 10
  small, 64
  two-dimensional echocardiographic view of, 209
Left ventricular aneurysm. See *Aneurysm, ventricular, left.*
Left ventricular cavity, 44
  small, 223
Left ventricular compliance, decreased, 65, 203, 206, 234
  in aortic stenosis, 106
Left ventricular contractility, hyperkinetic, with ventricular septal defect, 311
Left ventricular diastolic filling, impaired, 294
Left ventricular diastolic pressure, 200
  increased, 200
Left ventricular dilatation. See *Dilatation, of left ventricle.*
Left ventricular dimension, 48
  anteroposterior, 198
Left ventricular dysfunction, 220
  global, in congestive cardiomyopathy, 204
  in patients receiving Adriamycin, 208
  segmental, 69
Left ventricular ejection time, 13, 52, 53, 58
Left ventricular end-diastolic diameter, 121, 198
  definition of, 14
  dilated, 124
  normal, 14
Left ventricular end-diastolic dimension, enlargement of, in atheltes, 203
Left ventricular end-systolic diameter, 106, 121, 198
  dilated, 124
Left ventricular failure, 290
Left ventricular function, 197–202
  depressed, in aortic insufficiency, 108
  impaired, 124
  in coronary artery disease, 250–251
Left ventricular hypertrophy, 202–203, 215, 216, 217, 233, 316
  concentric, 203, 214
  eccentric, 203, 216
  idiopathic, 204
  in aortic stenosis, 106
  in athletes, 218
  in congestive cardiomyopathy, 204
  M-mode echocardiography for, 202
  physiologic, 202
  posterior wall thickness in, 14
  septal hypertrophy in, 204, 235
  two-dimensional echocardiography for, 202
Left ventricular inflow obstruction, 314
Left ventricular major axis dimension, normal, 15
Left ventricular mass, 199, 208
  calculation of, 211
  decreased, in anorexia nervosa, 208
  formulas for, with M-mode echocardiography, 199

Left ventricular mass (*Continued*)
  increased, 202
Left ventricular measurement, M-mode echocardiography with T-scan for, 197
  transducer position for, 197, 198
Left ventricular minor axis dimension, at chordae level, 15
  at papillary muscle level, 15
  in apical four-chamber view, 15
  normal, in parasternal long-axis view, 15
Left ventricular outflow tract, 2, 228, 238, 315, 320, 331, 332, 339
  calcium in, 343
  chordae tendineae in, 230, 231
  hypoplasia of, 316
  mass of echoes in, 162
  mural plaque in, 205
  narrowed, with complete endocardial cushion defect, 311, 312
  obstruction of, 314
  small, 206
Left ventricular posterior wall velocity, 84
Left ventricular pressure, end-diastolic, increased, 221
  formula for, 106
Left ventricular pseudoaneurysm. See *Pseudoaneurysm, of left ventricle.*
Left ventricular size, 197–202
  and function, in athletes, 203
    in M-mode and two-dimensional echocardiography, 197
    in systemic hypertension, 203
  decreased, during inspiration, 295
  small, 203
Left ventricular stroke volume, 83
Left ventricular systolic pressure, 201
Left ventricular thrombus, 208, 243, 244
  diastolic flutter with, 109
  flutter of, 125
Left ventricular tumor, 208
Left ventricular volume, area-length method for calculation of, 199, 210
  "bullet" method for calculation of, 199, 211
  D^3 method for calculation of, 198, 210
  derived, 198
  echocardiographic calculation of, 198
  length-diameter method for calculation of, 199, 210
  length-short-axis area method for calculation of, 199, 210
  Simpson's rule method for calculation of, 199, 211
Left ventricular volume overload, 78, 83, 84, 121, 129, 163, 313, 336
  in aortic insufficiency, 108
  in mitral insufficiency, 66
Left ventricular wall thickness, 25, 106
  increased, 202
  in athletes, 203
Left-to-right shunt, 313
  in patent ductus arteriosus, contrast echocardiography for, 314
Leiomyosarcoma, 281, 285, 286
  pathologic specimen of, 286
Length-diameter method, for calculation of left ventricular volume, 199, 210
Length-short-axis area method, for calculation of left ventricular volume, 199, 210
Lesion, trunk, main, left, false-positive, 256
  nonvisualization of, 256

Leukemia, 295
Levoversion, 308
Libman-Sacks disease, 207
Ligamentum arteriosum, 316
Lillehie-Kaster conduit, 179
Lillehie-Kaster prosthesis, 177
Löffler's endocarditis, 206
Long axis, of aorta, 34
  of aortic arch, 34
  of left ventricle, 50
  of right ventricle, 50
Long-axis dimension, of left ventricle, 198,
  209
Long-axis echocardiographic view, of left ventricle, 17, 18
Long-axis left parasternal view. See Long-axis
  view, parasternal, left.
Long-axis parasternal view. See Long-axis
  view, parasternal.
Long-axis section, aorta in, 2
  apex in, 2
  left atrium in, 2
  of heart, 2, 5
  posterior wall in, 2
  septum in, 2
Long-axis view, apical, 11, 30
  for segmental wall motion, 201
  transducer position in, 30
  M-mode, of left ventricle, 44
  of aortic arch, 11
  of aortic valve, 41
  of left ventricle, 16, 17
  apex in, 9
  of mitral valve, 38
  of right ventricular inflow tract, 10, 19
  parasternal, 15, 48
    aorta in, 15
    for segmental wall motion, 201
    in mitral stenosis, 72
    left, 9–10, 35
    left atrium in, 15
    left ventricular minor axis dimension in,
      15
    normal left ventricular minor axis dimen-
      sion in, 15
    normal right ventricular minor axis di-
      mension in, 15
    of ascending aorta, 131
    of endocardial cushion defect, 332
    right ventricular minor axis dimension in,
      15
    with lateral angulation, 212
    with medial angulation, 212
Long-term nonrheumatic mitral insufficiency,
  83
Low-profile prosthesis, in mitral stenosis, 65
Lumen, aortic, 316
  false, 128
  true, 128
Lumen size, decrease in, 255
  focal, 249
Lung, carcinoma of, 295
Lupus erythematosus, 207, 240
LVEDS, 106
LVET, 52. See also under Left ventricular ejec-
  tion time.
LVM, 199
LVV. See Left ventricular volume.
LVVen, 199

LVVep, 199
LVWTs, definition of, 106
Lymph node syndrome, mucocutaneous, 250
Lymphoma, 295
  Hodgkin's, 242
Lymphoma-induced pericardial effusion, 305
Lymphosarcoma, 244, 245

Main trunk, left, 254
Main trunk lesion, left, false-positive, 256
  nonvisualization of, 256
Main trunk stenosis, left, 255, 256
Major axis, of left atrium 15, 50
  of right atrium 15, 50
  normal measurement of, 15
Malignant carcinoid, as cause of tricuspid ste-
  nosis, 143
  pulmonic stenosis with, 152
Marfan's syndrome, 87, 107, 122, 128–130,
  139–142, 196, 255
  cardiovascular abnormalities of, 129
  echocardiographic findings of, 130
  lack of leaflet coaptation in, 108
Mass, ventricular, left. See Left ventricular
  mass.
Mechanical valve, classification of, 175t
Medial commissure, calcification of, 64
Melanoma, 295
Membranous aortic stenosis, 314
Membranous subvalvular aortic stenosis, dis-
  crete, 315–316, 343
Membranous ventricular septal defect, 310
  echo dropout with, 310
  echocardiographic views of, 327
Mesocardia, 308
Metastasis, pericardial, echocardiographic ap-
  pearance of, 295
Metastatic adenocarcinoma, 304
Mid-closure, of aortic valve, 224
  systolic, of aortic valve, 316
Mid-diastole, mitral valve in, 37
Mid-diastolic semiclosure, 63
Mid-late systolic click, 87
Mid-systolic aortic closure, 233, 234
Mid-systolic click, 85, 86
Mid-systolic closure, in pulmonary hyperten-
  sion, 151
  of aortic valve, 129, 140
  of pulmonic valve, 153, 154
Mid-systolic notching, of aortic valve, 206,
  222
Mid-systolic retraction, 237
Mid-systolic semiclosure, of aortic valve, 206
Minor axis, of left atrium, 15, 50
  of right atrium, 15, 50
  normal measurement of, 15
Minor axis dimension, ventricular, left, at
  chordae level, 15
Mitral and aortic Hancock valve, 192
Mitral and tricuspid caged-ball valve, echophonocardiography to identify, 186
Mitral and tricuspid stenosis, rheumatic heart
  disease with, 145
Mitral annulus, 77
  calcified, in mitral stenosis, 66
  description of, 69
  large, in mitral valve prolapse, 67

Mitral annulus calcification, 67, 69, *101–103*,
  130, *168*, *196*
  anterior, *103*
  behind posterior mitral leaflet, *102*
  echocardiographic appearance of, 69
  in front of posterior wall endocardium, *102*
  posterior, *103*
Mitral atresia, 314
Mitral caged-ball prosthesis, aortic and, *182*
Mitral Carpentier-Edwards prosthesis, *188*
Mitral cleft, isolated, 311
Mitral E to F slope, decreased, with inspira-
  ton, *295*
Mitral Hancock prosthesis, *188*
Mitral Hancock valve, *193*
Mitral insertion, in septum, *321*
Mitral insufficiency, 66, *83*, *88*, *99*, 130
  abnormal interatrial septal motion in, 66
  and papillary muscle dysfunction, 69
  aortic valve opening in, *83*
  causes of, 66
  early aortic valve closure in, 00
  increased E to F slope in, 66
  left atrial enlargement in, 66
  left atrial volume overload in, 66
  left ventricular volume overload in, 66
  mitral regurgitation in, 66
  nonrheumatic, long-term, *83*
  pulsation of left atrial wall in, 66
  rheumatic, 65, 67, 68, *84*, *85*
    M-mode echocardiographic appearance of,
      67
  secondary findings of, 69
  secondary to cleft mitral valve, in complete
    endocardial cushion defect, 312
  severe, *96*
Mitral leaflet, 316
  anterior, diastolic flutter of, *116*, *124*
  arcing of, *88*
  diastolic doming of, 63
  failure of, to reach peak systolic position, 69
  inferior, abnormal motion of, *333*
  posterior, diastolic flutter of, *80*
    mitral annulus calcification behind, *102*
  thickened, 63
Mitral leaflet motion, posterior, *79*
Mitral leaflet thickening, 63, *168*
  M-mode echocardiography for, 63
  two-dimensional echocardiography for, 63
Mitral leaflet vibration, septal and anterior,
  118
Mitral level, short-axis view at, *50*
Mitral position, caged-ball prosthesis in, *182*,
  183
  Carpentier ring in, *196*
  porcine valve in, *188–190*
Mitral regurgitation, *78*, *84*, *87*, *89*, *98*, *99*,
  167, *190*, *276*, *335*
  absent, in mitral stenosis, 65
  acute, *94*
  in mitral insufficiency, 66
  secondary echocardiographic abnormalities
    with, 66
Mitral ring, *88*
  calcified, *81*
  dilated, 130
Mitral ring size, 314
Mitral septal coaptation, *158*

Mitral Smeloff-Cutter prosthesis, *184*
  thrombosed, *184*, *185*
Mitral Starr-Edwards valve, normal, *185*
Mitral stenosis, 63–66, *70*, *72–79*, *81*, 143,
  145, 266
  a wave in, 63
  abnormal posterior leaflet motion in, *70*
  abnormal septal motion in, 64
  absence of calcium in, 65
  absent E to F slope in, *71*
  absent mitral regurgitation in, 65
  after commissurotomy, *79*, *80*
  anterior leaflet excursion in, *71*
  aortic insufficiency with, 66, 109
  apexcardiogram in, *82*
  before commissurotomy, *79*
  calcified mitral annulus in, 66
  commissurotomy for, 65
  confused with left atrial myxoma, 264
  congenital, 314
  decreased E to F slope in, 63, *70*, *71*
  differential diagnosis of, 65
  E to F slope in, 64
  early diastolic dip of interventricular sep-
    tum in, *74*
  echocardiographic findings in, 63
  graphics of, *82*
  left atrial myxoma in, 66
  left atrial thrombus in, 66
  long-axis parasternal view in, *72*
  low cardiac output in, 66
  low-profile prosthesis in, *83*
  mild, *76*
  normal posterior leaflet motion in, 65
  pseudo, *81*
  rheumatic carditis as cause of, 63
  septal vibration in diagnosis of aortic insuf-
    ficiency with, *81*
  severe, *75*
  severity of, 64
  surgical considerations in, 65
  two-dimensional echocardiographic view of,
    70
Mitral valve, *81*, *321*, *322*, *331*
  a wave in, *61*
  as reference for fourth heart sound, *57*
  anterior view of, *4*
  at end-systole, *36*
  cleft, 67, 309, *326*, *332*, *334–336*
    complete endocardial cushion defect and,
      echocardiographic findings in, 311–312
    confused with left atrial myxoma, 264
    echocardiographic examination of, 312
    in complete endocardial cushion defect,
      311, 312
    leaflet separation with, 312
    mitral insufficiency secondary to, in com-
      plete endocardial cushion defect, 312
    ostium primum septal defect with, 311
  closure of, early, in aortic insufficiency, 109
  diastolic flutter of, *81*, *107*, *117*, *120*, *126*,
    136, *139*, *163*
    in aortic insufficiency, 109
    without aortic insufficiency, *125*
  diastolic motion of, *61*
  diastolic vibration of, *117*
  doming of, *73*
  during diastole, *23*

Mitral valve (*Continued*)
  E to F slope of, 52, 57, *83*
  early closure of, *137*
  echocardiogram of, *53*
  echocardiographic appearance of, with alter-
    ation in heart rate, *59*
  echocardiographic examination of, 12, *35*
  flutter of, *352*
  gradient across, *81*
  hypermobile. 295
  in atrial systole, *37*
  in early diastole, *37*
  in four-chamber section, *2*
  in mid-diastole, *37*
  in systole, *38*
  long axis view of, *38*
  M-mode echocardiographic measurement of,
    13
  motion of, *9*
  normal, *36*
    effects of sinus arrhythmia in, *58*
  normal measurement of, *46*
  opening of, *272*
  pansystolic prolapse of, *164*
  "parachute", *314*
  pliable, *78*
  position of, *1*
  premature closure of, *122, 123, 171*
  presystolic closure of, 201
  redundant and elongated, *90*
  short-axis view of, *6, 23, 24, 38*
  systolic anterior motion of. See *SAM.*
  systolic bowing of, toward left atrium, 67
  systolic flutter of, *99*
    with ruptured chordae tendineae, 68
  thickening of, in rheumatoid arthritis, *241*
  with "shaggy" echoes, *162*
Mitral valve area, *75*
Mitral valve area index, 64
Mitral valve closure, 57
  and first heart sound, *53*
  in complete heart block, 51
  premature, *61*
    first-degree atrioventricular block and,
      108
    in aortic insufficiency, 108
Mitral valve closure index, 64
Mitral valve disease, 63–103, *159, 187*
  rheumatic, *152, 299*
    diastolic flutter of interventricular septum
      in, 107
Mitral valve echocardiogram, E to F slope of,
  56
Mitral valve echogram, *a* wave of, *52*
Mitral valve endocarditis, ruptured chordae
  tendineae in, *162*
Mitral valve excursion, *46*
  reduced, *218*
Mitral valve level, left ventricle at, *23*
  during diastole, *24*
  during systole, *24*
  short-axis left parasternal view at, *10, 212*
  short-axis echocardiographic view of left
    ventricle at, *23*
Mitral valve motion, *56*
  diastolic, *61*
  diastolic abnormalities of, *97*
  during cardiac cycle, *46*
  in premature ventricular contraction, *59*

Mitral valve opening, *120*
  absent E point with, 107
  decreased, 107
Mitral valve orifice area, in two-dimensional
  echocardiography, 65
Mitral valve orifice size, *76, 77*
  decreased, 64
  small, *219, 221*
Mitral valve prolapse, 67, 69, 85–88, *90, 91,*
  94, 99, 100, 130, 149, 150, 158
  apical view of, *89*
  before and after amyl nitrate inhalation, *92*
  conditions obscuring diagnosis of, 68
  confused with left atrial myxoma, 264
  diagnostic accuracy in, 67
  echocardiographic abnormalities in, 67
  echocardiographic examination of, 130
  holosystolic, *86, 92*
  hyperactive atrioventricular groove in, 67
  indistinguishable from ruptured chordae
    tendineae, 98
  inhalation of amyl nitrate in, 67
  into left atrium, *96*
  large mitral annulus in, 67
  late systolic, *92*
  leaflet thickening in, 67
  pansystolic, *87, 142*
  pseudo, *93, 293, 298, 299*
  redundant leaflet in, 67
  secondary, 68
  systolic, late, *93*
  transducer placement in chest in, 68
  transducer position for, *92*
  Valsalva maneuver in, 67
  with pulmonary hypertension, 152
  with ruptured chordae tendineae, 68
Mitral valve prosthesis, *194, 277*
  flutter of, *190*
  of caged-ball valve, 176
  Smeloff-Cutter, *182*
  thrombosed, *186*
Mitral valve replacement, 65, *88, 89, 195*
  diastolic flutter after, 109
Mitral valve stroke volume, 200
Mitral valve vegetation. See *Valve vegetation,*
  mitral.
Mitral valve vibration, in aortic insufficiency,
  116
Mitral-tricuspid alignment, *334*
Mitral-tricuspid continuity, *332*
M-mode echocardiogram, of ascending aorta,
  131
M-mode echocardiographic appearance, of
  rheumatic mitral insufficiency, 67
M-mode echocardiographic measurement,
  13–14
  of aorta, 13
  of aortic valve, 13
  of left atrium, 14
  of left ventricle, 14
  of pulmonic valve, 14
  of right ventricle, 14
M-mode echocardiographic view, of left ventricle, *209*
M-mode echocardiography, and two-dimensional echocardiography, combined,
  12–13
    left ventricular size and function in, 197
  for left atrial enlargement, 263

M-mode echocardiography (Continued)
    for left atrial myxoma, 263
    for left atrial thrombus, 264
    for left ventricular hypertrophy, 202
    for left ventricular pseudoaneurysm, 252
    for mitral leaflet thickening, 63
    for mural thrombus, 252
    for myocardial scar, 251
    for papillary muscle dysfunction, 252
    for valve ring abscess, 163
    for vegetation, 161
    for ventricular septal rupture, 252
    formulas for left ventricular mass with, 199
    in acute myocardial infarction, 251
    of left atrial myxoma, transducer position
        in, 275
    two-dimensional echocardiography versus,
        12
    with T-scan, for left ventricular measure-
        ment, 197
M-mode examination, of tricuspid valve pro-
    lapse, transducer position in, 144
M-mode long-axis view, of left ventricle, 44
M-mode short-axis view, of left ventricle, 44
Moderator band, 322
Mucocutaneous lymph node syndrome, 250
Mucopolysaccharidosis, 207
Multi-element cross-sectional transducer, 12
Mural plaque, in left ventricular outflow tract,
    205
Mural thrombus, 125, 258
    M mode echocardiography for, 252
    two-dimensional echocardiography for, 252
Murmur(s), 115
    diastolic, 115
    ejection, systolic, 110, 113, 114
    heart, 85
    heart sounds and, echocardiogram for evalu-
        ation of, 51
    high-frequency, holosystolic, 100
    holosystolic, 89
    late systolic, 87
    of aortic stenosis, 107
    presystolic, 82, 149
    systolic, early, 267
        late, 86
Muscle, papillary. See Papillary muscle.
Muscle dysfunction, papillary, 261
    M-mode echocardiography for, 252
    two-dimensional echocardiography for,
        252
Muscular dystrophy, Duchenne's 207
    progressive, 207
Muscular ventricular septal defect, 310
    echocardiographic views of, 328
Mycotic aneurysm, 161
Mymectomy, 319
Myocardial abscess, 161
Myocardial disease, coronary artery disease
        confused with, 204
    primary, 218, 220
Myocardial fiber hypertrophy, 205
Myocardial fibrosis, from radiation therapy,
    208
Myocardial hypertrophy, 202
Myocardial infarction. See Infarction, myocar-
    dial.
Myocardial scar, 251, 257, 258
    M-mode echocardiography for, 251
    two-dimensional echocardiography for, 251

Myocardial wall perforation, 282
Myocarditis, radiation-induced, 242
Myotonia atrophica, 107
Myxoma, atrial, calcified, 273
    left. See Left atrial myxoma.
    right. See Right atrial myxoma.
    atypical appearance of, 264
    echophonocardiography in diagnosis of, 264
    nonprolapsing, 264
    nonvisualization of, 264
    prolapse of, into left ventricle, 272
Myxomatous degeneration, as cause of rup-
    tured chordae tendineae, 68
Myxomatous valvular degeneration, infective
    endocarditis with, 162

Necrosis, valvular, in infective endocarditis,
    162
Neonates, and infants, septal hypertrophy in,
    204
Neurologic disease, 207
Neuromuscular disease, 207
Noncoronary cusp, 10, 39
    movement of, 12
    of aortic valve, 59
Noncoronary sinus of Valsalva, dilatation of,
    141
Nonobstructive hypertrophic cardiomyopathy,
    206, 231–233
    after amyl nitrate inhalation, 232
Nonpliable valve, 79
Nonprolapsing left atrial myxoma, 274, 275
Nonprolapsing myxoma, 264
Nonrheumatic mitral insufficiency, long-term,
    83
Nonvalvular endocarditis, 163
Normal saline solution, inferior vena cava be-
    fore and after injection of, 146
Normal sinus rhythm, after atrial fibrillation,
    60
Notching, mid-systolic, aortic valve, 206

o point, 82
Obstructive cardiomyopathy, hypertrophic.
    See Hypertrophic obstructive cardiomy-
    opathy.
Obstructive disease, vascular, pulmonary, 160
Opening click, of Björk-Shiley prosthesis, 187
    of caged-ball valve, 176
    of Smeloff-Cutter valve, 185
    of Starr-Edwards valve, 185
Opening snap, 53, 82
Organic tricuspid insufficiency, 143
    bacterial endocarditis in, 143
Orifice size, decreased, 72, 73
    in tricuspid stenosis, 143
    normal, 72
Orthogonal section, of heart, 5
Ostium primum atrial septal defect. See Atrial
    septal defect, ostium primum.
Ostium secundum atrial septal defect. See
    Atrial septal defect, ostium secundum.
Outflow tract, ventricular, left. See Left ven-
    tricular outflow tract.
    right. See Right ventricular outflow tract.

P₂, 52

P$_2$, 52
Pacemaker, cardiac, 281
    sequential, atrioventricular, DDD, *290*
Pacemaker endocarditis, 163, *173*
Pacemaker rhythm, *62*
Pacemaker wire, 281, *288*
Pacemaker wire malposition, *288, 289*
Pacemaker-induced thrombosis, 282
Pacer. See entries under *Pacemaker.*
Pacing, sequential, atrioventricular, *290*
        left atrial function in, 282
Pansystolic prolapse, of mitral valve, 87, *142,*
        164
Papillary muscle, 26, *307, 330*
    anterolateral, 69
    calcification of, 69
    fibrosis of, 69
    large, 203, *216*
    posteromedial, 69
    short-axis view of, *7*
Papillary muscle dysfunction, 67–69, *101,*
        261
    echocardiographic diagnosis of, 69
    M-mode echocardiography for, *252*
    two-dimensional echocardiography for, *252*
Papillary muscle function, mitral insufficiency
        and, 69
Papillary muscle level, *50*
    in short-axis left parasternal view, 10
    left ventricle at, *25*
    left ventricular minor axis dimension at, 15
    short-axis parasternal view at, *212*
"Parachute" mitral valve, 314
Paradoxic septal motion. See *Septal motion,*
        paradoxic.
Parasternal long-axis view. See *Long-axis*
        view, parasternal.
Parasternal short axis, 49
Parasternal short-axis view. See *Short-axis*
        view, parasternal.
Parasternal view, long-axis. See *Long-axis*
        view, parasternal.
        left. See *Long-axis view, parasternal, left.*
        short axis. See *Short-axis view, parasternal.*
        left. See *Short-axis view, parasternal, left.*
Parietal pericardium, 293
Partial atrioventricular canal, 309
Partial endocardial cushion defect, 311
Patent ductus arteriosus, 163, 313–314, *316,*
        319, 336, 337
    contrast echocardiography for left-to-right
        shunt in, 314
    echocardiographic findings in, 313–314
Peak systolic position, failure of mitral leaflet
        to reach, 69
    normal, of posterior leaflet, *101*
PEP, 52, *58*
Perforation, of leaflet, 161
Periarteritis nodosa, 207
Pericardial constriction, from radiation ther-
        apy, 208
Pericardial effusion, 93, 155, 208, 223, 230,
        239, 242, 293–294, 296–300, 302, 304
    echocardiography for, 293
    false-negative diagnosis of, 294
    false-positive diagnosis of, 294
    from radiation therapy, 208
    heart motion with, 293
    hemorrhagic, *306*
    in cardiac tamponade, 294

Pericardial effusion (*Continued*)
    in congestive cardiomyopathy, 204
    large, *298, 299*
    loculated, *303*
    lymphoma-induced, *305*
    pericardial fluid in, 293
    pleural and, echocardiographic differentia-
        tion between, 294
    pseudo prolapse caused by, 68
    SAM with, 206
    simulated, *132*
    surrounding heart, *297, 304*
Pericardial fibrosis, from radiation therapy,
        208
Pericardial fluid, 294
    in pericardial effusion, 293
Pericardial metastasis, echocardiographic ap-
        pearance of, 295
Pericardial window, *298*
Pericarditis, *351*
    constrictive. See *Constrictive pericarditis.*
    recurrent, 93
Pericardium, 295, *296, 301*
    diseases of, 293–306
    parietal, 293
    thickened, *305*
        in constrictive pericarditis, 295
    visceral, 293
Phonocardiogram, apexcardiogram, 51
Phonocardiographic, echocardiographic, and
        graphic recording, correlation of, *53*
Phonocardiography, in hypertrophic cardio-
        myopathy, before and after amyl nitrate
        inhalation, *238*
Physiologic left ventricular hypertrophy, 202
Plaque, mural, in left ventricular outflow tract,
        205
Pleural effusion, *299, 300, 301*
    and pericardial, echocardiographic differen-
        tiation between, 294
Pleural sarcoma, *300*
Pleuropericardial effusion, *301, 302*
Pliable mitral valve, 78
Pliable valve, 65
Polycythemia, *325*
Poppet motion, in caged-ball valve, 176
        echophonocardiography for, 176
    transducer position to evaluate, in caged-
        ball prosthesis, *182*
Porcine valve, 178
    echocardiographic appearance of, 178
    in aortic position, *187*
    in mitral position, *188, 189, 190*
    in tricuspid position, *188*
    stents in, *190*
    thrombosed, *191*
Porcine valve dehiscence, *192*
Porcine valve dysfunction, *190, 191*
Porcine valve vegetation, *192–194*
Portal vein, 313
Postductal coarctation, of aorta, *344*
Posterior leaflet, 36, 37
    diastolic anterior motion of, 63, 84, 314
    doming of, *72*
    flutter of, *80*
    normal peak systolic position of, *101*
Posterior leaflet motion, 84
    abnormal, in mitral stenosis, *70*
    normal, *80*
        in mitral stenosis, 65

Posterior leaflet thickening, 87, 91, 94
Posterior mitral annulus calcification, 103
Posterior mitral leaflet, diastolic flutter of, 80
  mitral annulus calcification behind, 102
Posterior mitral leaflet motion, 79
Posterior wall, absent motion of, 257
  in long-axis section, 2
  of left ventricle, 43
    movement of, 42
Posterior wall endocardium, mitral annulus
  calcification in front of, 102
Posterior wall hypertrophy, 234
Posterior wall motion, 46
  diastolic, early, 305
    slope of, in constrictive pericarditis, 295
  increased, 83
Posterior wall scar, 257
Posterior wall thickness, 48, 198
  definition of, 14
  end-diastolic, 47
  in left ventricular hypertrophy, 14
  normal, 14
Posterior wall velocity, diastolic, decreased,
  217
  left ventricular, 64
Posteromedial papillary muscle, 69
Poststenotic dilatation, 317
  in pulmonic stenosis, 152
PR AC interval, short, 200
PR interval, 54, 55
  length of, 51
Preductal coarctation, of aorta, 316, 344
Pre-ejection period, 52, 58
Premature aortic valve opening, 123
  in aortic insufficiency, 108
Premature closure, of mitral valve, 61, 122,
  123, 171
    first-degree atrioventricular block and,
    108
  in aortic insufficiency, 108
Premature opening, of pulmonic valve, 129
Premature ventricular contraction, 52, 59, 115
  mitral valve motion in, 59
  SAM after, 229
Pressure, diastolic, increased, in congestive
  cardiomyopathy, 204
    ventricular, left. See Left ventricular dia-
    stolic pressure.
  venous, central, elevated, 294
Presystolic closure, of mitral valve, 201
Presystolic murmur, 82, 149
Presystolic opening, of aortic valve, 201
Primary pulmonary hypertension, 68, 152,
  153, 157, 158
Progressive muscular dystrophy, 207
Prolapse, holosystolic, 68
  of left atrium, 294
  of mitral valve. See Mitral valve prolapse.
  of myxoma, into left ventricle, 272
  pansystolic, of mitral valve, 164
  pseudo, caused by pericardial effusion, 68
Prosthesis, aortic, of caged-ball valve, 176
  Björk-Shiley, 177
    aortic, 186, 187
    opening click of, 187
  caged-ball, aortic and mitral, 182
    in aortic position, 183
    in atrial fibrillation, 183
    in atrial systole, 182
    in mitral position, 182, 183

Prosthesis (Continued)
  caged ball, transducer to evaluate poppet
    motion in, 182
  Carpentier-Edwards, 181, 189
    mitral, 188
  dura mater, 178
  Hancock, 181, 187, 189
    mitral, 188
  Ionescu-Shiley, 178
  Lillehei-Kaster, 177
  low-profile, in mitral stenosis, 65
  mitral, flutter of, 190
    of caged-ball valve, 176
    thrombosed, 186
  Smeloff-Cutter, 184
    mitral, 184
      thrombosed, 184, 185
  St. Jude Medical, 177
  thrombus in, 176
  valve, mitral, 194, 277
Prosthetic leaflet, systolic flutter of, 191
Prosthetic valve, 175–196
  classification of, 175, 175t
  disc excursion in, 177
  St. Jude, 187
  ventricular volume overload with, 179
Prosthetic valve dehiscence, 176
Prosthetic valve endocarditis, 179
  Klebsiella in, 179
  Pseudomonas in, 179
  Staphylococcus in, 179
  Streptococcus in, 179
  valve dehiscence in, 179
Pseudo aortic override, 351
Pseudo bicuspid aortic valve, 342
Pseudo eccentric closure, 315
Pseudo left atrial mass, 303
Pseudo mitral stenosis, 81
Pseudo mitral valve prolapse, 93, 293, 298,
  299
Pseudo prolapse, caused by pericardial effu-
  sion, 68
Pseudo pulmonic stenosis, 345
Pseudo tunnel subaortic stenosis, 343
Pseudo vegetation, 68, 94
Pseudoaneurysm, of left ventricle, 252, 260,
  294
  M-mode echocardiography for, 252
  two-dimensional echocardiography for, 252
Pseudocoarctation, 316
Pseudomitral stenosis, 65
Pseudomonas, in prosthetic valve endocardi-
  tis, 179
Pseudosystolic anterior motion, 230, 231
Pseudotruncus arteriosus, 319
Pulmonary artery, 21, 317
  aneurysm of, 159
  anomalous origin of left coronary artery
    from, 250
  dilatation of, 152
  in short-axis section, 2
  pulmonic valve and, 151–160
  right, 128
  short-axis view of, 6
  shunt from aorta to, 313
Pulmonary artery bifurcation, 160, 337
Pulmonary artery dilatation, 160
  in increased pulmonary blood flow, 152
  in pulmonary hypertension, 152
  pulmonic valve in, 160

Pulmonary artery pressure, diastolic, increased, 151
Pulmonary atresia, with ventricular septal defect, 318, 319
Pulmonary blood flow, increased, pulmonary artery dilatation in, 152
Pulmonary embolism, *157*
Pulmonary hypertension, 64, 143, 151–152, *153–158, 159, 160*
　a wave amplitude in, 14
　abnormal septal motion in, *154*
　abnormalities of tricuspid valve in, 151
　absent *a* wave in, *153, 154*
　absent or diminished *a* wave in, 151–152
　amplitude of opening in, 14
　and right ventricular failure, *153*
　as cause of right ventricular hypertrophy, 282
　decreased E to F slope in, 151, *153*
　dilatation of right ventricle in, *154*
　distortion of left ventricle in, 151
　intracardiac shunt as cause of, 152
　mid-systolic closure in, 151
　mitral valve prolapse with, 152
　primary, 68, 152, *153, 157, 158*
　pulmonary artery dilatation in, 152
　systemic, *328*
Pulmonary trunk bifurcation, *21*
　in short-axis left parasternal view, 10
　short-axis view of, 6
Pulmonary vascular obstructive disease, *160*
Pulmonary vein, 313
　direct visualization of, to exclude anomalous venous connection, 313
Pulmonary venous chamber, common, 313
Pulmonary venous connection, anomalous, partial, 313
　total, 313, *336*
Pulmonary venous drainage, anomalous, 313
　atrial septal defect with, 313
Pulmonary venous return, anomalous. See *Anomalous pulmonary venous return.*
Pulmonic insufficiency, 152, *158, 159*
　causes of, 152
　diastolic flutter of tricuspid valve in, 152
　dilatation of valve ring as cause of, 152
　infective endocarditis as cause of, 152
　right ventricular volume overload in, 152
Pulmonic stenosis, 152, 235, 316–319, *346*
　a wave amplitude in, 14
　classification of, *345*
　infundibular, *291, 345, 349*
　poststenotic dilatation in, 152
　pseudo, *345*
　rheumatic, 152
　subvalvular, 317
　　as cause of right ventricular hypertrophy, 282
　　infundibular, 317
　　subinfundibular, 317
　supravalvular, 317, *345*
　valvular, 317, *345*
　　as cause of right ventricular hypertrophy, 282
　　congenital, 152
　with malignant carcinoid, 152
Pulmonic valve, 45, *58, 327*
　a wave of, 317
　and pulmonary artery, 151–160
　anterior view of, *4*
　as reference for ejection click, 51

Pulmonic valve (*Continued*)
　coaptation of, and aortic, 52
　doming of, 317
　echocardiographic examination of, 13
　flutter of, 317
　in complete heart block, *153*
　in pulmonary artery dilatation, *160*
　mid-systolic closure of, *153, 154*
　M-mode echocardiographic measurement of, 14
　normal, *47*
　position of, 1
　premature opening of, 129
　　in constrictive pericarditis, 295
　transducer position in examination of, 45
Pulmonic valve closure, in relation to second heart sound, 55
Pulmonic valve motion, 45
Pulmonic valve vegetation, 163, *172, 173*
Pulsatile inferior vena cava, dilated and, in tricuspid insufficiency, 144
Pulse, carotid. See *Carotid pulse.*
Pulse tracing, carotid, 51
Pulsus paradoxus, 294
PWT, 199

Q wave, 52, 107, 114
QP/QS ratio, *323, 325, 329*
QS$_2$, 52. See *Total electromechanical systole.*

Radiation carditis, *242*
Radiation therapy, endocardial fibrosis from, 208
　myocardial fibrosis from, 208
　pericardial constriction from, 208
　pericardial effusion from, 208
　pericardial fibrosis from, 208
Radiation-induced myocarditis, *242*
Raphe, 317
　confused with extra commissure, 315
Rapid filling period, *17*
Rapid filling phase, *36*
Rapid filling wave, *82, 100*
Rastelli Type A complete endocardial cushion defect, 311, *330*
Rastelli Type B complete endocardial cushion defect, 311, *330*
Rastelli Type C complete endocardial cushion defect, 311, *330*
Recurrent pericarditis, 93
Redundant and elongated mitral valve, *90*
Redundant leaflet, *93*
　in mitral valve prolapse, 67
References, 355–374
Regurgitant contrast material, in tricuspid insufficiency, 144
Regurgitation, aortic, 129
　mitral, *78, 84, 87, 89, 98, 99, 167, 190, 276, 335*
　　absent, in mitral stenosis, 65
　　acute, *94*
　　in mitral insufficiency, 66
　　secondary echocardiographic abnormalities with, 66
　tricuspid, *348*
Renal failure, *216, 296, 301, 302*
　chronic, *103*

Restricted leaflet motion, *111*
Restrictive cardiomyopathy, 206
  abnormal diastolic function in, 206
  causes of, 206
  echocardiographic findings in, 206
Rhabdomyoma, in right ventricular outflow tract, *291*
Rhabdomyosarcoma, atrial, left, *276*
Rheumatic aortic insufficiency, 107
Rheumatic aortic stenosis, 105
Rheumatic carditis, as cause of mitral stenosis, 63
  as cause of ruptured chordae tendineae, 68
Rheumatic heart disease, as cause of tricuspid stenosis, 143
  organic tricuspid insufficiency in, 143
  tricuspid insufficiency secondary to, *147*
  with mitral and tricuspid stenosis, *145*
Rheumatic mitral insufficiency, 65, 67, 68, *84, 85*
  E to F slope in, 65
  M-mode echocardiographic appearance of, 67
Rheumatic mitral valve disease, 152, *299*
  diastolic flutter of interventricular septum in, 107
Rheumatic pulmonic stenosis, 152
Rheumatic tricuspid insufficiency, *146, 148*
Rheumatic tricuspid stenosis, 143
  nodular, *241*
  thickening of mitral valve in, *241*
Rheumatoid arthritis, 200
  nodular, 241
  thickening of mitral valve in, 241
Rhythm, pacemaker, *62*
Rhythm, sinus, 62
Right aortic arch, 318
Right atrial enlargement, 281, *284*
Right atrial mass, 281, *284*
  two-dimensional echocardiography for, 281
Right atrial myxoma, 281, *286*
  prolapsing into right ventricle, *287*
Right atrial tumor, 163
Right atrial volume overload, in tricuspid insufficiency, 144
Right atrium, and right ventricle, 281–292
  dilatation of, 281
    in tricuspid insufficiency, 144
  major axis of, 15, *50*
  minor axis of, 15, *50*
  normal measurement of major axis of, 15
  normal measurement of minor axis of, 15
  vegetation in, *174*
Right bundle branch block, 52
Right coronary artery, 254, 255
  echocardiography of, 249
Right coronary cusp, *39*
  movement of, 12
  systolic flutter of, *233*
  thickening of, *110*
Right electromechanical systole, total, 58
Right pulmonary artery, 128
Right ventricle, 48
  dilatation of, 64, *111*, 143, *146*, *155*, *157*, *258*, 282, *321*, *322*, *331*, 336
    in pulmonary hypertension, 154
    with right ventricular thrombus, 283
  double outlet, 318, 320
  echocardiographic views of, *354*
  ventricular septal defect with, 320

Right ventricle (*Continued*)
  early systolic "notch" of, 295
  end-diastolic dimension of, 47
  enlarged, *159*
  increased end-diastolic pressure of, *290, 291*
  long axis of, *50*
  M-mode echocardiographic measurement of, 14
  position of, 1
  right atrium and, 281–292
  short axis of, *50*
  small, *348*
Right ventricular cavity, dilated, *347*
Right ventricular collapse, *304*
Right ventricular compression, in cardiac tamponade, 295
Right ventricular dilatation. See *Dilatation, of right ventricle.*
Right ventricular dimension, *48*
Right ventricular ejection time, 52, *53, 58*
Right ventricular end-diastolic diameter, 14
  in right ventricular volume overload, 14
  normal, 14
Right ventricular end-diastolic pressure, increased, 282
Right ventricular failure, 148, 291
  pulmonary hypertension and, *153*
Right ventricular free wall thickness, 282
Right ventricular hypertrophy, 282–283, *291*, 317, 318, 346, 349
  pulmonary hypertension as cause of, 282
  septal hypertrophy in, 204, *235*
  subvalvular pulmonic stenosis as cause of, 282
  valvular pulmonic stenosis as cause of, 282
Right ventricular infarction, echocardiographic findings in, 253
Right ventricular inflow tract, *148*
  long-axis view of, *10, 19*
Right ventricular major axis dimension, definition of, 15
  normal, 15
Right ventricular minor axis dimension, in apical four-chamber view, 15
  in parasternal long-axis view, 15
  normal, in apical four-chamber view, 15
  in parasternal long-axis view, 15
Right ventricular outflow tract, *21, 351*
  narrow, *350*
  rhabdomyoma in, *291*
  subcostal, 11
  subcostal view of, *33*
  transducer position for subcostal view of, *33*
Right ventricular pressure, end-diastolic, increased, 151
Right ventricular pressure overload, 154
Right ventricular thrombus, 283, *292*
  after cardiac contusion, 283, *291*
  dilated right ventricle with, 283
  with congestive cardiomyopathy, 283
Right ventricular tumor, 283
Right ventricular volume overload, *118, 129, 146, 159,* 282, *313, 323, 331*
  in pulmonic insufficiency, 152
  in tricuspid insufficiency, 144
  right ventricular end-diastolic diameter in, 14
  with complete endocardial cushion defect, 311, 312
  with prosthetic valve, 179

Right ventricular wall, posterior motion of, during diastole, 295
Right ventricular wall thickness, increased, 151
Right-to-left shunt, 330
  at atrial level, 309, 324
  contrast study of, 324
  exclusion of, 157
Ring abscess, 161, 179
  valve, 163
    M-mode echocardiography for, 163
    two-dimensional echocardiography for, 163
Root, aortic, dilatation of, 112
Rupture, septal, ventricular, 261
    M-mode echocardiography for, 252
    two-dimensional echocardiography for, 252
Ruptured chordae tendineae, 67, 68, 94, 96–100, 167, 168
  causes of, 68–69
    idiopathic, 68
  connective tissue disorders as cause of, 68
  diastolic flutter with, 109
  echocardiographic abnormalities with, 68
  echophonocardiography for, 69
  exaggerated leaflet motion with, 68
  flail leaflet with, 68
  in left atrium, 95
  in mitral valve endocarditis, 162
  infective endocarditis as cause of, 68
  mitral valve prolapse indistinguishable from, 98
  mitral valve prolapse with, 68
  myxomatous degeneration as cause of, 68
  rheumatic carditis as cause of, 68
  systolic flutter of, mitral valve with, 68
  trauma as cause of, 68
  tricuspid insufficiency with, 143
  with vegetation, 161
RVET, 52, 53, 58

S₁. See First heart sound.
S₂. See Second heart sound.
S₃. See Third heart sound.
S₄. See Fourth heart sound.
St. Jude Medical prosthesis, 177. See also St. Jude Medical valve and St. Jude prosthetic valve.
St. Jude Medical valve, 180. See also St. Jude Medical prosthesis and St. Jude prosthetic valve.
St. Jude prosthetic valve, 187. See also St. Jude Medical prosthesis and St. Jude Medical valve.
Saline solution, normal, inferior vena cava before and after injection of, 146
SAM, 68, 205, 206, 222–224, 234, 238, 316
  absent, after amyl nitrate inhalation, 235
  after amyl nitrate administration, 206, 229
  after premature ventricular contraction, 229
  at rest, 206
    in aortic insufficiency, 109, 126
  with pericardial effusion, 206
Sarcoidosis, 207
Sarcoma, 281
  pleural, 300

Scan, echocardiographic, 13
Scar, anteroseptal, 257
  myocardial, 251, 257, 258
    M-mode echocardiography for, 251
    two-dimensional echocardiography for, 251
  posterior wall, 257
Scleroderma, 207, 290
Sclerosis, aortic, 113
  tuberous, 207
Second heart sound, 52, 53, 55, 82
  aortic valve closure in relation to, 55
  pulmonic valve closure in relation to, 55
Secondary mitral valve prolapse, 68
Sector plane, to view aorta and left atrium, 22
Segmental left ventricular dysfunction, 69
Segmental wall motion, analysis of, 201
  apical four-chamber view for, 201
  apical long-axis view for, 201
  apical two-chamber view for, 201
  echocardiography for analysis of, 201
  long-axis parasternal view for, 201
  short-axis parasternal view for, 201
Semiclosure, of aortic valve, 83
  mid-systolic, 206
Semilunar valve, 52, 319, 354
  echocardiographic examination of, 308
Semilunar valve motion, 52
Senile fibrocalcific aortic stenosis, 105, 110
Septal and anterior mitral leaflet vibration, 118
Septal aneurysm, atrial. See Atrial septal aneurysm.
Septal aneurysm, ventricular, 311, 330
Septal coaptation, mitral, 158
Septal defect, atrial. See Atrial septal defect.
  interatrial, 318
    in Ebstein's anomaly, 317
  ostium primum, with cleft mitral valve, 311
  ventricular. See Ventricular septal defect.
  with tricuspid valve prolapse, 144
Septal excursion, 121
Septal hypertrophy. See Hypertrophy, septal.
Septal-mitral valve coaptation, 222
Septal-mitral valve distance, 13, 46
Septal motion, 84
  abnormal, 74, 121, 146, 151, 159, 270, 282
    in aortic insufficiency, 108
    in constrictive pericarditis, 295
    in mitral stenosis, 64
    in pulmonary hypertension, 154
  increased, 336
  interatrial, abnormal, in mitral insufficiency, 66
  paradoxic, 61, 62, 118, 305, 309, 313, 323, 331
Septal notch, 81
Septal rupture, ventricular, 261
    M-mode echocardiography for, 252
    two-dimensional echocardiography for, 252
Septal thickness, 198
  definition of, 14
  in asymmetric septal hypertrophy, 14
  in idiopathic hypertrophic subaortic stenosis, 14
  normal, 14
Septal vibration, in diagnosis of aortic insufficiency with mitral stenosis, 81

Septal wall hypertrophy, 234
Septal wall motion, increased, 83
Septal wall thickness, increased, 151
Septum, 48
    atrial, 311
        absent, 309
    flattened, 154–156
    flutter of, 352, 353
    in four-chamber section, 2
    in long-axis section, 2
    interatrial. See Interatrial septum.
    interventricular. See Interventricular septum.
    mitral insertion in, 321
    thickened, 223, 225
    tricuspid insertion in, 321
Sequential pacemaker, atrioventricular, DDD, 290
Sequential pacing, atrioventricular, 290
Short axis, aortic valve in, 22
    of aorta, 34
    of left ventricle, 50
    of right ventricle, 50
    parasternal, 49
Short-axis echocardiographic view, of left ventricle, at mitral valve level, 23
Short-axis parasternal view. See Short-axis view, parasternal.
Short-axis section, left ventricle in, 2
    of aorta, 2
    of heart, 2, 5
    pulmonary artery in, 2
Short-axis view, at mitral level, 50
    M-mode, of left ventricle, 44
    normal aortic valve in, 22
    of aortic arch, 12
    of aortic valve, 41
    of descending aorta, 134
    of heart, 20
        transducer position in, 20
    of mitral valve, 23, 24, 38
    parasternal, 15, 48
        aorta in, 10, 15
        at apical level, 212
        at mitral valve level, 10, 212
        at papillary muscle level, 212
        for segmental wall motion, 201
        left, 10, 35
            of descending aorta, 134
        left atrium in, 10, 15
        of ascending aorta, 132
        of descending aorta, 134
        of left ventricle, 10
        pulmonary trunk bifurcation in, 10
Shunt, at ventricular level, contrast echocardiography for, 311
    bidirectional, 329
    from aorta to pulmonary artery, 313
    left-to-right, 313
        in patent ductus arteriosus, contrast echocardiography for, 314
    right-to-left, 330
        atrial level, 324
        exclusion of, 157
Sick sinus syndrome, 103
Silastic ball, 180
Simpson's rule method, for calculation of left ventricular volume, 199, 211
Single ventricle, 320, 354

Sinus, aortic, 316
    coronary, 264–265, 313
        dilated, 264
        left superior vena cava draining into, 278, 279
        movement of, 133
Sinus arrhythmia, 52, 58, 59
    a wave in, 58
    effects of, in normal mitral valve, 58
Sinus of Valsalva, 105, 127
    noncoronary, dilatation of, 141
Sinus of Valsalva aneurysm, 128, 129, 138, 139
Sinus rhythm, 62, 97
    normal, after atrial fibrillation, 60
Sinus tachycardia, 52, 59
Sinus venosus, echocardiography in, 309
Sinus venosus atrial septal defect, 323
Sinus venosus defect, 308
Situs inversus, 308
Situs solitus, 308
Slope, E to F. See E to F slope.
Smeloff-Cutter prosthesis, 184. See also Smeloff-Cutter valve.
    mitral, 182, 184
        thrombosed, 184, 185
Smeloff-Cutter valve, 180. See also Smeloff-Cutter prosthesis.
    closing click of, 185
    opening click of, 185
Spondylitis, ankylosing, 107, 130, 208
Staphylococcus, in prosthetic valve endocarditis, 179
Staphylococcus aureus, in tricuspid valve infection, 163
Starr-Edwards caged-ball valve, 180
Starr-Edwards valve, mitral, normal, 185
    opening click of, 185
Stellite ring, in Hancock valve, 178, 181
Stenosis, aortic. See Aortic stenosis.
        valvular. See Aortic stenosis, valvular and Valvular aortic stenosis.
    artery, coronary, echocardiography of, 249
    infundibular, 318
    mitral. See Mitral stenosis.
    pseudomitral, 65
    pulmonic. See Pulmonic stenosis.
    subaortic, hypertrophic, idiopathic. See Idiopathic hypertropic subaortic stenosis.
    tunnel, 314
        pseudo, 343
    subvalvular, 64
        fibromuscular, 316
    tricuspid. See Tricuspid stenosis.
    trunk, main, left, 255, 256
    valvular, 318
Stenotic tricuspid valve, 184
Stenotic valve, 63
Stent, Delrin, 181
    in porcine valve, 190
Stomach, 321
Straddling atrioventricular valve, 312
    ventricular septal defect in, 312
Streptococcus, in prosthetic valve endocarditis, 179
Stroke volume, 200
    decreased, 59, 200
        in congestive cardiomyopathy, 204
    increased, in athletes, 203

Stroke volume (*Continued*)
  left ventricular, *83*
  valve, mitral, 200
Strut, motion of, in caged-ball valve, 176
Subaortic stenosis, hypertrophic, idiopathic.
    See *Idiopathic hypertrophic subaortic stenosis.*
  tunnel, 314
    pseudo, *343*
Subclavian artery, left, 316
  origin of, 128
Subcostal area, 1
Subcostal four-chamber view, 11, *32*
  transducer position in, *32*
Subcostal right ventricular outflow tract, 11
Subcostal transducer position, 11, *31*
  hepatic vein with, 11
  inferior vena cava with, 11
Subcostal view, of right ventricular outflow
    tract, *33*
  transducer position for, *33*
Subinfundibular subvalvular pulmonic stenosis, 317
Subpulmonary conus, 320
Subvalvular aortic stenosis, 314–316, *337*
  fibromuscular, 314–316
  membranous, discrete, 315–316, *343*
Subvalvular pulmonic stenosis, 317
  as cause of right ventricular hypertrophy, 282
  infundibular, 317
  subinfundibular, 317
Subvalvular stenosis, 64
  fibromuscular, 316
Subxiphoid region, *31*
Sulcus, atriopulmonary, 163
Superior vena cava, left, draining into coronary sinus, *278, 279*
    two-dimensional echocardiography for, 265
Supraclavicular area, 1
Supracristal ventricular septal defect, 310, *327*
Suprasternal area, 1
Suprasternal region, *34*
Suprasternal transducer position, 11, *33, 34*
Supravalvular aortic stenosis, 314, 316, *337, 344*
  membranous type, 316
Supravalvular pulmonic stenosis, 317, *345*
Supravalvular ring, 314
Surgical considerations, in mitral stenosis, 65
Suture ring, of caged-ball valve, 176
Swan-Ganz catheter, 281, *288*
Syphilitic aortic aneurysm, 128
Syphilitic aortitis, 107
Systemic disease, cardiac involvement in, 207–208
  physical and toxic causes of, 208
Systemic hypertension, *215*
  echocardiographic abnormalities in, 203
  ventricular size and function in, 203
Systole, aortic valve in, *40*
  atrial, 17
    caged-ball prosthesis in, *182*
    mitral valve in, *37*
  electromechanical, right, total, 58
    total, 58
  left ventricle at mitral valve level during, *24*
  left ventricle in, *43*
  mitral valve in, *38*
  ventricular, 17

Systolic anterior motion, *86, 93, 226–229*
  of mitral valve. See *SAM.*
Systolic bowing, of mitral valve, toward left atrium, 67
Systolic click, mid-late, *87*
Systolic ejection click, 115
Systolic ejection murmur, *110, 113, 114*
Systolic flutter, *99*
  of mitral valve, *99*
    with ruptured chordae tendineae, 68
  of prosthetic leaflet, *191*
  of right coronary cusp, *233*
  of tricuspid valve, 282
Systolic mid-closure, of aortic valve, 316
Systolic mitral valve prolapse, late, *92, 93*
Systolic murmur, early, *267*
  late, *86, 87*
Systolic "notch," early, of right ventricle, 295
Systolic position, peak, failure of mitral leaflet to reach, 69
  normal, of posterior leaflet, *101*
Systolic time interval, 52, *58*
  right-sided, 52, *58*
Systolic vibration, *99*

Tachycardia, sinus, 52, *59*
  ventricular, 52, *61, 247*
Tamponade, cardiac, 294–295, *304–305*
  pericardial effusion in, 294
  right ventricular compression in, 295
Teflon cloth sewing ring, *180*
Tendon, false, *246, 247*
  of left ventricle, 208
Tetralogy, Fallot's. See *Fallot's tetralogy.*
Third heart sound, 52, *56, 57, 100*
Thrombosed mitral prosthesis, *186*
Thrombosed porcine valve, *191*
Thrombosis, of caged-ball valve, *184*
  pacemaker-induced, 282
Thrombus, *260, 281*
  atrial, left. See *Atrial thrombus, left.*
  in prosthesis, 176
  mural, *125, 258*
    M-mode echocardiography for, 252
    two-dimensional echocardiography for, 252
  ventricular, left. See *Left ventricular thrombus.*
    right. See *Right ventricular thrombus.*
  with heterograft, 178
Tilting-disc valve, 177
  classification of, 175t
  echocardiographic appearance of, 177
Tissue degeneration and calcification, with xenograft, 178
Tissue valve, classification of, 175t
Tomographic anatomy, of heart, 1–2
Total electromechanical systole, *58*
Total electromechanical time, 52
Total right electromechanical systole, *58*
Trabeculae carneae, prominent, 203, 217
Transducer, multi-element cross-sectional, 12
Transducer placement, in chest, in mitral valve prolapse, 68
Transducer position, and eccentric closure of aortic valve, *342*
  apical, 10, *27*
  for left ventricular measurement, 197, 198

Transducer position (*Continued*)
  for mitral valve prolapse, *92*
  for poppet motion in caged-ball prosthesis, *182*
  for subcostal view, of right ventricular outflow tract, *33*
  in apical five-chamber view, *281*
  in apical long-axis view, *30*
  in apical two-chamber view, *29*
  in coronary artery visualization, 249
  in examination of pulmonic valve, *45*
  in examination of tricuspid valve, *45*
  in M-mode echocardiography of left atrial myxoma, *275*
  in M-mode examination of tricuspid valve prolapse, 144
  in short-axis view of heart, *20*
  in subcostal four-chamber view, *32*
  left parasternal, *9, 16, 17*
  subcostal, *11, 31*
    hepatic vein with, *11*
    inferior vena cava with, *11*
  suprasternal, *11, 33, 34*
Transposition, 308
  contrast echocardiography for, 308
  of great arteries, 319–320, *354*
    echocardiographic examination of, 319
    echocardiographic views of, *353*
  of great vessels, 318
    corrected, *322, 323*
      contrast study of, *323*
Trauma, as cause of ruptured chordae tendineae, 68
  in tricuspid insufficiency, 143
  to chest, cardiac contusion from, 208
Tricuspid annulus, 317
Tricuspid atresia, 318, *348, 349*
Tricuspid caged-ball valve, mitral and, echophonocardiography to identify, *186*
Tricuspid cleft, isolated, 311
Tricuspid insertion, in septum, *321*
Tricuspid insufficiency, 143–144, 146–149, *172*
  contrast study of, *146, 147*
  dilated and pulsatile inferior vena cava in, 144
  dilated right atrium in, 144
  echocardiography for, 143
  in common atrioventricular canal, 143
  in Ebstein's anomaly, 143
  in tricuspid valve prolapse, 143
  inferior vena cava in, *147*
  organic, 143
    bacterial endocarditis in, 143
  regurgitant contrast material in, 144
  rheumatic, *146, 148*
  right ventricular volume overload in, 144
  secondary to rheumatic heart disease, *147*
  thickened leaflet in, 144
  trauma in, 143
  with ruptured chordae tendineae, 143
  with tricuspid valve vegetation, 163
Tricuspid leaflet, diastolic flutter of, *159*
Tricuspid-mitral alignment, with complete endocardial cushion defect, 311, 312
Tricuspid position, porcine valve in, *188*
Tricuspid regurgitation, *348*
Tricuspid stenosis, 143, *145, 149*
  causes of, 143
  congenital disease as cause of, 143

Tricuspid (*Continued*)
  decreased diastolic slope in, 143
  decreased orifice size in, 143
  diastolic doming in, 143
  echocardiographic abnormalities in, 143
  endocardial fibroelastosis as cause of, 143
  malignant carcinoid as cause of, 143
  mitral and, rheumatic heart disease with, *145*
  rheumatic, 143
  rheumatic heart disease as cause of, 143
Tricuspid valve, 45, *286, 321, 322, 327, 331*
  abnormalities of, in pulmonary hypertension, 151
  anterior, E to F slope of, *318*
  anterior view of, *4*
  arcing of, *150*
  carcinoid heart disease involving, 144
  closed, *19*
  closure of, delayed, *318*
  displaced, *346, 347*
  domed, *148*
  echocardiographic examination of, 13
  hypermobile, *295*
  in four-chamber section, *2*
  position of, *1*
  prominent, *347*
  prominent B notch in, *290, 291*
  stenotic, *184*
  systolic flutter of, *282*
  transducer position in examination of, *45*
Tricuspid valve area, 143
Tricuspid valve closure, delayed, *347, 348*
  in relation to first heart sound, *53*
Tricuspid valve disease, 143–150
Tricuspid valve excursion, *347*
  excessive, *282*
Tricuspid valve infection, in intravenous drug user, *163*
  Staphylococcus aureus in, 163
Tricuspid valve motion, 13
Tricuspid valve opening excursion, increased, 309
Tricuspid valve prolapse, 144, *149, 150*
  definition of, 144
  septal defect with, 144
  transducer position in M-mode examination of, 144
  tricuspid insufficiency in, 143
Tricuspid valve vegetation, *163, 172*
  tricuspid insufficiency with, 163
True apex, *18, 30*
True lumen, 128
Truncus arteriosus, incompetent, *351, 353*
  persistent, 318, 319
    septal flutter in, 319
    Type I, 319
    Type II, 319
    Type III, 319
    Type IV, 319
Trunk, main, left, *254*
Trunk lesion, main, left, false-positive, *256*
  nonvisualization of, *256*
Trunk stenosis, main, left, *255, 256*
T-scan, M-mode echocardiography with, for left ventricular measurement, 197
Tuberosclerosis, *291*. See also *Tuberous sclerosis*.
Tuberous sclerosis, 207. See also *Tuberosclerosis*.

Tumor, atrial, left, confused with left atrial myxoma, 264
    right, 163
    extracardiac, 208, 244–246
        after chemotherapy, 245
    ventricular, left, 208
        right, 283
"Tumor notch," 277
"Tumor plop," 276, 277
Tunnel aortic stenosis, 315, 316
Tunnel subaortic stenosis, 314
    pseudo, 343
Two-chamber view, apical, 11, 29
    for segmental wall motion, 201
    transducer position in, 29
Two-dimensional echocardiographic findings, in constrictive pericarditis, 295
Two-dimensional echocardiographic measurements, 15
Two-dimensional echocardiographic view, of left ventricle, 209
    of mitral stenosis, 70
Two-dimensional echocardiography, 9–12
    contrast, for left superior vena cava draining into coronary sinus, 265
    for aortic valve vegetation, 162
    for left atrial enlargement, 263
    for left atrial myxoma, 263
    for left atrial thrombus, 264
    for left ventricular aneurysm, 251
    for left ventricular hypertrophy, 202
    for left ventricular pseudoaneurysm, 252
    for mitral leaflet thickening, 63
    for mural thrombus, 252
    for myocardial scar, 251
    for papillary muscle dysfunction, 252
    for right atrial mass(es), 281
    for valve ring abscess, 163
    for ventricular septal rupture, 252
    in acute myocardial infarction, 251
    mitral valve orifice area in, 65
    M-mode and, combined, 12–13
        left ventricular size and function in, 197
    of anterior wall, 202
    of apex, 202
    of interventricular septum, 202
    of lateral wall, 202
    versus M-mode, 12

U time, 107

Valsalva, sinus of. See Sinus of Valsalva.
Valsalva maneuver, in mitral valve prolapse, 67
Valve, atrioventricular. See Atrioventricular valve.
    autograft, 178
    bileaflet, 177–178
        classification of, 175t
        echocardiographic appearance of, 177–178
    Björk-Shiley, 180
    bovine, 178
    caged-ball. See Caged-ball valve.
    caged-disc. See Caged-disc valve.
    cardiac. See Cardiac valve.
    Carpentier-Edwards, 178

Valve (Continued)
    eustachian, 290
        and Chiari network, 282
    Hancock, 178
        mitral, 193
            and aortic, 192
    mechanical, classification of, 175t
    mitral. See Mitral valve.
    nonpliable, 79
    pliable, 65
    porcine, 178
        echocardiographic appearance of, 178
        in aortic position, 187
        in mitral position, 188, 189
        in tricuspid position, 188
        stent in, 190
        thrombosed, 191
    prosthetic, 175–196
        classification of, 175t
        St. Jude, 187
        ventricular volume overload with, 179
    pulmonic. See Pulmonic valve.
    St. Jude Medical, 180
    semilunar, echocardiographic examination of, 308
    Smeloff-Cutter, 180
        closing click of, 185
        opening click of, 185
    Starr-Edwards, mitral, normal, 185
        opening click of, 185
    stenotic, 63
    tilting-disc. See Tilting-disc valve.
    tissue, classification of, 175t
    tricuspid. See Tricuspid valve.
Valve area, 76
Valve area index, mitral, 64
Valve closure, aortic, 138
    early, 83
        in mitral insufficiency, 66
    mitral, 57
        premature, 61
    tricuspid, delayed, 347, 348
Valve closure index, mitral, 64
Valve coaptation, septal-mitral, 222
Valve dehiscence, 178
    in prosthetic valve endocarditis, 179
    porcine, 192
    prosthetic, 176
Valve disease, aortic, 105–126
    mitral, 63–103, 159, 187
        rheumatic, 299
    tricuspid, 143–150
Valve dysfunction, porcine, 190, 191
Valve endocarditis, mitral, ruptured chordae tendineae in, 162
Valve excursion, 79
    aortic, decreased, 124
    definition of, 13
    mitral, 46
        reduced, 218
    tricuspid, 347
        excessive, 282
Valve leaflet thickening, mitral, 168
Valve motion, 51
    aortic, 59
    atrioventricular, 52
    mitral, diastolic, 61
        during cardiac cycle, 46
        in premature ventricular contraction, 59
    semilunar, 52

Valve opening, aortic, premature, in aortic insufficiency, 108
  mitral, *120*
Valve orifice, aortic, narrowing of, 105
Valve orifice area, mitral, in two-dimensional echocardiography, 65
Valve orifice size. See also under *Valve area.*
  mitral, small, *219*, *221*
Valve prolapse, aortic, as cause of aortic insufficiency, 107
  in aortic insufficiency, 108
  mitral. See *Mitral valve prolapse.*
  tricuspid. See *Tricuspid valve prolapse.*
Valve prosthesis, mitral, *194*, *277*
  Smeloff-Cutter, *182*
Valve replacement, aortic, 88
  in aortic insufficiency, 108
  causes of recurrent symptoms after, 175
  mitral, 65, 88, *195*
    diastolic flutter after, 109
Valve ring, dilatation of, as cause of pulmonic insufficiency, 152
Valve ring abscess, 163
  M-mode echocardiography for, 163
  two-dimensional echocardiography for, 163
Valve stroke volume, mitral, 200
Valve vegetation, aortic, 162, *170*, *171*
  two-dimensional echocardiography for, 162
  mitral, 162, *164–167*
    change in, 162
    confused with left atrial myxoma, *166*, 264
    from aortic valve, *167*
    prolapsing into left atrium, *166*
  porcine, *192–194*
  pulmonic, 163, *172*, *173*
  tricuspid, 163, *172*
    tricuspid insufficiency with, 163
Valvular aortic insufficiency, causes of, 107
Valvular aortic stenosis, 105–107, 314, *337*
Valvular degeneration, myxomatous, infective endocarditis with, 162
Valvular heart disease, vegetation with, 161
Valvular necrosis in, infective endocarditis, 162
Valvular pulmonic stenosis. See *Pulmonic stenosis, valvular.*
Valvular stenosis, 318
Valvuloplasty, 315, *338*
Valvulotomy, congenital aortic stenosis after, *338*
Vascular obstructive disease, pulmonary, *160*
Vascular wall, focal reflectivity of, 249
Vegetation, 89, 281
  from aortic valve, 162
  healed, *169*
  in infective endocarditis, 161
  in right atrium, *174*
  M-mode echocardiography to detect, 161
  prolapsing into left atrium, 162, *168*, *169*
  pseudo, 68, *94*
  ruptured chordae tendineae with, 161
  valve. See *Valve vegetation.*
Vein, hepatic. See *Hepatic vein.*
  innominate, left, 313
  portal, 313
  pulmonary, 313
    direct visualization of, to exclude anomalous venous connection, 313

Vena cava, inferior, with subcostal transducer position, 11
Vena cava, inferior. See *Inferior vena cava.*
Vena cava, superior, left, draining into coronary sinus, *278*, *279*
    two-dimensional echocardiography for, 265
Venous catheter, 281–282
Venous chamber, pulmonary, common, 313
Venous circulation, 323
Venous connection, anomalous, direct visualization of pulmonary vein to exclude, 313
  pulmonary, anomalous, partial, 313
    total, 313, *336*
Venous drainage, pulmonary, anomalous, 313
  atrial septal defect with, 313
Venous pressure, central, elevated, 294
Venous return, pulmonary, anomalous. See *Anomalous pulmonary venous return.*
Ventricle, echocardiographic examination of, 307
  left. See *Left ventricle.*
  right. See *Right ventricle.*
  single, 329, 354
Ventricular aneurysm. See *Aneurysm, ventricular.*
Ventricular apex, *213*
Ventricular bigeminy, *59*
Ventricular cavity, left, small, *223*
Ventricular collapse, right, *304*
Ventricular complex, *122*
Ventricular compliance, left, decreased, 65, 203, 206, 234
Ventricular compression, right, in cardiac tamponade, 295
Ventricular contractility, left, hyperkinetic, with ventricular septal defect, 311
Ventricular contraction, premature, 52, *59*, *115*
  mitral valve motion in, *59*
  SAM after, *229*
Ventricular diastolic filling, left, impaired, 294
Ventricular diastolic filling rate, 295
Ventricular diastolic pressure, left. See *Left ventricular diastolic pressure.*
Ventricular dilatation. See *Dilatation, of left ventricle* and *Dilatation, of right ventricle.*
Ventricular dimension, 47
  left, anteroposterior, 198
Ventricular dysfunction, left, *220*
  global, in congestive cardiomyopathy, 204
  in patients receiving Adriamycin, 208
  segmental, 69
Ventricular ejection, *62*
Ventricular ejection time, *46*
  left, *53*
  right, *53*
Ventricular end-diastolic diameter, left, *121*, *198*
  dilated, *124*
Ventricular end-diastolic dimension, left, enlargement of, in athletes, 203
Ventricular end-diastolic pressure, right, increased, 282
Ventricular end-systolic diameter, left, *121*, *198*
  dilated, *124*
Ventricular enlargement, *323*

Ventricular failure, left, *290*
  right, *148*, *291*
    pulmonary hypertension and, *153*
Ventricular free wall thickness, right, 282
Ventricular function, left, 197–202
    depressed, in aortic insufficiency, 108
    impaired, *124*
    in coronary artery disease, 250–251
Ventricular hypertrophy, left. See *Left ventricular hypertrophy.*
  right. See *Right ventricular hypertrophy.*
Ventricular infarction, right, echocardiographic findings in, 253
Ventricular inflow obstruction, left, 314
Ventricular inflow tract, right, *148*
Ventricular inversion, 308
Ventricular level, contrast echocardiography for shunt at, 311
Ventricular mass, left. See *Left ventricular mass.*
Ventricular measurement, left, transducer position for, 197, 198
Ventricular minor axis dimension, left. See *Left ventricular minor axis dimension.*
Ventricular outflow tract, left. See *Left ventricular outflow tract.*
  right. See *Right ventricular outflow tract.*
Ventricular pacing, 52
Ventricular pressure, 200
    left, end-diastolic, increased, *221*
    formula for, 106
    right, end-diastolic, increased, 151
Ventricular pressure overload, right, *154*
Ventricular pseudoaneurysm, left. See *Pseudoaneurysm, of left ventricle.*
Ventricular septal aneurysm, 311, *330*
Ventricular septal defect, 129, *160*, 173, 316, 319, *332*, 348, 351, 353
    atrioventricular canal, 311, *335*
    classification of, 310
    conotruncal, 311, 318, *349*
    contrast study of, *328–330*
    hyperkinetic left ventricular contractility with, 311
    in straddling atrioventricular valve, 312
    inlet, 311
    left atrial dilatation with, 311
    left ventricular dilatation with, 311
    membranous, 310
      echo dropout with, 310
      echocardiographic views of, *327*
    muscular, 310
      echocardiographic views of, *328*
    pulmonary atresia with, 318, 319
    supracristal, 310, *327*
    with double outlet right ventricle, 320
Ventricular septal rupture, 261
    M-mode echocardiography for, 252
    two-dimensional echocardiography for, 252

Ventricular size, and function, left, in M-mode and two-dimensional echocardiography, 197
    in systemic hypertension, 203
  left, 197–202
    decreased, during inspiration, 295
    small, 203
Ventricular systole, *17*
Ventricular tachycardia, 52, *61*, 247
Ventricular thrombus, left. See *Left ventricular thrombus.*
  right. See *Right ventricular thrombus.*
Ventricular tumor, left, 208
  right, 283
Ventricular volume, left. See *Left ventricular volume.*
Ventricular volume overload, left. See *Left ventricular volume overload.*
  right. See *Right ventricular volume overload.*
Ventricular wall thickness, 346
  left, increased, 202
    in athletes, 203
  right, increased, 151
Vessels, great. See *Great vessels.*
Vibration, diastolic, of interventricular septum, *118, 119*
    of mitral valve, *117*
  mitral valve, in aortic insufficiency, *116*
  septal and anterior mitral leaflet, *118*
Visceral pericardium, 293

Wall hypertrophy, posterior, *234*
  septal, *234*
Wall motion, 52
  posterior. See *Posterior wall motion.*
  segmental. See *Segmental wall motion.*
  septal. See *Septal wall motion.*
Wall motion abnormalities, exercise-induced, ischemia with, 250
  regional, during dynamic ergometry, 250
    during isometric exercise, 250
Wall scar, posterior, 257
Wall thickness, free, ventricular, right, 282
  ventricular, 346
    left, *25*, 106
Wave pattern, in atrial fibrillation, *60*
Whipple's disease, 94
Wolff-Parkinson-White syndrome, 52
  type B, *62*

Xenograft. See also under *Heterograft.*
  Angell-Shiley, *181*
  classification of, 175t
  tissue degeneration and calcification with, 178

Cardiac Cycle — Period from the beginning of one beat of the heart to the beginning of the succeeding beat, including systole, Contraction of atria & ventricles propelling the blood onward, and the diastole, the period during which the cavities are being refilled w/ blood. The atria contract immediately before the ventricles. The ordinary cycle lasts 0.8 seconds w/ the heart beating approx 60-85 times a minute in the adult at rest. The atrial systole lasts 0.1 sec. ventricular systole " 0.3 sec. and diastole 0.4 sec. Thus even though the heart seems to be working continuously, it actually rests for a good portion of each cardiac cycle.

Cardiac Cycle

Systole typically is defined as the segment of the cardiac cycle from mitral valve closure to aortic valve closure. The onset of systole is defined by (EKG) as ventricular depolarization (onset of QRS) complex, with the end of systole occurring after repolarization (end of T wave) In terms of ventricular pressure and volume curves over time, systole begins when left ventricular diastolic pressure exceeds left atrial pressure, resulting in closure of the mitral valve. Mitral valve closure is followed by isovolumic contraction, during which the cardiac muscle depolarizes, calcium influx. & myosin-actin shortening occur and ventricular pressure ↑ rapidly at a constant ventricular volume. When ventricular pressure exceeds aortic pressure, the aortic valve opens. During ejection (aortic valve opening to closing), left ventricular volume falls rapidly as blood flows from the left ventricle to the aorta. Left ventricular pressure exceeds aortic pressure for approximately the first half of systole, corresponding to rapid acceleration of blood flow and a small pressure difference from ventricle to the aorta. In the normal heart, pressure crossover occurs in midsystole, so during the second half of systole, aortic pressure exceeds left ventricular pressure resulting in continued forward blood flow but at progressively slower velocities (deceleration) Aortic valve closure occurs at the dicrotic notch of the aortic pressure tracing immediately following end-ejection. In sum, systole includes isovolumic contraction and ventricular ejection (acceleration & deceleration) phases. Ventricular volume ranges from a maximum at end-diastole (or onset of systole) to a minimum at end systole.

Pg 221 - (B-notch)

Ascending Aorta — pg 131. (Fig 6.1)

pacemaker wire — pg. 288

endocardium serous lining membrane of inner surface & cavities of the heart

epicardium — The inner or visceral layer of the pericardium. which forms a serous membrane forming the outermost layer of the wall of the heart.

pericardium — double membranous fibroserous sac enclosing the heart, It is composed of an inner serous layer (visceral pericardium) or epicardium) and an outer fibrous layer (parietal pericardium) The space between the two constitutes the pericardial cavity, which normally filled with a small amt of serous fluid.

Normally — pericardium contains a thin serous fluid (<20cc)
less than

Pg. 296 / 298 — { P.E. pericardial effusion.
"swinging Heart" P.E.

(Pg 371)